Decision-Making in Veterinary
Practice

Decision-Making in Veterinary Practice

Barry Kipperman, *DVM, DACVIM, MSc, DACAW*
Instructor, Veterinary Ethics, University of California at Davis, School of Veterinary Medicine, Davis, CA, USA;
Adjunct Associate Professor, University of Missouri College of Veterinary Medicine, Columbia, MO, USA

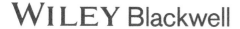

Library of Congress Cataloging-in-Publication Data applied for
Paperback ISBN: 9781119986348

Cover Design: Wiley
Cover Images: © BLOOM image/Getty Images; Kriangkrai Thitimakorn/Getty Images

Set in 9.5/12.5pt STIXTwoText by Straive, Pondicherry, India

SKY10061277_112923

Contents

Contributors

Jim Clark, DVM, MBA
Instructor, Professional Skills
University of California at Davis
School of Veterinary Medicine
Davis, CA, USA

Kathleen Cooney, DVM, CHPV, DACAW resident
Companion Animal Euthanasia Training Academy
Loveland, CO, USA

Acknowledgments

I'm thankful to all the students, interns, veterinarians, technicians, clients, and patients I've learned from during my career. To Dr. Lori Goeders, who was the smartest vet I'd ever worked with when I was in vet school and who inspired my career path as an internist. To those I worked with during my internship at the Animal Medical Center and in my residency at UC Davis, where I learned more in three years than I ever could have imagined. To Dr. Bill DeHoff for being my first employer in referral practice and who gave me confidence that I knew what I was doing.

To Dr. Fritha Langford for accepting me into the master's program at the University of Edinburgh, which inspired my transition from clinical practice to academia that sharpened my writing skills. I'm appreciative of the time, expertise, and knowledge of the contributing authors Drs. Jim Clark and Kathy Cooney. I am grateful to my colleagues Drs. Larry Gilman, Rene Gandolfi, Naomi Barnea, Anne Quain, and Bea Monteiro, for their thoughtful ideas and feedback. I'm appreciative of Dr. Ritu Bose and the editors at Wiley for supporting the idea for this book and seeing it to its fruition. Finally, to all the animals I've loved and shared my life with: Missy, Sheba, Whitney, Toby, Lillie, Galen, Winston Puggy Pugster, and Buttercup. You inspired me to be the best vet I could be.

Introduction: Why a Book on Decision-Making in Veterinary Practice?

During my 33 years as a small animal internal medicine specialist and 17 years as a practice owner interacting with patients, clients, associates, technicians, and referring veterinarians, and teaching students and interns, I realized that there is an absence of principles or strategies to guide veterinary practitioners in the process of decision-making. This sometimes results in decisions that, when examined retrospectively, appear to be illogical or difficult to justify based on the information in medical records. McKenzie observes that "There is nothing we do as often or that is ultimately as central to clinical medicine as making decisions. However, veterinarians and veterinary students receive little, if any, formal training in decision-making, and there is little explicit discussion in the veterinary literature about this critical activity" [1].

In my experience, each hospital has a unique culture that profoundly influences the way in which its clinicians make decisions. These influences are known as the "hidden curriculum," where clinicians are implicitly expected to adopt systems and behaviors that align with the philosophy of the practice. For example, a specific practice may customarily send patients home shortly after surgery or advise hospitalization overnight. Some practices encourage their clients to pursue diagnoses in sick patients while others prioritize therapeutic trials. At some practices, clinicians perceive pressure to proceed with euthanasia requests they find ethically problematic, while other practices support declining euthanasia requests on moral grounds.

To mitigate cognitive dissonance and interpersonal conflicts, clinicians may unknowingly modify their behaviors to conform with their practice's expectations. Doing what is expected of you or what your employer has done preceding you is quite understandable. But when scrutinized, this practice may discourage care shaped by sound principles and evidence in lieu of adhering to historical precedents or hospital protocols.

The goal of this book is to examine veterinary decision-making. Many unique considerations that influence clinical outcomes will be addressed, including how to obtain a patient history, why the time of day and the day of the week matter, why patient weight should be an important determinant of course of action, how to render a prognosis, when it is reasonable to perform a therapeutic trial, and interpreting results of diagnostic tests and treatment outcomes.

Other questions relevant to decision-making that often differ between practices and clinicians that will be covered in this book include:

- What standard should be utilized to assess clinician success?
- How should a veterinarian balance client or patient advocacy?
- How should veterinarians balance paternalistic or shared decision-making?
- Should clients be offered all available options, only those the practice can provide, or those that the clinician believes the client can afford?
- Should practitioners be compensated based on their production?

- How should economic concerns influence clinician decisions?
- When should veterinarians refer cases?
- Should clinicians disclose medical errors to clients?
- What factors should influence whether, when, and how a diagnosis should be pursued?
- How should veterinarians balance the desire to make a diagnosis with client requests for therapeutic trials?
- What considerations should dictate whether a patient is admitted to the hospital or managed at home?
- What circumstances should inform when treatment should stop?
- How should veterinarians balance the need to effectively manage postoperative pain versus client desires to have their companion at home?

One of the recurrent themes in this book is that *reflective* thinking by veterinary clinicians is challenged by the standard of modern-day practice in which the short duration of consultations does not accommodate such deliberation. This often results in *reflexive* decisions being made "on the fly," analogous to a myotatic reflex, limiting not only the capacity to make good decisions for patients but also acquisition of informed consent from our clients. In veterinary school, students spend hours writing extensive and impressive patient medical records, then discover after graduation that medical records are characterized by their brevity.

For most of my career in practice, my consultations were 60 minutes in duration. I typically spent about 10 minutes reviewing patient records; 10 minutes creating a list of patient problems, differential diagnoses, and a potential diagnostic plan; and spent the remaining 40 minutes in the exam room with my clients. While I appreciate that applying this time frame for appointments in general practice may be untenable, there is no doubt that the quality of veterinary decision-making would improve dramatically if consultation times and fees for sick patients both doubled. Barring this type of paradigm shift, a clinician who wishes to apply some of the counsel provided in this book will need to spend decision-making time before or after consultations have been completed.

Normative ethics is a branch of philosophy where one seeks to determine principles of good and bad, or right and wrong behaviors and attitudes, i.e. what one *ought* to do. We should be able to ask *why* one made a clinical decision and examine the process in hindsight, much as we are trained to perform a patient autopsy to determine what disease we may have missed. The absence of discrete principles for clinical decision-making often has far greater consequences for our patients than our knowledge of medicine or surgery.

My intention in this book is to improve the quality of veterinary clinical reasoning and thoughtfulness. Tables and figures will be utilized to offer guidance, and case studies will be provided for context and to encourage reflection. At my hospital I established a tradition in which in exchange for my efforts in passing on my advice and teaching, the interns would present me with a top-10 list of what they learned during their internship. These lists taught me lessons as well.

Veterinary clinicians should provide their clients and their animals with the benefit of not only our compassion, but also our wisdom, manifested by judicious decisions. It's my hope that passing on what I have learned and considered, including my mistakes, will help you make better decisions resulting in improved patient outcomes. Let's begin examining some of the most important topics relevant to veterinary decision-making.

Reference

1 McKenzie, B.A. (2014). Veterinary clinical decision-making: cognitive biases, external constraints, and strategies for improvement. *Journal of the American Veterinary Medical Association* 244 (3): 271–276.

Section 1

Fundamental Concepts in Making Clinical Decisions

1

How to Define Your Success as a Clinician

Barry Kipperman

Abstract

This chapter considers finding a suitable criterion by which to assess success in clinical veterinary practice and why this is important. It discusses the limitations of satisfying varied practitioner interests including those of referring veterinarians, performing advanced treatments or procedures, financial compensation, conforming to employer expectations, pleasing animal owners, and achieving desired patient outcomes as benchmarks for success. Case studies are used to illustrate these examples. The Principle of Patient Advocacy is defined and introduced as the ideal means by which to determine clinician success.

Keywords: *success, moral stress, referring veterinarian, compensation, employer, advanced care, clients, owners, patient advocacy*

As this book is devoted to veterinary decision-making, perhaps one of the most meaningful decisions is how to define one's success as a clinician. During my career, numerous interns and students have asked me, "How do you know whether you are a good veterinarian or had a successful day?" I had no answer to this profound question when it was first posed, but significant introspection since then has allowed me to gain clarity, which I hope to provide in this chapter.

Why is the answer to this question so vital? Because whatever criterion one uses to measure success will inevitably guide one's practice philosophy and behaviors that may endure over the course of an over 30-year career in the profession. Another reason grappling with this question is so important relates to the mental health of veterinarians. There has been increasing research interest in examining the occurrence of stress within the veterinary profession. Many factors have been cited to cause stress, including ethical dilemmas, client financial limitations affecting patient care, work overload, client complaints, and dealing with death and errors [1].

Two recent investigations discovered that 50% [2] and 31% [3] of veterinarians had high burnout scores. A study of small animal veterinarians found that 49% reported a moderate to substantial level of burnout [4]. In another report, when North American veterinarians were asked "How often have you felt distressed or anxious about your work?", 52% responded "often" or "always" [5]. It's apparent that work-related stress is a significant challenge for the veterinary profession. The effects of work-related stress on mental health are well documented and include emotional exhaustion, anxiety, and depression [6, 7]. Numerous studies have documented higher rates of suicidal ideation and suicide in the veterinary profession compared with those in the general population and other healthcare professionals [8–11].

If one applies a standard of success that becomes unfulfilling, too difficult, or impossible to attain, it's likely that moral (dis)stress may be experienced. Moral distress has been defined as "The experience of psychological distress that results from engaging in, or failing to prevent, decisions or behaviors that transgress ... personally held moral or ethical beliefs" [12]. Moral stress is therefore recognized as a consequence of experienced conflicts involving work-related obligations or expectations that do not coincide with one's values [13, 14]. Studies in veterinary medicine have suggested or documented that moral distress is inversely associated with wellbeing and correlates with career dissatisfaction and attrition [15, 16].

To consider the question of how to assess your success, let's systematically examine the numerous interests veterinary clinicians are expected to serve and the viability and limitations of satisfying each of these as a benchmark to evaluate clinical success.

Referring Veterinarian

To meet the demand that medical care for animals rival that of humans, the number of referral and emergency veterinary practices in the United States has increased dramatically in the last three decades [17]. Of the estimated 119 000 US veterinarians [18], 11% are board-certified specialists [19]. These veterinarians have the same diverse obligations as those of the referring veterinarian (RDVM), but in addition must satisfy the perceived or real demands of the RDVM.

Just as general practitioners (GPs) are economically dependent on the animal owner for their livelihood, the veterinary specialist is dependent on present and future referrals from their colleagues. As most pet owners are not aware of the existence of specialists [20], the GP is considered the gatekeeper to the referral process. While GPs are careful not to offend pet owners, specialists feel the same way toward RDVMs due to concern over losing referrals and their associated income.

As a result of these forces, the veterinary specialist may feel conflicted in satisfying their varied duties (Case Studies 1.1 and 1.2).

Case Study 1.1 A Dog with Chronic Vomiting Referred for Endoscopy

You are an internist in a referral practice. Bella, a nine-month-old dog, is referred for endoscopy for evaluation of chronic vomiting. Novel diet trials have not been performed and appetite is normal. Lab work and radiographs are within normal limits. Physical examination reveals Bella to be in good body condition with no abnormalities. Based on Bella's young age and the evaluation, you advise a novel diet trial for food allergy/intolerance, with endoscopy and biopsies to follow if vomiting does not improve within a few weeks.

The client seems confused and explains that endoscopy was advised by her veterinarian. You inform the client that approximately 50% of cases like Bella's will respond to diet change, supporting the recommendation to delay the cost and anesthetic risk of endoscopy and the need for medications that may have undesirable side effects. The RDVM calls you later in the day to express his displeasure with the agreed course of action, stating, "You showed me up to the client because I wanted an endoscopy. Now I'll refer her to someone else who will do the endoscopy."

In this case, there is conflict between what the specialist perceives to be in the best interest of the patient and the expressed desire of the GP. Ideally, this problem can be sufficiently resolved via a professional conversation. If not, should the specialist comply with the request for the endoscopy? This procedure is benign, commonly performed, and will enhance the income of the specialist, but may be unnecessary for the patient.

Case Study 1.2   A Dog with Abdominal Distension

Sydney, an 11-year-old male German shepherd, is seen by a local GP on Wednesday for lethargy and poor appetite of 1–2 days' duration. The medical record confirms abdominal distention. Sydney is sent home while a mobile ultrasound is scheduled. On Friday, ultrasound reveals a splenic mass. Sydney is sent home for the weekend and arrives at your referral practice Monday morning in a moribund, life-threatening condition, with a packed cell volume (PCV) of 17%. Sydney undergoes emergency splenectomy for abdominal bleeding and dies postoperatively from oliguria and coagulopathy. Should you inform the client or the GP of your concern that surgery should have been advised before 5 days had passed after initial presentation? Should you report this colleague to the state board?

While in many cases the interests of the GP, specialist, client, and patient are aligned, conflicts can occur. Unfortunately, attempts by the specialist to constructively discuss with the RDVM what could have been done better sometimes result in a punitive loss of future referrals. If satisfying the RDVM is viewed as a measure of success, then the specialist may either modify their standards of practice to conform with GP expectations, or may not attempt to provide constructive feedback to GPs to improve their standards of practice. Both choices are detrimental to promoting animal welfare. Conversely, a GP should also feel they can discuss concerns about shared patient care with the specialist. While striving to satisfy RDVMs may seem appropriate as an indicator of success, these examples suggest that in some cases doing so can be self-serving and disregard obligations to the client, the patient, and the profession.

Veterinarian

Veterinary clinicians have an interest in career satisfaction. Professional self-esteem may be linked to learning and performing novel or advanced procedures or treatments [21]. The increased demand of animal owners for advanced care and the rise in availability of emerging technologies and advanced imaging create a recipe for futile or non-beneficial interventions. As noted by Durnberger and Grimm [22]: "Undoubtedly, veterinarians have a positive duty to help animals – but at what point do they run the risk of violating the negative duty not to harm animals?" In considering this issue of when well-intended interventions cause unwarranted harm, studies show that veterinarians are sometimes requested to provide treatment that they consider futile [5, 23].

Emotionally driven factors are often associated with decisions to pursue advanced care (Case Study 1.3). Taylor [24] has noted that "a question being increasingly asked is whether there are many clinicians who currently view euthanasia as a failure rather than a considered, considerate

---

Case Study 1.3   My Pug with Collapsing Bronchi

Winston was a 13-year-old pug with progressive exercise intolerance and episodes of cyanosis and syncope associated with wheezing. My perception was that his quality of life was worsening. Imaging evaluations confirmed collapsing bronchi as the cause, likely secondary to chronic inspiratory dyspnea from brachycephalic obstructive airway syndrome. While the surgeons at my practice were adept at inserting tracheal stents as a salvage procedure for dogs with collapsing trachea with good short-term outcomes, bronchial stenting at that time was considered experimental. My love for Winston, fear of losing him, and the hope of finding some means of resolution clouded my medical judgment. I called the closest university teaching hospital and was informed no one there performed bronchial stenting. I called the company that produces tracheal stents and discovered it had recently began producing bronchial stents, but very few colleagues were trained in placing them. Out of desperation, I purchased several different-sized stents and requested my other internist and surgeon assist me in trying this for Winston. I arranged real-time remote access to an expert in this procedure, and with his guidance we worked for hours to properly implant the stents via bronchoscopy.

Winston spent the next few days in the hospital receiving sedatives and antitussives to mitigate risks such as stent migration or fracture. When I brought Winston home, it was clear that his condition was worse, and he could barely move without having to honk and wheeze. I let him go the day after Christmas. In hindsight, the risk–benefit ratio for this procedure was quite poor, and in addition to my own sense of guilt and moral stress for putting him through this, I likely also contributed to the same negative emotions for my staff involved in this procedure.

---

option for a struggling animal." Moral stress is one of the potential consequences of participating in procedures or treatments that one feels are prolonging a poor quality of life or are worsening welfare [21].

Defining one's success by the number or nature of advanced treatments or procedures performed is clearly not a desirable standard.

Financial Compensation

In human medicine, the idea that fee-for-service payment models incentivize recommending highly compensated procedures has been considered [25]. A systematic review of 18 studies concluded that 83% discovered an association between oncologists' care and compensation consistent with influence by financial incentives [26]. A recent review of financial performance incentives in US health systems found that while most primary care and specialist compensation methods included incentives based on performance, they averaged less than 10% of compensation [27].

Veterinarians in practice are commonly compensated based on a proportion of their revenues [28]. Although such systems are purportedly intended to reward those seeing many patients and to discourage discounting and pro bono work, these also create an incentive for the veterinarian to advise costly testing, procedures, hospitalization, and surgery. Consequently, an implicit conflict of interest exists that may influence veterinary recommendations (Case Studies 1.4 and 1.5), contributing to unnecessary, inappropriate, or delayed interventions [29]. After my practice purchased a computed tomography (CT) scanner, I would be dishonest not to recognize the influence of the potential economic benefits to me and my practice for advising this procedure.

Case Study 1.4   Request to Postpone Emergency Surgery

Herbie, a 10-year-old large-breed dog, is referred to you at a 24-hour referral practice at 7 p.m. for evaluation of weakness and anemia. An ultrasound study reveals a splenic mass and hemo-abdomen. Herbie's PCV is 20%. You call the RDVM to provide an update and to inform them that emergency splenectomy will be advised. The RDVM requests that surgery not be offered, and that Herbie be medically stabilized on intravenous (IV) fluids overnight and transferred back, so that the surgery can be performed at their practice the following morning. You are concerned that delaying surgery may result in death or the need to provide a blood transfusion to facilitate Herbie's survival for the next 14 hours.

What should you do? Acquiesce to the request? Ignore the request? Decline the request? Inform the client of the conflict? Is there a valid medical rationale for this request, or is financial remuneration influencing it?

Case Study 1.5   Workup for Young Cat with an Abscess

A two-year-old cat presents for lethargy. Physical examination confirms fever and a fluctuant swelling on the lateral thorax. The attending veterinarian advises a complete database of testing to include a complete blood count (CBC), chemistry, urinalysis, feline leukemia virus/feline immunodeficiency virus (FeLV/FIV) test, and radiographs prior to surgery to lance the presumed abscess. You are the practice owner reviewing this medical record as part of your usual evaluation of associate performance. Is this diagnostic recommendation excessive and unnecessary or in keeping with quality medicine? The tests enhance practice revenues and are not risky or painful. Should you confront the attending doctor about this or let it go?

This conflict of interest is perceived by clients, as 30% of pet owners agreed that veterinarians advise additional services to make money [30]. This issue has also been raised regarding veterinary clinicians profiting from dispensing medications, in contrast to the medical profession, which abrogates this concern by relegating the prescribing and selling of medications to outside pharmacies [31, 32].

When I owned my practice, each month I provided associate doctors with a spreadsheet that included numbers of patients seen, average transaction fees, and revenue generated for all staff doctors. At the time, I would have asserted that my motivations included transparency and to inspire good medical care. In retrospect, I believe that this data promoted competition among doctors to raise their revenues, resulting in unnecessary medical procedures and a race to be the "highest performer." I suspect this also caused poor self-esteem for "lower-producing" staff. This approach also appears to be common within corporate veterinary practices to encourage competition [33].

For a portion of my career, I based my success on practice revenue and my gross income. In fact, I recall my accountant writing a personal note of congratulations when my income reached a certain milestone. As many practice owners frequently evaluate such metrics, it's easy to fall prey to this criterion as a benchmark for success. During my career, I have been told by numerous colleagues that the justifications for their medical recommendations included "I've got a house to pay for" and "I've got kids to send to college." It should be apparent that utilizing income as an arbiter of success is tempting, but also can become self-serving and can quickly empty one's soul in the process, leading you away from what inspired you to become a veterinarian and a caregiver.

Practice Owner/Employer

As I was a practice owner, I can attest that the profitability of the practice is a prominent concern of employers. This may arise from laudable desires, including ensuring the staff are paid well and receive adequate benefits and aspiring to have the latest equipment to facilitate excellent patient care. Conversely, if financial gain becomes the primary driver of behavior for practice owners, a preeminent concern with ensuring perceived client satisfaction may ensue, resulting in harm to animal welfare, violations of the duty to obtain informed consent, and moral stress concerns for staff (Case Studies 1.6 and 1.7)

These cases illustrate that an important expectation of many employers for their associates is to generate income for the practice and retain clients. The associate veterinarian may feel vulnerable and may also be influenced by economic pressures, such as jeopardizing their job security and status within the practice if their behavior does not conform with their employer's requests or demands. Performing convenience surgeries is a source of moral conflict, challenging the concept

---

Case Study 1.6   Employer Request Not to Disclose Patient Obesity

You have been working as a new graduate in a small animal general practice. You see Samantha Smith, a four-year-old female golden retriever, for acute-onset unilateral hindlimb lameness. On exam, Sam is markedly obese and is minimally weight-bearing on the affected limb. You cannot find any notation in her medical record that weight gain has been discussed with Mrs. Smith despite increasing body weights documented in the past two years. You suspect a ruptured cruciate ligament in the knee as the most likely cause. As this is your first diagnosis of this condition, you meet with your employer, Dr. A, and discuss your plan of action, which includes:

- Discuss with Mrs. Smith why Sam is lame, and the need for surgery to resolve the condition.
- Discuss with Mrs. Smith how Sam's obese state contributed to this condition and formulate options to facilitate weight loss to prevent the same injury to her other knee.
- Lab work as presurgical screen including thyroid test.
- Send Sam home on an analgesic and limited activity until surgery can be performed.
- Provide an estimate for the orthopedic repair.

When you present this plan, Dr. A shares with you that all of Mrs. Smith's dogs have been overweight over the years. She has tried to discuss this topic with Mrs. Smith in the past, but no ameliorative measures were taken. Dr. A approves of your plan except for disclosing Sam's obesity, which she strongly prefers you not discuss. She maintains that your efforts are likely to be ineffective at achieving weight loss, and notes numerous liabilities of your proposal, including:

- Mrs. Smith is one of the hospital's best clients and may be offended and take her pets to another practice. The practice may lose the income from the surgery and significant future income.
- Mrs. Smith is active in the golden retriever community, and the practice could lose other clients if she is unhappy or offended.
- It is possible the orthopedic injury is independent of Sam's obese state.

What should you do?

Case Study 1.7   Request for Declawing a Cat
You are a small animal veterinarian. Mrs. Jones, a long-term client, calls to tell you that her indoor, one-year-old cat Fluffy is scratching furniture, which concerns and upsets her. There is a dog in the house as well. Her family is pressuring her to either relinquish Fluffy to a shelter or have you arrange declawing. She requests your professional opinion to guide her decision. You consult with your employer, who suggests you schedule Fluffy for a declaw procedure. Bear in mind that convenience surgeries or medically unnecessary surgeries are those performed to benefit humans rather than veterinary patients [34]. Onychectomy is associated with acute and chronic pain, and increased risk of unwanted behaviors including urinating and defecating outside the litter box, excessive grooming, biting, and aggression [35]. Elective onychectomy is opposed by the American Association of Feline Practitioners and the American Animal Hospital Association. These organizations encourage veterinarians to educate cat owners about normal feline behavior and provide alternatives to onychectomy [36, 37]. What should you do?

of the veterinarian as patient advocate [34]. It should be clear that an absolute dedication to satisfy one's employer is not an ideal standard by which to measure one's success.

Animal Owner/Client

Veterinarians must respect client autonomy regarding decisions related to veterinary care. While many clients seek and pursue the best care for their animals, exceptions to this ideal are common. A fundamental ethical problem in veterinary practice is whether veterinarians should give primary consideration to the animal or to the animal owner/client. Rollin makes the distinction between two models of veterinarians: the pediatrician model characterized by patient advocacy, and the model of the mechanic, beholden to client requests and demands regarding the disposition of their legal property [13]. Veterinarians may seek to promote client autonomy in lieu of patient interests. One might believe that the fundamental responsibility of a veterinarian is to obey client decisions even at the detriment of the medical interests of patients (short of breaching cruelty laws). Moreover, any interventions legally and ethically require informed consent from the client.

Morris's ethnographic study of small animal veterinarians concludes: "Because animals are legally considered property and veterinarians depend on clients for income, veterinary medicine is more client oriented than patient oriented" [15]. Many clinicians are praised by their supervisors for receiving positive letters, cards, or social media posts written by clients, and many practices solicit positive reviews from their clients. I have a box of client letters and cards in my office expressing appreciation for my efforts. I admit reading these during times when my self-esteem needed a boost.

Unfortunately, all owners do not meet their moral and legal duties to take care of their animals. Some clients may choose not to pursue treatment of a patient with a good prognosis or may elect euthanasia for reasons that may violate the ethos of the veterinarian. For example, the client might assert that the animal is simply too old, too costly, or the care is too burdensome. Other clients may request ongoing treatment when the prognosis is very poor. Conversely, attempting to save animals through expensive treatment may be perceived as profiteering and clients may characterize the clinician as incompetent or exploitative if the animal dies. They may try to make the veterinarian feel guilty for not offering free or subsidized treatment [38].

Clients may neglect or abuse their animal(s). They may threaten reprisals or loss of business for reporting suspected animal maltreatment, may request not using analgesics for a painful procedure to save money, or may choose to take their suffering animal home instead of pursuing humane euthanasia. Vets might also be criticized for seeming to "coerce" owners into or against euthanasia [38].

It should be apparent that always acquiescing to the requests of animal owners may result in outcomes that may be detrimental to animal welfare, violating the veterinary oath. Consequently, allegiance to client satisfaction is not an adequate arbiter to guide clinician success.

Patient

Outcomes

One of the main reasons I pursued a career in veterinary medicine was to help and heal sick animals. I'm not alone. In a report of veterinary students, helping animals was the most common reason identified for wanting to become a veterinarian [39]. In veterinary school we are taught about diseases, afflictions, and infections, and as clinicians we focus on ways to achieve the best possible patient outcomes as measured by remission rates, discharge from hospital, weight gain, clinical resolution of symptoms, and owner perceptions of improvement (see Chapter 24). While in some cases we can "cure" patients (gastric dilatation-volvulus, extraction of gastrointestinal foreign bodies), in other cases we can only achieve palliation of symptoms (lymphoma, hemolytic anemia).

For a significant portion of my career, I viewed my job as "defeating the reaper"; i.e. warding off death in my patients. In fact, I sometimes would tell my patients that I wouldn't let them down and I'd protect them from death. While this posture of devotion to my patients' outcomes may seem admirable, it shouldn't take long to predict the liabilities. I recall sending a young dog to surgery for relief of an intestinal obstruction seen on radiographs, emphasizing to the owners the likelihood of a curable foreign body when, in fact, a mast cell tumor was identified. The same thing happened with a one-year-old cat that had a mass related to feline infectious peritonitis. I was devastated, feeling I had misled my clients, and had trouble coping with the reality that what appeared to be a promising outlook was now a bleak picture. I remember breaking down and crying when a cute shih tzu I'd gotten emotionally attached to with immune-mediated hemolytic anemia (IMHA) developed a thromboembolic event and died, or when a Labrador developed IMHA days after surgical removal of an ingested corn cob when a good prognosis had been provided.

In some cases, our attempts to diagnose or improve patient condition instead cause harm: I recall several patients in hepatic failure who died days after anesthesia for laparoscopic liver biopsies. These cases taught me painful but valuable lessons as I tried to assess which patients could survive and benefit from this procedure. I spent considerable time during my career trying to reconcile the indirect association between my efforts and patient outcomes, and navigating how to keep an emotional distance from patient survivals or deaths while still not losing my desire to help all patients I see.

The lesson to be learned here is that while caring about your patient's improvement and doing all you can toward this goal are commendable, there are many factors that influence patient outcomes that are beyond your control, including patient age and co-morbidities, patient body condition, extent and timing of client compliance with your recommendations, other individuals involved in patient care, economics, etc. As patients may (and too often do) fail despite you doing everything correctly medically to achieve a positive result, attaching your success to patient outcomes is a recipe for emotional devastation and possibly career attrition. Let's find a better standard to connect your devotion to patients with perceived success.

Advocacy

Revisiting the fundamental question regarding to whom the veterinarian owes their allegiance, it is assumed by animal owners and by society that veterinarians are advocates for animals. Rollin [40] asserted that "It is ... a major part of veterinary medicine to defend the interests of animals." One of the main impediments to animal advocacy is that veterinarians are hired and paid by humans, not by animals. In this paradigm, the veterinarian is a medical counselor who forms a relationship with, and works on behalf of, the animal owner. Veterinarians need to contend with clients' desires and wishes. What is the responsibility of the veterinarian when they believe the decision the owner reaches is not in the animal's best interest? It can be difficult and uncomfortable for veterinarians to confront owners in these circumstances; some may not consider this as within their purview.

Numerous studies assessing the advocacy behaviors of veterinarians document that a client-centered orientation is more prevalent than a patient-focused orientation [5, 41–43]. Substantiating this conclusion and drawing distinctions between the ideals of students and practitioners, 92% of veterinary students indicated that veterinarians should prioritize patient interests when the interests of clients and patients conflict, whereas 84% of students reported that veterinarians most often prioritize client interests in these circumstances [39]. This data suggests that while those aspiring to be veterinarians see their role as patient advocate, realizing this role in practice is challenging.

Several ethicists have proposed a "best interest" or patient advocacy model for veterinary medicine [13, 44, 45]. Coghlan implores veterinarians to pursue "strong patient advocacy" (SPA), suggesting that this is a philosophy of practice:

> What distinguishes SPAs ... is the *preparedness* to engage in the full gamut of justifiable advocacy options required for preventing harm to patients. Strong patient advocacy involves a disposition and a moral stance orientated toward the goal of improved patient wellbeing and an embrace of the range of justifiable ethical means and resources veterinarians have at their disposal. [46]

Limitations of enacting patient advocacy include the following:

- Acquiring informed consent from the owner requires knowledge and is time consuming (see Chapter 3).
- Discussing all the available alternatives for the patient with the client, advising the option believed to provide the best chance for a positive result, and having the client regularly choose another option that the practitioner believes compromises patient outcome or prolongs poor quality of life can be emotionally draining and onerous (Case Study 1.8). Consequently, pursuing a "patient best interest" model may be a metaphorical weight that becomes too heavy to lift for veterinarians over time, contributing to moral stress.
- Attempts to effect changes in practices regarding patients, such as advocating for management of patient obesity via dietary modifications or for earlier recognition of patient illness (Case Study 1.9), may be perceived by clients as offensive or confrontational.

Case Study 1.8   A Geriatric Dog with Metastatic Cancer

You see Molly, a 12-year-old large-breed dog, for anorexia and weight loss. Physical examination reveals cachexia and abdominal distension. Abdominal ultrasound confirms a splenic mass and numerous hepatic nodules consistent with metastases. You discuss the findings and bad news with the owner and express your condolences. You advise humane euthanasia as the best option for Molly, as she is suffering, there is no effective treatment given the extent of the cancer, and the efficacy of palliative treatment is doubtful. Molly's owner tells you: "This is a terrible time to receive this news. My daughter will be home from college in two weeks, so can you give me medication to help Molly, and we'll bring her back then?"

Should you accept this decision without further discussion? Should you dispense analgesics and/or appetite stimulants? Might dispensing medication prolong Molly's suffering and the interval before she is returned for euthanasia by masking symptoms the owner may recognize as concerning? Should you offer referral to an expert in hospice/palliative care? Should you describe in more detail what Molly is experiencing, advocating that a more appropriate timetable for consideration of euthanasia should be measured in hours or days rather than weeks? Is doing so patient advocacy or client coercion? Should you be concerned about potential repercussions such as a negative social media review?

Case Study 1.9   Client with Many Cats That Present for Advanced Weight Loss

---

Mrs. J is one of your best clients and is considered one of the top clients (by money spent) in your practice. She has about a dozen cats in an indoor setting. She sees you exclusively, pursues all diagnostics you suggest, always complies with your treatment recommendations, and consistently informs your employer how happy she is with your care. You've noticed that in the past few months her cats are being brought to you in a more advanced stage of illness than before. Whereas in the past her cats had lost 10% of their weight at presentation, now this has risen to 25–30% of weight lost. You are concerned that something has changed at home to cause a delayed recognition or action regarding symptoms of illness in the cats. You are also concerned that weight loss of this degree imposes a poorer prognosis for the cats.

Should you address your concern with Mrs. J? With her family? Might this jeopardize your standing or the practice's relationship with Mrs. J? Might this reflect a change in the household's financial capacity that the family may wish not to disclose? Should you instead encourage they purchase a cat scale and advise weighing all the cats regularly and bringing them in if 5% weight loss is noted (see Chapter 11)? Should you simply do the best you can for the cats that are presented?

- A veterinarian's capacity to pursue a "best interest" posture may reasonably be associated with their perception of autonomy within the culture and hierarchy of a particular practice.
- Excellent communication skills are required.

Hernandez et al. [47] assert that animal advocacy requires courage and speaking up:

> Advocating for animal welfare may not be comfortable and may, at times, require courage but is necessary … to improve human regard for animals. [Failure to do so] … can lead to an

inability or difficulty in speaking up about concerns with clients and ultimately, failure in their duty of care to animals, leading to poor animal welfare outcomes.

To revisit the question at the start of this chapter, "How do you know whether you are a good veterinarian or had a successful day?" My response is simple: "Did I advocate for each of my patients to the best of my ability?" Or to use Coghlan's term [46], was I a "strong patient advocate"? I will refer to this concept throughout the book as the Principle of Patient Advocacy. Enacting the Principle of Patient Advocacy should enhance patient outcomes, is free, and is within your control to utilize in your practice via effort, intention, and courage.

Veterinarians manifest ambivalence as they navigate ethical conflicts involving clients, patients, employers, and self-interest. Having a sense of clarity regarding one's professional identity can act as a moral compass, helping to assuage the contextual inconsistencies inherent in veterinary practice. You can apply the Principle of Patient Advocacy regardless of economic considerations or many of the other limitations discussed in this chapter. Now let's discuss opportunities and methods for how you can incorporate the Principle of Patient Advocacy in your practice.

References

1 Pohl, R., Botscharow, J., Böckelmann, I. et al. (2022). Stress and strain among veterinarians: a scoping review. *Irish Veterinary Journal* 75: 15. https://doi.org/10.1186/s13620-022-00220-x.

2 Ouedraogo, F.B., Lefebvre, S.L., Hansen, C.R. et al. (2021). Compassion satisfaction, burnout, and secondary traumatic stress among full-time veterinarians in the United States (2016–2018). *Journal of the American Veterinary Medical Association* 258 (11): 1259–1270.

3 Volk, J.O., Schimmack, U., Strand, E.B. et al. (2022). Executive summary of the Merck Animal Health Veterinarian Wellbeing Study III and Veterinary Support Staff Study. *Journal of the American Veterinary Medical Association* 260 (12): 1547–1553.

4 Kipperman, B.S., Kass, P.H., and Rishniw, M. (2017). Factors influencing small animal veterinarians' opinions and actions regarding cost of care and effects of economic limitations on patient care, outcomes and professional career satisfaction and burnout. *Journal of the American Veterinary Medical Association* 250 (7): 785–794.

5 Moses, L., Malowney, M.J., and Boyd, J.W. (2018). Ethical conflict and moral distress in veterinary practice: a survey of North American veterinarians. *Journal of Veterinary Internal Medicine* 32 (6): 2115–2122.

6 Ganster, D.C. and Rosen, C.C. (2013). Work stress and employee health: a multidisciplinary review. *Journal of Management* 39 (5): 1085–1122.

7 Oh, Y. and Gastmans, C. (2015). Moral distress experienced by nurses: a quantitative literature review. *Nurse Ethics* 22 (1): 15–31.

8 Nett, R.J., Witte, T.K., Holzbauer, S.M. et al. (2015). Risk factors for suicide, attitudes toward mental illness, and practice-related stressors among US veterinarians. *Journal of the American Veterinary Medical Association* 247 (8): 945–955.

9 Volk, J.O., Schimmack, U., Strand, E.B. et al. (2018). Executive summary of the Merck Animal Health Veterinary Wellbeing Study. *Journal of the American Veterinary Medical Association* 252 (10): 1231–1238.

10 Witte, T.K., Spitzer, E.G., Edwards, N. et al. (2019). Suicides and deaths of undetermined intent among veterinary professionals from 2003 through 2014. *Journal of the American Veterinary Medical Association* 255 (5): 595–608.

11 Tomasi, S.E., Fechter-Leggett, E.D., Edwards, N.T. et al. (2022). All causes of death among veterinarians in the United States during 1979 through 2015. *Journal of the American Veterinary Medical Association* 260 (9): 1–10.

12 Crane, M.F., Bayl-Smith, P., and Cartmill, J. (2013). A recommendation for expanding the definition of moral distress experienced in the workplace. *Australian and New Zealand Journal of Organizational Psychology* 6: e1. https://doi.org/10.1017/orp.2013.1.

13 Rollin, B.E. (2006). *An Introduction to Veterinary Medical Ethics*, 2e. Ames, IA: Blackwell Publishing.

14 Fawcett, A. and Mullan, S. (2018). Managing moral distress in practice. *In Practice* 40 (1): 34–36.

15 Morris, P. (2012). *Blue Juice: Euthanasia in Veterinary Medicine*. Philadelphia, PA: Temple University Press.

16 Chun, M.S., Joo, S., and Jung, Y. (2019). Veterinary ethical issues and stressfulness of ethical dilemmas of Korean veterinarians. In: *Sustainable Governance and Management of Food Systems: Ethical Perspectives* (ed. E. Vinnari and M. Vinnari), 193–202. Wageningen: Wageningen Academic Publishers.

17 Kipperman, B., Block, G., and Forsgren, B. (2022). Economic issues. In: *Ethics in Veterinary Practice*, ch. 8 (ed. B. Kipperman and B.E. Rollin). Chichester: Wiley-Blackwell.

18 American Veterinary Medical Association (AVMA). (2020). US veterinarians 2020. https://www.avma.org/resources-tools/reports-statistics/market-research-statistics-us-veterinarians (accessed May 10, 2022).

19 American Veterinary Medical Association (2020). Veterinary specialists 2020. https://www.avma.org/resources-tools/reports-statistics/veterinary-specialists-2020 (accessed May 10, 2022).

20 Buechner-Maxwell, V. and Byers, C. (2013). ACVIM member engagement and brand assessment survey corona insights survey results summary. *Journal of Veterinary Internal Medicine* 27 (5): 1287.

21 Quain, A., Ward, M.P., and Mullan, S. (2021). Ethical challenges posed by advanced veterinary care in companion animal veterinary practice. *Animals* 11: 3010. doi: 10.3390/ani11113010.

22 Dürnberger, C. and Grimm, H. (2022). Companion animals: futile intervention. In: *Ethics in Veterinary Practice*, ch. 10 (ed. B. Kipperman and B.E. Rollin). Chichester, Wiley-Blackwell.

23 Peterson, N.W., Boyd, J.W., and Moses, L. (2022). Medical futility is commonly encountered in small animal clinical practice. *Journal of the American Veterinary Medical Association* 260 (12): 1475–1481.

24 Taylor, N. (2021). Just because we can, should we? *Veterinary Record* 189: 294.

25 Khullar, D., Chokshi, D.A., Kocher, R. et al. (2015). Behavioral economics and physician compensation—promise and challenges. *New England Journal of Medicine* 372 (24): 2281–2283.

26 Mitchell, A.P., Rotter, J.S., Patel, E. et al. (2019). Association between reimbursement incentives and physician practice in oncology: a systematic review. *JAMA Oncology* 5 (6): 893–899.

27 Reid, R.O., Tom, A.K., Ross, R.M. et al. (2022). Physician compensation arrangements and financial performance incentives in US health systems. *JAMA Health Forum* 3 (1): e214634.

28 Opperman, M. (2019). Pro on ProSal. *Today's Veterinary Business*, February/March. https://todaysveterinarybusiness.com/pro-on-prosal (accessed May 10, 2022).

29 Rosoff, P.M., Moga, J., Keene, B. et al. (2018). Resolving ethical dilemmas in a tertiary care veterinary specialty hospital: adaptation of the human clinical consultation committee model. *American Journal of Bioethics* 18 (2): 41–53.

30 Brown, B.R. (2018). The dimensions of pet-owner loyalty and the relationship with communication, trust, commitment and perceived value. *Veterinary Sciences* 5 (4): 95.

31 Ramey, D.W. (2022). Equines. In: *Ethics in Veterinary Practice*, ch. 13 (ed. B. Kipperman and B.E. Rollin). Chichester: Wiley-Blackwell.

32 Blackwell, T.E., Perrin, S., and Walker, J. (2022). Food animals. In: *Ethics in Veterinary Practice*, ch. 12 (ed. B. Kipperman and B.E. Rollin). Chichester: Wiley-Blackwell.

33 Edling, T. (2022). Corporate veterinary medicine. In: *Ethics in Veterinary Practice*, ch. 17 (ed. B. Kipperman and B.E. Rollin). Chichester: Wiley-Blackwell.

34 Quain, A. (2022). Companion animals: convenience surgeries. In: *Ethics in Veterinary Practice*, ch. 10 (ed. B. Kipperman and B.E. Rollin). Chichester: Wiley-Blackwell.

35 Martell-Moran, N.K., Solano, M., and Townsend, H.G. (2018). Pain and adverse behavior in declawed cats. *Journal of Feline Medicine and Surgery* 20 (4): 280–288.

36 American Association of Feline Practitioners (AAFP) (2017). AAFP position statement: declawing. *Journal of Feline Medicine and Surgery* 19: NP1–NP3.

37 American Animal Hospital Association (2021). AAHA position statements and endorsements: declawing. https://www.aaha.org/about-aaha/aaha-position-statements/declawing (accessed May 9, 2022).

38 Yeates, J.W. (2022). Death. In: *Ethics in Veterinary Practice*, ch. 21 (ed. B. Kipperman and B.E. Rollin). Chichester: Wiley-Blackwell.

39 Kipperman, B., Rollin, B., and Martin, J. (2020). Veterinary student opinions regarding ethical dilemmas encountered by veterinarians and the benefits of ethics instruction. *Journal of Veterinary Medical Education* 48 (3): 330–342.

40 Rollin, B. (2004). The broken promise; ethics and the human animal-bond. Part 2. *Veterinary Forum* Feb. 22–29.

41 Kipperman, B., Morris, P., and Rollin, B. (2018). Ethical dilemmas encountered by small animal veterinarians: characterisation, responses, consequences and beliefs regarding euthanasia. *Veterinary Record* 182 (19): 548. https://doi.org/10.1136/vr.104619.

42 Quain, A., Mullan, S., McGreevy, P.D. et al. (2021). Frequency, stressfulness and type of ethically challenging situations encountered by veterinary team members during the COVID-19 pandemic. *Frontiers in Veterinary Science* 8: 647108. https://doi.org/10.3389/fvets.2021.647108.

43 Springer, S., Sandoe, P., Grimm, H. et al. (2021). Managing conflicting ethical concerns in modern small animal practice—a comparative study of veterinarian's decision ethics in Austria, Denmark and the UK. *PLoS One* 16 (6): e0253420. https://doi.org/10.1371/journal.pone.0253420.

44 Grimm, H., Bergadano, A., Musk, G.C. et al. (2018). Drawing the line in clinical treatment of companion animals: recommendations from an ethics working party. *Veterinary Record* 182 (23): 664.

45 Kipperman, B. (2022). Veterinary advocacies and ethical dilemmas. In: *Ethics in Veterinary Practice*, ch. 7 (ed. B. Kipperman and B.E. Rollin). Chichester: Wiley-Blackwell.

46 Coghlan, S. (2018). Strong patient advocacy and the fundamental ethical role of veterinarians. *Journal of Agricultural and Environmental Ethics* 31 (3): 349–367.

47 Hernandez, E., Fawcett, A., Brouwer, E. et al. (2018). Speaking up: veterinary ethical responsibilities and animal welfare issues in everyday practice. *Animals* 8 (1): 15.

2

How to Obtain a Patient History

Barry Kipperman

Abstract

This chapter discusses how to acquire an accurate and thorough patient history, which is fundamental to fulfilling the Principle of Patient Advocacy. Included are the components of a veterinary consultation, requirements of a patient history, a flow chart for obtaining a patient history, and examples of written medical histories. Patient histories should be directed by the veterinary clinician using closed-ended questions. History-taking should not be performed concurrently with patient examination. With practice, a thorough patient history can be completed in 5–10 minutes. A consultation for a sick patient should be a minimum of 30 minutes' duration to sufficiently complete the necessary components.

Keywords: *patient history, consultation, preliminary questions, contemporary questions, ancillary questions, client-centered, veterinarian-directed, consultation duration, patient advocacy*

For many veterinary clinicians, the first opportunity to apply the Principle of Patient Advocacy is during the consultation with clients and their ill animals. Several pivotal responsibilities are required at this time, outlined in Table 2.1.

It should be apparent on considering the steps in Table 2.1 that sufficiently completing these tasks within the typical median duration of office visits in general practice of 10–15 minutes is untenable. Appointment times for sick patients should be extended to at least 30 minutes. This chapter will focus on the first three components in Table 2.1. Informed consent will be discussed in Chapter 3.

Introduction

It is important that veterinary clinicians take a moment to introduce themselves to their clients and to acknowledge their patients in a positive manner. This should not require behaviors that are insincere (i.e. "I just love [insert any breed name here]!"), nor does this step entail the need to learn about the client's vocation, hobbies, etc. To be an advocate for animals, one must establish trust

Table 2.1 Components of a veterinary consultation.

Introduction
Explain the process
Obtain a patient history
Physical examination
Informed consent/client education
Create an estimate for care
Present the estimate to the client
Modify the estimate as needed
Approve the estimate and care plan
Document findings, options presented, and client decision in the medical record

and have the client see you as both a knowledgeable and caring figure. As all veterinarians possess these qualities, this step should be easy to master. You should dress professionally. While societal norms for dress are relaxing (I wore a tie for the first half of my career), ripped jeans, T-shirts, sweatpants, and shorts are not advised.

An example of an introduction can simply include the following:

- Introduce yourself.
- Make eye contact with client(s) and shake hands.
- Acknowledge the patient, i.e. "This is Buster," "Hi Winston," etc.

Explain the Process

Taking a moment to explain to clients what will transpire during their visit eases the uncertainty and anxiety associated with veterinary consultations. This also conveys a perception that you are organized and thorough and inspires confidence: "Mrs. Smith, before I examine [patient name], I want to ensure I understand what your concerns are. I'm going to ask you specific questions that will help me to help you and [patient name]. I'll then perform an examination and discuss my findings, concerns, and recommendations, including costs. Is that OK?"

Obtain a Patient History

One of the barriers to acquiring a history in veterinary patients is that we can't communicate directly with them to discern their feelings and concerns: we are dependent on the animal caretaker/owner acting as a proxy to provide this information. This presents several challenges:

- If the client is emotionally upset by their animal's illness, this can influence their capacity to provide a reliable history. Caregiver burden and emotional exhaustion may result in a more pessimistic portrayal of the patient's condition.
- The client may be unable to tell you what happened ("I came home from work and found this").
- There may be disparities between family members regarding what is happening with the animal.
- The client with the needed information may be unavailable when the patient is presented.

- Economic concerns may cause clients to render a more optimistic perspective than is warranted to attempt to reduce the chances of your advising testing.
- To cope with feelings of guilt or inadequacy for delaying presentation of the animal, some clients may provide information implying the animal's illness is less severe or of a shorter duration than is true.
- Clients with medical knowledge may attempt to make diagnoses for you that can be misleading ("I'm not a veterinarian, but ...").

Obtaining an accurate, concise patient history is an art. Unfortunately, this skill is a lost art, perhaps due to the short time frames of veterinary visits or because few textbooks devote chapters to this subject (comparatively, chapters on performing patient examinations are plentiful). An accurate history is at least as important as conducting a proper examination to guide a diagnostic and treatment plan for patients, if not more so. When I entered exam rooms to begin consultations, many clients picked up their pets and placed them on the exam table to facilitate examination before I could even greet them. I presume this reflects their experience with veterinarians where history-taking and examinations were performed concurrently, ostensibly to save time. When I would thank them and explain that my examination would take place after discussion with them regarding their pet, I often received puzzled looks.

Countless times, my history revealed profound differences from that of the referring veterinarian, often with important ramifications for patient plans and prognosis. These disparities sometimes related to the nature of the problem, but more often to its duration and progression, with my history frequently revealing a more protracted illness requiring a more aggressive approach. Given the importance of obtaining an accurate patient history, your full attention should be devoted to this. This step should not be combined with patient examination. Taking a history exclusively is more likely to provide a more accurate understanding of patient problems and client concerns. Additionally, noting client expressions and body language when they are answering questions can be quite informative. With practice, an accurate and succinct history should take 5–10 minutes to complete.

Despite instructing my interns at the beginning of their internships that they had 15 minutes to obtain patient histories, I would often have to retrieve them from the exam room after 20 minutes because their task had not been completed. The main reason their process took so long was that they asked clients open-ended questions, then spent considerable time writing down each word the client said. By the time we met in my office and they presented their history, it was typically very unfocused. While they had many words written down, they often were unable to provide a brief presentation of what was wrong with the patient or what the client's concerns were.

While the trend in academia is to teach students to ask clients open-ended questions [1] because clients value a conversational approach to history taking [2], in my experience this strategy with sick patients commonly results in meandering notes that do not meet the ideal requirements of a patient history noted in Table 2.2.

Asking open-ended questions such as "What's going on with Max today?" or "How can I help you and Buster?" allows the client to lead the discussion. While this may please the client, clients

Table 2.2 Ideal requirements of a patient history.

What is/are the patient's problem(s)?
What are the onset, duration, and progression of these problems?
What is/are the client's most important concern(s)?

are not trained to provide patient histories. For example, when asked "What's going on with Max today?" or "What can I do for you?" clients often discuss one problem, then divert to a second problem before the first problem has been adequately described, then discuss concerns that are irrelevant to the history (i.e. "I then cleaned up the mess using disinfectant"). A client may tell you that Max vomited a few times, but fail to mention whether dietary indiscretion was associated with those events or what the vomitus looked like. Refocusing clients when asking open-ended questions is inevitable, may require interrupting them to stay on time, and often results in inadequate histories. Therefore, I suggest that clinicians ask closed-ended questions, and gently refocus clients when their responses meander off topic.

A flow chart for obtaining a medical history is outlined in Figure 2.1. I suggest that new graduates bring this flow chart (or an alternate template of questions) with them during consultations to refer to until it is no longer needed.

Preliminary Questions

If your patient's condition is stable, begin history-taking by asking a series of preliminary questions. These address basic information and retrieving responses should take a minute or two. While you and the client may be eager to start with discussion of the patient's current problem(s), doing so may result in the clinician forgetting to address responses to these questions. For example, if your patient presents for acute vomiting and the client tells you that he has undergone two procedures to remove gastrointestinal (GI) foreign bodies, that's valuable information! As another example, if the client tells you that they spend a portion of their time with the animal in the desert, then you might consider screening for Valley fever as the cause of the patient's cough.

Contemporary Questions

By asking the first question in this subset of inquiries (see Figure 2.1), you are determining both the main problem(s) and when they began. If clients blend two separate problems together in their response, simply say that you'd like to discuss one problem first so you can properly address that, then discuss the other concern. At the completion of this step, you should understand the nature of the patient's problem(s), when it/they started, and whether they are improving, progressing, or remaining static. The remaining questions address the most common and important internal medicine symptoms of most ill veterinary patients.

Ancillary Questions

Ancillary questions are dictated by the patient problems that arise from contemporary questioning. These questions allow the clinician to (i) validate the problem, i.e. that vomiting is the concern rather than something rarer such as regurgitation, or that a cat is coughing and not vomiting; (ii) attempt to characterize potential etiologies for the problem, such as ingestion of a fatty meal that would suggest pancreatitis or of a steak bone that would suggest a GI foreign body; and (iii) evaluate the severity of the problem, which influences the clinical approach. Note that severity should consider the perspective of the patient and the client. For example, vomiting five times daily is clearly detrimental to patient welfare, while keeping an owner up at night with patient coughing is detrimental to both the patient's and the client's welfare.

Of all the questions listed in this section (which are by no means exhaustive), the most important relate to patient appetite. As declining appetite is the most common symptom

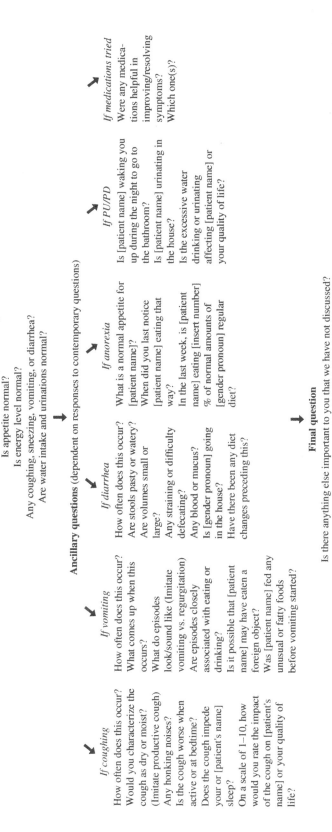

Preliminary questions

How long have you lived with [patient name]?
Where did you acquire [gender pronoun] from?
Has [patient name] experienced any major illnesses or surgeries in the past? When?
Diet? Travel? Vaccination status? Indoor/Outdoor/Both?
Medications and doses? Duration?
Other animals?

Contemporary questions

When did you first notice something was different with [patient name]?
Discuss Problem #1: Onset, duration, progression
Discuss Problem #2, #3, etc. as needed
[Delete below as needed if already cited by client as a problem]
Is appetite normal?
Is energy level normal?
Any coughing, sneezing, vomiting, or diarrhea?
Are water intake and urinations normal?

Ancillary questions (dependent on responses to contemporary questions)

If coughing
How often does this occur?
Would you characterize the cough as dry or moist? (Imitate productive cough)
Any honking noises?
Is the cough worse when active or at bedtime?
Does the cough impede your or [patient's name] sleep?
On a scale of 1–10, how would you rate the impact of the cough on [patient's name] or your quality of life?

If vomiting
How often does this occur?
What comes up when this occurs?
What do episodes look/sound like (Imitate vomiting vs. regurgitation)
Are episodes closely associated with eating or drinking?
Is it possible that [patient name] may have eaten a foreign object?
Was [patient name] fed any unusual or fatty foods before vomiting started?

If diarrhea
How often does this occur?
Are stools pasty or watery?
Are volumes small or large?
Any straining or difficulty defecating?
Any blood or mucus?
Is [gender pronoun] going in the house?
Have there been any diet changes preceding this?

If anorexia
What is a normal appetite for [patient name]?
When did you last notice [patient name] eating that way?
In the last week, is [patient name] eating [insert number] % of normal amounts of [gender pronoun] regular diet?

If PU/PD
Is [patient name] waking you up during the night to go to the bathroom?
Is [patient name] urinating in the house?
Is the excessive water drinking or urinating affecting [patient name] or your quality of life?

If medications tried
Were any medications helpful in improving/resolving symptoms? Which one(s)?

Final question

Is there anything else important to you that we have not discussed?

Figure 2.1 Flow chart for obtaining a patient history.

associated with serious patient illness, accurate characterization of patient appetite is imperative to guide proper diagnostic and therapeutic plans. Statements in medical records such as "poor appetite," "subnormal appetite," "not eating well," and "anorexia" are insufficient. Preferred descriptions would include "Eating 10% of normal food intake in past five days" or "Appetite down 50% in past two days." While both patients have reduced appetites, the need for a rapid diagnosis (and probably nutritional support) is much more compelling for the patient with the more protracted anorexia. I have found that when I ask clients to tell me when their pet last ate a normal amount of food, the actual duration of patient anorexia is much longer than the client initially reported.

Documenting Patient Histories

Documenting your patient's history in medical records should transcribe a summary of client concerns and responses and should not include a complete description of everything the client stated during the consultation. Lengthy and protracted narratives make it more difficult for you and your peers to extract the essence of the patient's problem(s). These are some examples of histories (using common abbreviations and acronyms):

1) Past hx: None.
   Current h/x: Declining appetite/lethargy × 10 days; progressive. Eating 10% of normal in past three days. Vomiting once daily in past three days; bile. No c/s/d/PU/PD. No known diet changes or dietary indiscretion. No meds. No toxins/travel. Indoor only. Diet; dry. Vax; current.
2) Past hx: Heart murmur documented in June 2022.
   Current h/x: Cough × 2 weeks; worse at night and with activity. Coughs multiple times daily; static. O rates 6/10 impact on QOL. Impedes sleep. Exercise intolerance? No s/v/d/syncope/dyspnea. Normal appetite. No meds. No toxins/travel. Indoor only. Diet; dry. Vax; current.
3) Past hx: None
   Current hx: Collapsing episodes × 1 week. Usually 1–2×/day. Rapid recovery. O notes noisy breathing associated with all episodes which are related to activity/exertion/heat exposure. Reduced frequency since O limited duration of walks and outdoor access. No sz activity suspected. Normal appetite. No c/s/v/d/PU/PD. Meds: Carprofen BID × 1 year. No toxins/travel. Indoor/Outdoor. Diet; dry. Vax; current.

Conclusion

This chapter discusses how to acquire an accurate and thorough patient history, which is fundamental to fulfilling the Principle of Patient Advocacy. Using the format in Figure 2.1, questioning is veterinarian directed using closed-ended questions, to which clients provide responses. Clients are given the opportunity to discuss anything else important to them in the last phase of history-taking. While this model does not focus on client-centered dialogue, many of your clients will remark how thorough they perceive you are, and this will translate to their belief that you are an advocate for their animal.

References

1 Clark, J.J. and Linder, C.M. (2022). Evaluation of a novel communication and consultation skills model (WISE COACH) on dog owner perceptions of veterinarians and projected spending on veterinary care. *Journal of the American Veterinary Medical Association* 260 (2): 257–268.

2 Shaw, J.R., Barley, G.E., Broadfoot, K. et al. (2016). Outcomes assessment of on-site communication skills education in a companion animal practice. *Journal of the American Veterinary Medical Association* 249 (4): 419–432.

3

Informed Consent

Barry Kipperman

Abstract

This chapter discusses why veterinarians should obtain informed consent from their clients and outlines the goals, owner expectations, and ideal components of informed consent. Issues associated with acquisition of informed consent are discussed, including requirements for legitimate consent, how many options should be presented, who should present the information including costs, risk disclosure, use of verbal and written communication, and visit duration. Examples of client education are provided. Recommendations are made as to how veterinarians can meet the ideal goals of informed consent. Finally, the effectiveness of informed consent is considered.

Keywords: *informed consent, goals, owner expectations, client education, visit duration, capacity, risk, novel treatments, clinical trials, communication*

Acquisition of informed consent is fundamental to applying the Principle of Patient Advocacy. To be an advocate for animals, we must do our best to ensure that their owners and caretakers understand the nature of their animals' problems and the options available to address them. This step is enacted after history-taking and physical examination. At this point in the consultation, the clinician should formulate a list of patient problems, differential diagnoses, and a diagnostic and/or therapeutic plan of action tailored to the patient. I suggest new graduates leave the exam room to conduct research as needed so you are prepared prior to discussing this with clients. Even experienced practitioners may wish to do this when encountering a patient problem that they have little experience with.

Reasons to Obtain Informed Consent

Doctors, veterinarians, and other professionals are thought to have knowledge that is beyond the understanding of the average person, with such knowledge often referred to as the "mysteries of the learned professions" [1]. Because the average person is not expected to know and understand these "mysteries," the courts impose a special duty on members of these professions, requiring them to inform their clients and patients of the facts concerning their medical care. Animals are for legal purposes considered property and cannot provide consent. Thus, animal owners enjoy certain property rights, and the power to consent or deny consent to a medical procedure is one of those rights.

Ethical guidance is found in the American Veterinary Medical Association (AVMA) Principles of Veterinary Medical Ethics, which require veterinarians to "respect the rights of clients," while stipulating that veterinarians have a "responsibility to inform the client of the expected results and costs, and the related risks of each treatment regimen" [2]. Therefore, informed consent is both a legal and an ethical obligation of veterinarians. Finally, owner approval of the proposed plan of action serves as a basis for a contract to agree to perform work.

Goals of Informed Consent

The objective of informed consent is that "Owners be provided adequate information so they can make the right decision for their pet and for themselves" [3]. This both achieves a patient and client advocacy posture and protects the clinician, as observed by Gray and Favre:

> The acquisition of consent to the treatment of an animal patient requires careful balancing of respect for the client's wishes and protection of the best interests of the animal patient. The purposes of informed consent ... can therefore be defined as threefold: it should protect the patient from inappropriate or harmful treatment or excessive risk, it should protect the client from unexpected costs, and it should protect the veterinary professional from complaints and claims by evidencing the client's agreement to proceed. [4]

As an example, providing both medical and surgical treatment options for a 14-year-old dog with insulinoma-induced hypoglycemic symptoms allows the client to decide whether to assume the risks for the patient associated with partial pancreatectomy and the affiliated costs, and ensures that clinician liability for litigation or grievances is diminished based on documentation of these choices and their potential consequences in the medical record.

Owner Expectations Regarding Informed Consent

A focus group study found that pet owners expected their veterinarian to communicate (i) information in both verbal and written formats; (ii) a range of options for care; (iii) in understandable terms; (iv) a prognosis or expectation about patient quality of life; and (v) respect for their decisions [5]. A more recent study discovered that pet owners wanted their veterinarian to (i) respect their understanding of their pets; (ii) acknowledge their thoughts and opinions, including both listening to what they say verbally and evaluating body language to assess their emotional state; (iii) recognize the level of information sought by each client; (iv) explain things in a way that they understood; and (v) be honest about their pet's prognosis [6]. Veterinary clinicians should endeavor to meet all these goals, and the remainder of this chapter will provide guidance and discuss some of the practical limitations of providing informed consent.

Components of Informed Consent

The good news is that owner expectations are aligned with the most important components of informed consent, as outlined in Table 3.1.

Table 3.1 The most important components of informed consent in veterinary practice.

Medical concerns and possible or probable diagnoses

Diagnostic and treatment options

Rationale for tests and treatments

Benefits and risks of tests and treatments

Outcomes/prognosis/lifespan/quality of life

Referral options

Costs

Owner expectations excluding costs

Source: Adapted from [1, 4].

Medical concerns and diagnoses relate to informing clients of the possible or probable causes of the patient's symptom(s) based on the problem(s) and differential diagnosis list. Diagnostic and treatment options include discussing choices that serve the patient's best interest, and rationale for tests and treatments includes explaining why the tests or treatments you advise are warranted. Inability to adequately explain the reason tests are necessary is one of the most common reasons for poor client compliance with clinician recommendations. While veterinarians may assume that abdominal imaging to screen for causes of vomiting in a young dog is the first reasonable step, clients need to understand *why* this is valuable to gain their approval: "X-rays and possibly ultrasound of Max's abdomen are very valuable methods for diagnosing pancreatitis, gastrointestinal foreign body, and dietary indiscretion, which are the most likely causes for Max's vomiting that we just discussed. I advise starting with x-rays as these are less costly. If x-rays are inconclusive, then the combination of x-rays and ultrasound should provide close to a 100% diagnostic rate for identifying the cause."

Benefits and risks of tests and treatments include discussing the chances of success and the associated risks of each choice. For example, "Because Buddy the cat is having difficulty breathing, x-rays of his chest are the most valuable test to try to ascertain the cause, which can lead to a more refined and successful treatment approach. The main risk is that the stress to Buddy may worsen his breathing and could even result in death. Because Buddy is a young cat and is having extreme difficulty breathing, and asthma is considered the most likely cause, I suggest we prioritize treatment and give Buddy an hour or two to receive oxygen and medication and to adapt to being in the hospital with minimal handling. Once his breathing improves, then we can more safely take confirmatory x-rays if this is feasible after the costs of treatment are accounted for. If his condition worsens at any time or he does not improve, then I'd request permission to sedate him to perform x-rays and a cursory ultrasound. While these would still entail risks, in my experience the risk of inaction would exceed the small risk of imaging while he is sedated, and the potential benefits of finding the cause could be very high."

For a dog with idiopathic epilepsy, one may elect to inform an owner: "As lab testing was normal, I suspect Ricky has epilepsy. We can usually manage the seizures with lifelong medication(s), and these usually reduce the frequency, severity, and duration of the seizures, but these are not curative, and some seizures are likely to persist. Some of the medications used to control seizures have side effects, which can include sedation and excessive appetite. These may affect your perception of his quality of life. In most dogs, we can find a balance between medication-induced concerns and seizures. Regular checkups and blood tests will be needed to reduce the chances of recurrent seizures."

Outcomes and prognosis include discussing survival versus mortality rates (and providing quantitative estimates if this data is available), expected lifespan, and defining what success or failure looks like (see Chapter 20). Use of the terms "good prognosis" or "poor prognosis" alone is discouraged, as these are vague and suggest that the veterinarian is defining what is "good or bad" rather than the client. Better yet, state: "With lifelong treatment of hypoadrenocorticism almost all patients live a normal quality of life and normal lifespan" or "Most cats with kidney failure respond to supportive care in the hospital after 2–4 days and have improved and acceptable quality of life as perceived by their owners, with lifelong care at home including daily administration of fluids under the skin. Unfortunately, almost all will experience progression of their disease and die from this condition. In a recent report, the median survival time after diagnosis is about one year. This means that about half of cats will live for less than one year and half of cats with this disease will exceed one year survival time" [7]. These discussions should also address impacts on patient quality of life, for example any anticipated lifestyle limitations such as reduced exercise or activity or the need to eat a special diet.

Referral options involve informing the client of their right to seek a second opinion, especially if referral may improve the probability of enhanced patient outcome or survival (see Chapter 7). Costs relate to addressing the fees for the various options, often presented to clients in a formal estimate of care. These should also address any long-term expenses such as the need for serial veterinary visits, tests, medications, etc.

Finally, non-economic expectations of owners as caretakers should be discussed. Examples include the need to extract blood samples and use a glucometer to evaluate patient glucose measurements, giving subcutaneous fluids, administering lifelong medications, assistance with walking, etc. These concerns should be addressed so that owners can decline such measures if these expectations exceed their capabilities. The concept of client caregiver burden associated with providing care for companion animals with protracted illness has been documented and should be acknowledged by the empathic practitioner [8].

Pertinent Issues Associated with Obtaining Informed Consent

This chapter has discussed why obtaining informed consent from clients is important, and the ideal goals and components of informed consent. Now, let's discuss putting these principles into action in practice. For many of these issues, there is little guidance for practitioners in codes of conduct or textbooks.

Requirements for Legitimate Consent

It is inevitable that someone will request medical information about a patient or claim to be the decision-maker for the patient, when it is either apparent (i.e. the individual is underage) or doubtful (the individual is not the animal owner or a family member) that divulging such information is appropriate. As I'm a veterinarian and not an attorney, I will discuss this from an ethical and practical perspective, but keep in mind that there are client confidentiality and privacy rights to be respected when considering to whom medical information should be imparted.

The owner of the animal is typically the person who should provide consent for veterinary care. In some cases this is straightforward, while in other cases several family members may make this claim. This can be frustrating for the clinician, as they are often asked to disclose medical information to multiple parties on separate occasions, which is time consuming. This also tends to delay decisions for the patient, as the time frame for three people to agree on a course of action often exceeds that needed by one individual. In circumstances where multiple parties claim to be the animal owner, I suggest all decision-makers be available at once for the discussion with the clinician. If this is not feasible, then ask to speak to whomever is most likely to be responsible for the final decision. They can then share the disclosed information with the others.

In some settings, the financially responsible person may delegate the decision about the animal's veterinary care to a caretaker. This person is designated as the agent of the owner and is granted the power to provide consent. This concept is illustrated by Gray and Favre: "In veterinary practice, agency includes those with whom the owner has a contract for the provision of boarding or training services (for example, kennel or stable proprietors, or trainers of sporting animals) but also friends and family of the animal owner" [4]. To reduce misunderstandings, it is ideal if the decision-maker on behalf of the animal is also the person paying the bill. It has been my experience that the person responsible for payment often expects a direct conversation with the veterinarian, even if they have delegated agency to another person.

The client must be deemed to have the "capacity" to make judgments based on the information presented, in order for them to grant permission [4]. Capacity is legally defined as the ability to understand information relevant to a decision, to retain that information, to use or weigh that information as part of the process of making the decision, and to communicate the decision [9]. In situations in which an animal is suffering from an acute illness (i.e. thromboembolic event) or trauma, some owners may be so emotionally distraught that they are unable to assimilate complicated information or decide between multiple options. In such cases guidance is unclear, as the AVMA Principles of Veterinary Medical Ethics do not consider the issue of client capacity [2]. In these situations, having a team member console the client and reassure them that the medical staff are doing their best to provide life-saving care (if necessary) and comfort can allow time for the client to regain their composure. Meanwhile, the patient can be provided with analgesics, intravenous fluids, oxygen, etc. as medically indicated.

Finally, the veterinarian might also need to confirm the client's age in addition to determining capacity. Most codes of professional conduct establish the age of consent as 18 years, the minimum age below which veterinarians must get parental or guardian consent [4].

Who Should Present the Information?

The veterinary clinician is typically responsible for discussing all the components of informed consent in Table 3.1. Some practices attempt to remove the clinician from all financial discussions with clients, ostensibly to associate the image of the veterinarian with medical decisions and to discourage the perception of the clinician as an income generator. The problem with this approach is that unlike in human medicine where most patients have health insurance, which insulates them from the costs of medical care and bills are due after services have been provided, only about 2% of companion animals in North America have health insurance [10]. Veterinarians in practice utilize a fee-for-service model of income, with clients paying out of pocket, usually before and after services are rendered.

Consequently, medical decisions in veterinary practice are inherently tied to their costs. It is commonplace for a practitioner to present an estimate of desired care to a client, and to have the client request that the plan be modified to reduce the costs. If a veterinary technician, customer service representative, or hospital manager is in the exam room, they are not as qualified as the veterinarian to know which items (if any) are most suitable to be withdrawn or postponed. To address this, some clinicians will create estimates where certain items are designated as "desirable but not essential" by placing the quantity for that service as 0 or 1 in the estimate.

Veterinary clients are knowledgeable enough to recognize that all medical professionals have economic incentives that may influence their recommendations. They also hope that their clinicians will abide by their respective code of ethics to nullify or minimize this tendency. The veterinarian should be responsible for negotiating with clients when necessary to modify a diagnostic or treatment plan.

How Many Options Should Be Presented? In What Order?

Should clients be offered all available options for their animals? Let's consider an example of a young cat presented for multiple bouts of acute vomiting with no known cause. A clinician could support each of the following considerations (or combinations of these):

- Supportive care and observation at home.
- Supportive care in hospital.
- Radiographs only.
- Radiographs and laboratory testing.
- Upper gastrointestinal series.
- Abdominal ultrasound.

This illustrates one of the challenges veterinary clinicians face, which is ensuring that our recommendations are comprehensive while not overwhelming our clients. Even with excellent communication skills, I believe that most clients would feel inundated if they were expected to choose among six or more options. One could argue that the presentation of too many options might encourage clients to ask their veterinarian to choose what is best for them, i.e. a paternalistic posture, rather than one of shared decision-making. While shared decisions are desirable for many reasons, the AVMA Principles of Veterinary Medical Ethics state that "Attending veterinarians are responsible for choosing the treatment regimen for their patients" [2], suggesting a paternalistic posture. Pet owners in a recent study emphasized that a paternalistic approach to communication by their veterinarian left them with negative feelings and increased the likelihood that they would seek care from another veterinarian [6].

If we are going to limit the number of choices presented to clients, which ones should be presented and in what order? One could consider the following criteria:

- Best for patient.
- Best for veterinarian.
- Most to least costly.
- Least to most costly.
- Only those the practice can provide.
- Only those the clinician believes the client can afford.

The Principle of Patient Advocacy compels veterinarians to advise the option(s) deemed to be in the best interest of each individual patient. A "one size fits all" diagnostic approach to patients with identical problems should be eschewed. While this seems like an obvious approach, my experience has been that clinicians are influenced by economic factors when advising clients, especially if they are compensated based on generated revenues. Veterinarians also appear to routinely make judgments about their clients, including categorizing them as "good" or "bad" in terms of inclination to pursue treatments or pay the fees [11]. Therefore, if a veterinarian presumed that a client could not afford diagnostic testing or would not pay for it, testing might not be offered. A study corroborates this, finding that approximately a third of small animal veterinarians indicated that they do not offer ideal diagnostic or treatment options in the list of alternatives provided to all clients [12]. Limiting provision of options due to classification of clients can compromise both patient advocacy and the veterinarian's capacity to promote animal welfare.

I can recall many times during my career when I left an exam room to create an estimate for the ideal plan for the patient plagued with doubt that the clients would consent, only to be pleasantly surprised. One case I'll never forget was an older, large-breed dog with gastric dilatation-volvulus. This is a painful and life-threatening disease that requires surgery to resolve. With surgery, the condition is cured. Based on the costs and older age of many dogs with this condition, economic euthanasia is an all too common outcome. When I presented the $5000 estimate for surgery and postoperative care expecting the worst, the family looked at me and said, "Well, Doc. She's given us a lifetime of companionship, so we owe this to her. We'll find a way to make this work. We want to proceed." I was on the verge of tears when I admitted that dog to the hospital, moved by the power of the human–animal bond.

Veterinarians should always present the best option for each patient and discuss this first (including why it is preferred). As pet owners in one report noted that they were more likely to feel that their veterinarian's recommendation was financially motivated when only one option was provided [6], secondary and tertiary options that may be less optimal should also be presented and discussed (when feasible). While some veterinarians in that study expressed the need to provide options only when the cost of the ideal care was not feasible for the client, participating pet owners suggested multiple options should be provided upfront with cost as one of several aspects of discussing options. As an example, one might advise surgical repair of a long-bone fracture in a cat, but also inform the client of non-surgical options including rest and splints/bandages.

Risk Disclosure

In human medicine, risk disclosure involves giving the patient information about material risks that would be required by a "reasonable person" or "particular patient" deciding about treatment [4]. In veterinary medicine, Gray and Favre note a practical concern about discussing risks:

> a common concern is how many risks need to be disclosed for a particular procedure? Veterinarians may be concerned that they must mention every single risk, no matter how rare, and that disclosing too much information may scare the client and reduce the likelihood that they will pursue the procedure. Any risks that are common to the proposed treatment ... or that would be regarded as serious (for example, the small but devastating risk of death with general anesthesia) should be discussed. [4]

A retrospective study identified the mortality rates associated with general anesthesia in primary care veterinary practice as 0.05% for dogs and 0.11% for cats [13]. I have never heard of a veterinarian disclosing to a client that a patient's risk of dying under anesthesia was 5 in 10 000. Most colleagues consider these risks as so remote as to not require informing clients. Based on what occurs in practice, clinicians discuss some risks considered to be "reasonably common." Where this line should be drawn is unclear. As examples, I suspect that most surgeons discuss risks including infection and dehiscence. In my practice, the potential side effects of chemotherapy including nausea, reduced appetite, and neutropenia increasing risks of infection were routinely discussed with clients. Veterinary clinicians tend to minimize risk disclosure. This will be discussed further in Chapter 4.

Novel or Experimental Treatments and Clinical Trials

Ethical concerns associated with the recommendation of unproven or experimental treatments or entering patients into clinical trials include the fact that the practitioner may be influenced by extraneous factors besides the patient's interest, including self-esteem, reputational, or financial benefits. Consequently, animal owners should be provided sufficient information to make decisions about whether their animals should participate. This should include available evidence, risks and benefits, and the number of patients that have been treated with the proposed protocol. The client's vulnerability should be considered, especially if they are desperate to heal their pet and cannot afford traditional therapy [14]. Also, unlike human research, animal subjects do not have the ability to remove themselves from a treatment trial. Although owners may be able to withdraw their animals from a trial, they are not routinely provided with the results of interim analyses to consider such a decision [15] (Case Study 3.1). Finally, oversight concerns to protect animal welfare of veterinary patients are poorly regulated, in contrast with research conducted on humans and laboratory animals.

Written and Verbal Communication

Many years ago, a mundane experience had profound implications for how I discussed the components of informed consent with my clients in the latter half of my career. I was picking up my car from a repair shop after the main staff and mechanics had left. I was told that the car had been repaired and paid my bill. The only paperwork I received was the credit card receipt. I inquired as to what was wrong that had cost $750 and was told "A [insert instrument name here] rod, and [insert instrument name here] gasket was replaced." When I got home, my girlfriend asked me what was wrong with the car. Despite being told the names of the defective parts, I had no recollection of these an hour later, and could only reply, "I don't know. Maybe a Johnson rod and Giggety gasket."

My failure to remember, much less comprehend, what I had been told in "mechanic speak" inspired a revelation: "So this must be what my clients feel like when I speak to them!" After this event, I committed that my client education in exam rooms would include both verbal and written

---

Case Study 3.1 Clinical Trial for Chylothorax Treatment

You refer Bo, a canine patient, to a referral hospital for evaluation of idiopathic chylothorax. At that time, the standard of care was to perform surgical thoracic duct ligation and partial pericardiectomy, with good success rates [16]. After Bo underwent thoracoscopic ligation only, you learn from the client that she enrolled Bo in a subsidized clinical trial to evaluate whether both procedures were warranted, or whether one of the two procedures alone could be sufficient to resolve the problem. Unfortunately, the pleural effusion persisted, resulting in the need for multiple emergency visits due to episodes of dyspnea and cyanosis requiring centesis to remove the thoracic fluid. Weeks later, Bo had to undergo a second thoracic surgery for the pericardiectomy, which fortunately resolved the issue.

While Bo was lucky to have an owner this committed, for many dogs in this trial death or euthanasia was a likely outcome, as many owners would not be willing to endure (emotionally and financially) continued episodes of dyspnea in their pet and a second, painful thoracic surgery. Did this owner truly understand the ramifications of a failed first procedure? Should you express your concerns about this trial to either the client or the teaching hospital?

communication. The change was immediate. Rather than feeling insecure about whether my clients understood what I was saying while they nodded their head affirmatively when I'd ask "Is that clear?", now my clients asked more insightful questions reflecting an understanding of the discussion, took less time to make decisions, were more committed to their decisions, and seemed much more pleased with the consultation than when I only communicated verbally. If my client was uncertain of what to do, they sometimes would take photos of what I had written and text or email it to those they wanted counsel from. Many clients would point to select sections of tables or figures created during their visit, proclaiming "We want option number 2." A focus group study of pet owners corroborates my experience: owners discussed their difficulty comprehending new information when it was only conveyed verbally, and mentioned that they found using a visual aid alongside a verbal explanation an effective method for their veterinarian to share information with them [6].

While on rare occasions I would bring in a preexisting table, in almost all cases I would stand by the examination table with the client(s) and create a table or flow chart unique to each patient's set of problems. Examples of written client education I've used are noted in Tables 3.2 and 3.3 and in Figure 3.1. I prefer to order lists documenting the causes I believe are most likely for the patient at the top and those considered least likely at the bottom.

Handouts are another useful tool to augment client understanding. In one study, pet owners conveyed appreciation for receiving informational handouts to review on their own time because it allowed them to reflect on what was discussed during their appointment [6]. In the author's practice, client handouts on topics such as seizures, diabetes mellitus, and cancer chemotherapy were routinely given to clients and were utilized to supplement the discussion in the exam room.

Table 3.2 Example of client education for a dog with acute vomiting and anorexia.

Causes	Tests	Treatment	Prognosis
Dietary indiscretion	History	Symptomatic care	Excellent
Pancreatitis	History, lab tests, ultrasound	Supportive care in hospital	Good
GI foreign body/obstruction	X-rays, ultrasound	Endoscopy/surgery	Excellent
Metabolic	Lab tests	Supportive care in hospital	Guarded–poor

GI, gastrointestinal.

Table 3.3 Example of client education for a dog with chronic diarrhea and good appetite.

Causes	Tests	Treatment	Prognosis
Dietary intolerance/allergy	Dietary trial	Dietary trial	Excellent
Antibiotic-responsive enteropathy	?	Antibiotic trial	Excellent
Inflammatory bowel disease	Ultrasound, endoscopy and biopsies vs. medication trials	Medications	Guarded
Exocrine pancreatic insufficiency	Blood test	Enzyme supplementation	Excellent
Parasites	Fecal tests	Medication	Very good

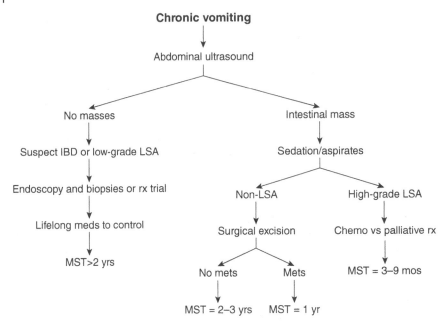

Figure 3.1 Example of client education for a geriatric cat with chronic vomiting, weight loss, and normal lab results. Chemo, chemotherapy; IBD, inflammatory bowel disease; LSA, lymphoma; mets, metastases; MST, median survival time; rx, therapeutic.

Visit Duration

Veterinarians have mentioned time constraints as their primary concern in meeting the expectation of information exchange [6]. In a report from the United Kingdom, consultations for patients with health problems were 15 minutes in duration [17], which aligns with visit times in older investigations [18, 19]. It is very difficult (if not impossible) to acquire a thorough history as outlined in Chapter 2, complete a physical examination, and acquire informed consent based on the components in Table 3.1 in consultation times of 15 minutes or less. Increased consult length has been associated with increased veterinarian satisfaction [17]. Consultation times for sick patients should be at least 30 minutes with commensurate fees. This would enhance the quality of veterinary care and your capacity to fulfill your role as patient advocate. While some may claim that clients will not pay for consults of this duration, this contention is undermined by the success of referral practices where consultation times are often 30 minutes or longer (my consults were 60 minutes' duration).

Informed versus Consent

While this chapter has discussed obtaining "informed consent" to characterize one of the most pivotal responsibilities of the veterinary clinician, far too often in practice the emphasis is placed on achieving "consent" via a signature on a form, rather than on the term "informed," which connotes client understanding. If the components noted in Table 3.1 are not met, then client consent cannot be considered to be "informed." Countless times in my career, a client would be unable to tell me why their animal companion was receiving a medication prescribed by their veterinarian. The most common response was "My vet said he needed it."

Gray and Favre provide guidance on the distinction between information and consent:

> The veterinary healthcare consent process could ... be regarded as a mixture of a consent process for treatment and a contract for payment for this treatment. Most forms seem designed to provide authorization for treatment rather than to substantiate or facilitate client comprehension. The presence ... of a signed consent form does not in itself confirm the validity of any associated consent. Good practice requires that the client is provided with written evidence of the discussion that has taken place between veterinarian and client. Consent is more than just a signature on a form: it requires sharing of information, ensuring mutual understanding and collaborative decision-making. [4]

How Effective Is Informed Consent in Veterinary Practice?

There are very few empirical studies examining the question of how effective veterinarians are in acquiring informed consent from the perspective of their clients. In a survey of clients from a referral hospital in the United Kingdom (note that these appointment times are usually longer than in general practice) whose animals were admitted for surgery, 96% were satisfied with the amount of time provided to consider the surgery before approving, and 90% felt adequately informed [20]. Unfortunately, 60% of these clients did not read the form, 66% reported being confused about the purpose of the consent form they were asked to sign, and 53% were not reassured by the process. The authors concluded that there was limited understanding of the purpose of consent and advised that the profession modify the consent process "to ensure that the professional and contractual objectives of consent are met." A study observing consent discussions for elective neutering procedures concluded that these contained most of the information that comprises informed consent, but the essence of these conversations was not documented on an accompanying consent form [21]. Of course, meeting the criteria for consent for gonadectomy is far less demanding than when discussing care options for an ill patient.

References

1 Flemming, D.D. and Scott, J.F. (2004). The informed consent doctrine: what veterinarians should tell their clients. *Journal of the American Veterinary Medical Association* 224 (9): 1436–1439.

2 American Veterinary Medical Association (n.d). Principles of veterinary medical ethics of the AVMA. https://www.avma.org/KB/Policies/Pages/Principles-of-Veterinary-Medical-Ethics-of-the-AVMA.aspx (accessed February 26, 2023).

3 Fettman, M.J. and Rollin, B.E. (2002). Modern elements of informed consent for general veterinary practitioners. *Journal of the American Veterinary Medical Association* 221 (10): 1386–1393.

4 Gray, C. and Favre, D. (2022). Veterinary ethics and the law. In: *Ethics in Veterinary Practice*, ch. 5 (ed. B. Kipperman and B.E. Rollin). Hoboken, NJ: Wiley-Blackwell.

5 Coe, J.B., Adams, C.L., and Bonnett, B.N. (2008). A focus group study of veterinarians' and pet owners' perceptions of veterinarian-client communication in companion animal practice. *Journal of the American Veterinary Medical Association* 233 (7): 1072–1080.

6 Janke, N., Coe, J.B., Bernardo, T.M. et al. (2021). Pet owners' and veterinarians' perceptions of information exchange and clinical decision-making in companion animal practice. *PLoS One* 16 (2): e0245632.

7 Conroy, M., Brodbelt, D.C., O'Neill, D. et al. (2019). Chronic kidney disease in cats attending primary care practice in the UK: a VetCompass TM study. *Veterinary Record* 184 (17): 526.

8 Spitznagel, M.B., Jacobson, D.M., Cox, M.D. et al. (2017). Caregiver burden in owners of a sick companion animal: a cross-sectional observational study. *Veterinary Record* 181 (12): 321.

9 Mental Capacity Act 2005 (UK), Section 3.1. https://www.legislation.gov.uk/ukpga/2005/9/section/3 (accessed August 10, 2023).

10 North American Pet Health Insurance Association (NAPHIA). State of the pet insurance industry in North America, 2021. https://naphia.org/industry-data (accessed February 26, 2023).

11 Morgan, C.A. (2009). Stepping up to the plate: animal welfare, veterinarians and ethical conflicts. PhD thesis, University of British Columbia, Vancouver, BC, Canada.

12 Kipperman, B.S., Kass, P.H., and Rishniw, M. (2017). Factors that influence small animal veterinarians' opinions and actions regarding cost of care and effects of economic limitations on patient care and outcome and professional career satisfaction and burnout. *Journal of the American Veterinary Medical Association* 250 (7): 785–794.

13 Matthews, N.S., Mohn, T.J., Yang, M. et al. (2017). Factors associated with anesthetic-related death in dogs and cats in primary care veterinary hospitals. *Journal of the American Veterinary Medical Association* 250 (6): 655–665.

14 Regan, D., Garcia, K., and Thamm, D. (2018). Clinical, pathological, and ethical considerations for the conduct of clinical trials in dogs with naturally occurring cancer: a comparative approach to accelerate translational drug development. *ILAR Journal* 59 (1): 99–110.

15 Habing, G.G. and Kaneene, J.B. (2011). Stopping rules in veterinary randomized controlled trials. *Journal of the American Veterinary Medical Association* 239 (9): 1197–1199.

16 Mayhew, P.D., Steffey, M.A., Fransson, B.A. et al. (2019). Long-term outcome of video-assisted thoracoscopic thoracic duct ligation and pericardectomy in dogs with chylothorax: a multi-institutional study of 39 cases. *Veterinary Surgery* 48 (S1): O112–O120.

17 Corah, L., Mossop, L., Dean, R. et al. (2020). Measuring satisfaction in the small animal consultation and its relationship to consult length. *Veterinary Record* 187 (11): 446.

18 Shaw, J.R., Adams, C.L., Bonnett, B.N. et al. (2008). Veterinarian-client-patient communication during wellness appointments versus appointments related to a health problem in companion animal practice. *Journal of the American Veterinary Medical Association* 233 (10): 1576–1586.

19 Robinson, N.J., Dean, R.S., Cobb, M. et al. (2014). Consultation length in first opinion small animal practice. *Veterinary Record* 175 (19): 486. https://doi.org/10.1136/vr.102713.

20 Whiting, M., Alexander, A., Habiba, M. et al. (2017). Survey of veterinary clients' perceptions of informed consent at a referral hospital. *Veterinary Record* 180 (1): 20.

21 Gray, C.A. (2019). The role of informed consent in the veterinary clinic: a case study in companion animal neutering. PhD thesis, University of Birmingham. https://etheses.bham.ac.uk//id/eprint/9029 (accessed February 26, 2023).

4

Risks, Benefits, and Ageism

Barry Kipperman

Abstract

This chapter considers types of patient and client harms, framing of benefits and risks, and issues associated with discussing risks. Lack of access to reliable data about the risks associated with veterinary procedures, biases toward framing procedures the clinician is familiar with more optimistically, and concern about upsetting clients may limit the veterinarian's capacity to provide clients with accurate knowledge of patient risks. The concepts of risk aversion and ageism are presented. Risk aversion likely influences veterinarian decisions and may contribute to ageism. Ageism may be as prevalent in veterinary medicine as in the human medical profession, if not more so due to the capacity to elect for euthanasia.

Keywords: *risks, harms, benefits, framing, evidence, data, biases, risk aversion, ageism*

Risks versus Harms

During consideration of informed consent in Chapter 3, one of the most important components was discussion of the benefits and risks of potential tests and treatments. There are numerous issues related to this obligation that are worth exploring further. Let's examine the term "risks." A recent paper suggests that physicians should replace use of the time-honored word "risks" with "harms" [1]. The term "harms" seems more relevant to the welfare of our patients, as not all risks are harms. As an example, let's consider an abdominal ultrasound. One risk may be that I do a lousy job of clipping hair, and the remaining hair is uneven. While this is a risk of this procedure, it's not a harm to the patient. Alternatively, if my clipping is too aggressive, the patient may get "clipper burn" or a painful rash on their belly. This is a risk that accompanies a patient harm. Conversely, not all harms are associated with risks. While it is common knowledge that hypertension is a risk factor for a stroke or vascular event, not all patients with stroke are hypertensive. In fact, some stroke patients may have had no risk factors at all.

While these semantic distinctions may be interesting, the popular use of the term "harms" suggests intentionality. One legal definition defines harms as a "term for any wrong or harm done by one individual to another individual's body, rights, reputation, or property" [2]. Therefore,

I suggest veterinary clinicians use the term "risks" rather than "harms" in discussions with clients, where risks are defined as unintentional harms to patients that are not associated with medical errors (see Chapter 10).

Types of Harms

Seven domains of potential harms to human patients receiving a test or treatment have been recognized [3]. Of these domains, those relevant to veterinary practice are physical impairment; psychological distress; social disruption; financial impact; and treatment burden – the workload from managing healthcare conditions.

While most clinicians are apt to consider harms through a medical lens (such as decline in patient condition, medication-induced side effects, or death), it is equally important to bear in mind the emotional experiences or affect of our patients. Doing all we can to reduce the need for stressful visits to the hospital (such as incorporating telemedicine appointments), using anxiolytics before warranted visits as needed, and utilizing evidence-based methods to alleviate stress in the hospital – including gentle handling and restraint, use of sedation, enrichment such as hiding boxes in cages for cats, and minimizing noise – are all important steps to mitigate patient anxiety. Veterinarians also have an ethical and medical duty to prevent, diagnose, and treat pain (see Chapter 25), because pain causes negative emotions and negative emotions enhance pain perception [4].

Animal patients may have robust social lives, which can include daily hikes or walks with other family pets or the animal companions of friends or neighbors, play dates with other dogs, visits to dog parks, etc. Many medical problems such as surgical recoveries, orthopedic conditions, and cardiopulmonary diseases are likely to disrupt these social patterns temporarily, or even permanently. Helping our clients find creative means to minimize these disruptions or alternative substitutes for patients should be considered.

In my experience, clinicians seldom inquire as to the implications for the client of the costs associated with tests or treatment. We rely on clients to inform us when there are financial limitations, and we do our best to tailor care to each client's budget. In a spectrum of care practice philosophy, veterinarians would attempt to find out about a client's financial capacity *before* a plan and estimate are proposed to better align care with budgets (K. Jankowski, personal communication, 2022).

Finally, the emotional burden of caregiving on our clients is an important factor that should be considered in decision-making. For example, the well-known tendency of polypharmacy (prescribing multiple medications for patients) should be viewed skeptically for multiple reasons (those related to the patient will be discussed in Chapter 22). Many times, during an initial consultation I'd ask a client what medications their animal was receiving. In response, they would open a bag filled with medication vials, and spill 4–8 different vials on the exam table. Most of these were to be administered 2–3 times a day. Let's do the math here: 6 medications $\times$ 2.5 administrations = 15 doses per day. Often, to a cat!

When one of my cats developed chronic kidney failure and I gave him daily subcutaneous fluids by myself, I developed a newfound appreciation for what I had routinely expected my clients to do. Additionally, when my cat Whitney required daily medications for his chronic enteropathy, I quickly acquired empathy when my clients would complain that medicating cats was difficult. The need to seek emergency care for patients suffering from recurrent episodes of dyspnea, seizures, etc. should be considered traumatic events for both the patient and the client. Emotional exhaustion is a common and underappreciated reason why clients elect euthanasia of veterinary patients. Empathy for the burden of treatment on our clients is warranted to address this harm associated with treating patients.

Ideally, veterinary clinicians and clients making collaborative decisions about care should consider all these domains of harms, which should enhance communication about this component of informed consent.

Framing of Benefits and Risks

During my career I paid little attention to how I discussed benefits and risks with my clients. I suspect that if I believed that a procedure, surgery, or medication caused minimal risk, I'd emphasize success or survival rates. If I thought that my patient would endure something likely to cause harm, decline, or death, I'd discuss mortality or failure rates. One of the most notable cognitive biases is the framing effect, discovered by Tversky and Kahneman [5]. It occurs when people respond differently to a particular choice depending on whether it is framed as a gain or a loss. Some studies in the human medical field have concluded that patients' decisions are shaped by whether outcomes were referred to as something that was positive or negative.

One report found that patients receiving information about angioplasty were more likely to consent to the procedure when it was framed as 99% safe, compared to those who were told there was a 1% complication rate [6]. In another study, physicians who recommended immediate treatment for prostate cancer (vs. active surveillance) used fewer words related to losses and significantly fewer words related specifically to death from cancer [7]. In a review of the medical literature on framing, the authors concluded that the influence of framing information with compliance with health recommendations is unclear [8].

Veterinary clients may be more likely to pursue recommendations for care if outcomes are discussed citing success or survival rates instead of failure or mortality rates. To avoid framing bias on client decisions, success and failure rates should be discussed.

Pertinent Issues Associated with Discussing Risks in Veterinary Practice

Insufficient Data

One of the difficulties in adequately discussing risks with our clients is the dearth of rigorous evidence from randomized clinical trials or empirical studies addressing the prevalence of major harms. In the United Kingdom and Australia, the VetCompass™ program is a voluntary database of health information related to patients under primary care [9]. A recent report of commonly diagnosed conditions from this database evaluated over 900 000 dogs at 886 veterinary clinics [10]. Another report from the same database investigated survival times post diagnosis in over 350 000 cats with chronic kidney disease [11]. This program has revealed very useful epidemiologic data for select conditions on large numbers of dogs and cats. Two well-established insurance databases, Pet Protect from the United Kingdom and Agria from Sweden, have been utilized for epidemiologic research on the causes of morbidity and mortality in insured dog populations [12]. No comparable databases in the United States are currently reporting data on veterinary patient risks or mortality rates.

When I conducted a literature search for mortality rates of small animal veterinary diseases and procedures, only a few retrospective studies of relatively uncommon conditions appeared.

One study documented a 10% mortality rate in dogs with pyometra when euthanasia cases were included [13]. Other studies reported a 12% mortality rate in dogs with gastric dilatation-volvulus [14], a 5% mortality rate in dogs undergoing gastrointestinal (GI) surgery [15], and a 15% mortality rate associated with canine adrenalectomy [16]. While this is valuable information, it's important to note that the number of cases in these studies varied from 40 to 700. A more useful paper discovered mortality rates associated with anesthesia of over 3500 dogs and cats of 0.12% for healthy animals and 5% for sick animals [17].

As a result of the scarcity of data on mortality rates in veterinary patients (considered to be the most significant harm a client would be concerned about), and the confounding influence of euthanasia as a contributing cause of patient deaths, veterinarians are left either hoping this information will be available and accessible, or more likely are providing clients with their best estimates of risks based on their experience. Veterinary clinicians need greater access to evidence-based data of the benefits and harms of interventions to facilitate informed consent.

Biases

During my career, I was always intrigued as to why one of my emergency doctors would see a client and complain that they would not pursue advanced diagnostics, yet when I consulted with the same client the next day, they would often agree to move forward with testing. Some of my referring veterinarians confided that they had a difficult time convincing their clients to be referred for diagnostic endoscopy. Yet, I had little trouble achieving client compliance for the same procedure. On further reflection, my client compliance rate to treat cancer with chemotherapy (which I offered and felt comfortable performing) far exceeded my ability to get my clients to consider radiation treatment (which I did not offer and felt less knowledgeable about).

If we exclude financial, self-esteem, or reputational practitioner interests in performing tests or treatments, it is plausible that veterinary clinicians may be more likely to persuade their clients to pursue interventions they are more familiar with or knowledgeable about because the client perceives more confidence with the information being imparted. Conversely, if clients believe that the clinician lacks conviction regarding a procedure, non-compliance would be more likely. I believe that our clients can perceive whether we believe in a recommendation we are making. Alternatively, veterinarians may project an overly optimistic rendition of benefits compared to risks for recommended procedures. As there is no scientific data on this subject in veterinary medicine, let's look at data on these potential biases in human medicine.

Studies of human general practitioners revealed significant inaccuracies in their knowledge of the benefits and harms of proposed treatments [18, 19]. In one study, clinicians were asked to estimate the probability of adverse disease outcomes and expected effects of therapies for diseases common in primary care [20]. These clinicians consistently overestimated the chance that treatments would benefit a patient compared with scientific evidence. Clinicians whose overestimations were greater were more likely to report using that treatment for patients in their practice. In a systematic review of physician expectations of the benefits and harms of medical interventions, they more often overestimated benefits and underestimated harms [18]. One study comparing two specialties found that clinicians overwhelmingly recommended the intervention that they provide [21]. These results and my observations in veterinary medicine provide some support for the existence of "therapeutic illusion," defined as "an unjustified enthusiasm for treatment" [22].

Potential reasons that veterinary clinicians may be more likely to frame interventions they perform more optimistically include lack of time to adequately research up-to-date information on procedures they are not familiar with, economic incentives for offering tests or treatments provided by the practice, and commission bias, the tendency toward action rather than inaction [18]. Consequences of these biases can include inappropriate or excessive use of interventions and a disinclination to refer patients for procedures unfamiliar to the practitioner. In a recent report, only 55% of equine veterinarians in Sweden referred patients for integrative medicine services [23]. These services, such as acupuncture and botanical medicine, are seldom taught in veterinary school and are likely to be less understood by practitioners not providing these services.

Concern about Upsetting Clients

Another potential reason for reluctance to discuss risks is the concern that the client may be dissuaded from proceeding with a beneficial procedure for the patient by such disclosure. As examples, if a clinician's last words to a client were "Oh, and by the way, he has a 0.05% chance of anesthetic-related death; just stop at the front desk and we'll take it from here" or "I forgot to mention, the urethrostomy procedure is quite painful," this could be problematic for patient advocacy. I'm reminded of an episode from the TV show *Seinfeld*, where Elaine is about to receive a rabies vaccine and asks the doctor, "Is this going to hurt?" He responds, "Yes, very much!", then immediately jabs her arm!

As with so many communication issues, how the content is imparted means everything. For conveying risk associated with routine anesthesia in a healthy patient one might say: "There are risks associated with anesthesia. He will be closely monitored using state-of-the-art equipment to warn us of any problems. I'll call you if necessary. Very serious concerns such as death are very, very uncommon. The most common issues relate to being sedated with a diminished appetite for 12–24 hours, which may require restricted activity and close monitoring." For a painful procedure one could state: "While a bone marrow aspirate is painful, she will receive both a local anesthetic and a narcotic to address this. You may note she favors that leg for the next 12–24 hours, then all should be fine." Even better, if the risks can be discussed before the day of the procedure, then providing informational handouts that clients can review is encouraged.

Lack of access to reliable data about the risks associated with veterinary procedures, biases toward framing procedures the clinician is familiar with and performs in an optimistic light, and concerns about distressing clients may limit the veterinarian's capacity to provide clients with accurate knowledge of patient risks.

Risk Aversion

Distinct from not disclosing or underestimating patient risks, some clinicians may conversely be unwilling to accept certain risks. Risk aversion is "the tendency to avoid uncertain large risks by choosing another option with a more certain, but less beneficial, expected outcome" [24]. Some veterinary clinicians may be more concerned with making perceived errors of commission rather than omission to avoid accountability for undesirable patient outcomes. In this paradigm, a natural death is deemed less problematic by clients than if a patient dies while or shortly after performing a procedure. This may be a contributing factor to choosing therapeutic trials (see Chapter 22) instead of testing or a more definitive intervention. A suitable analogy may be a financial advisor recommending a client invest in bonds or cash rather than stocks, to mitigate complaints associated with the larger losses of equities in down markets.

I recall treating a cat with congestive heart failure, pleural effusion, and renal disease. The cat was doing well on low doses of cardiac medications and effusion was minimal. At one recheck, the blood urea nitrogen had risen to double the high end of the reference range, and I was concerned that this might be a warning sign of imminent decline from kidney disease. I advised reducing the dose of diuretic, and a week later the cat had to have a large volume of effusion removed from its chest cavity due to dyspnea from recurrence of heart failure. As soon as I walked into the exam room to see the client after the procedure, I knew what I'd be confronted with: "He was doing so well, and since we saw you and changed the medication, now this!" Of course, I felt bad and responsible for this relapse.

Many times in my career, I'd see a patient receiving phenobarbital, an anti-convulsant medication. When I asked, these clients would sometimes tell me that the patient's last seizure was many years ago. Given the potential adverse effects of long-term drug therapy, attempted withdrawal of medication is reasonable in animals that are seizure free for 1–2 years [25]. When I asked if there was ever an attempt to taper off the medications, I was told "My vet said he needs to stay on these for life." Is it conceivable that these veterinarians chose not to attempt a medication taper to avoid the risk of seizure recurrence so as not to experience what I did after tapering the diuretic dose in the cat? I often saw self-referred clients who told me that their veterinarian discouraged them from pursuing intervention for a declining patient condition based on a low probability of survival.

With a rising emphasis on public reporting of patient outcomes in human hospitals, a recent report evaluated the association between risk-averse practices and outcomes via publicly available data on patients having cardiac surgery [26]. High-risk surgery was defined as predicted risk of mortality ≥5%. The rate of high-risk cases decreased from 18% to 13% over a 14-year period. Significant risk aversion was seen in 39% of hospitals, which had a 59% decrease in high-risk volume. Another review of interventional cardiology procedures concluded that there is consistent and compelling evidence for withholding high-risk cardiovascular care because of public reporting [27].

While veterinary clinicians need not be concerned with public reporting of patient outcomes (this is not required and is not done, to the best of my knowledge), an analogous concern is for one's reputation. For twenty-first-century practitioners, this concern is heightened by the influence of social media reviews and comments. Yet a century ago, Codman challenged concerns of risk aversion and not offering treatment to high-risk patients in practice: "But if we think too much about mortality, shall we not fail to do desperate operations which we should do?" [28] (Case Study 4.1).

Case Study 4.1   A Dog with an Adrenal Gland Mass

Jazzy, a 14-year-old shih tzu, presents for lethargy and "something is just not right." Physical exam, lab work and radiographs are unremarkable. Abdominal ultrasound reveals a unilateral adrenal gland mass. You discuss that this finding may be the cause of the vague symptoms or could be incidental. You inform the client that brain disease could also be the cause, but requires anesthesia and magnetic resonance imaging to assess. The owners request treatment for the adrenal mass. Hormonal testing suggests a pheochromocytoma. You inform the owners that medical management may be helpful, but adrenalectomy is the only definitive means of treating this condition. You discuss a 15% mortality rate associated with this surgery and remind the client that symptoms may not improve or resolve after the mass is removed. The owners affirm that they feel Jazzy's quality of life is poor and they are willing to accept an 85% survival rate and the uncertainty, if there is a chance that this improves her energy and alertness. Jazzy survives the surgery with no complications. At the time of suture removal, the owners bring you a gift of appreciation and tell you "She's acting like a puppy again!"

Shahian et al. expand on the concept of risk aversion:

> For some severe diseases and conditions, the only hope for cure may be treatments that have a high-risk of failure, complications, or death. Risk aversion ... refers to the denial of interventions to high-risk patients who might have benefited, specifically when that decision is motivated by fear that worse outcomes among such patients will affect a provider's reputation, [or] referrals. For ... patients with a particular disease to have optimal outcomes, it is necessary that some very high-risk patients receive interventions, and some will likely not survive. [27]

Of course, in some cases risk aversion may be beneficent, reflecting a genuine concern for unacceptable or insurmountable patient harms, preventing some patients and their families having the ordeal of a futile intervention. However, as noted earlier in this chapter, balancing an accurate estimation of harms with the family's goals for care may prove challenging in very high-risk cases. Risk aversion likely influences veterinarian decisions and may contribute to ageism.

Ageism

On numerous occasions, I have seen veterinarians make judgments about patients based primarily on their age (Case Studies 4.2 and 4.3). Such statements included "Well, she's 16 years old, so we need to be conservative," "I don't think I'd invest the costs into this procedure given his age," or "I'm not sure he will live long enough after this procedure to make it worthwhile." In fact, some textbooks use a random geriatric age as a cutoff for when surgery should no longer be considered.

Ageism refers to "stereotypes, prejudice, and discriminatory behaviors against older adults [patients]" [29]. In a satirical novel by a psychiatrist, *The House of God* [30], the derogatory acronym GOMER (Get Out of My Emergency Room) was popularized, referring to older patients with incurable conditions. A qualitative study concluded that there is ample evidence for ageism among physicians in diagnostic procedures, treatment of older patients, and interactions with older patients [29]. In another report, older patients with lung cancer were less likely to be referred for surgery despite clinical evidence that postoperative recovery outcomes are not dependent on age [31]. Another investigation found that institutional ageism was manifested as either (i) exclusion of older patients from high-cost treatments; (ii) postponement of interventions; or (iii) proposal of less definitive treatments [32]. Discriminatory patterns have also been noted regarding provision of medications to older patients [33].

Sometimes treatable conditions are diminished or ignored because they are deemed to be "normal" problems in old age. Veterinary conditions that may be subject to "selective neglect" include obesity, degenerative joint disease/arthritis, coughing, and cognitive decline. Studies have identified that veterinary professionals are less likely to discuss obesity when animals are older compared to younger animals [34, 35]. Due to ageist views, withholding invasive medical interventions from geriatric patients may be perceived as compassionate care rather than undertreatment [29].

Veterinary clinicians should attempt to assess the geriatric patient's quality of life before clinical signs of illness arose, to guide clients through the difficult process of making informed decisions, including whether to elect for aggressive intervention, palliative care, or euthanasia. If the client reports that declining ambulatory status, vision, hearing, or other problems have resulted in a notably poor quality of life before the presenting symptoms (and these concurrent problems cannot be improved), then palliation or euthanasia is a reasonable course of action. Conversely,

---

Case Study 4.2   Whether to Perform an Endoscopy for a Geriatric Cat

Whitney was my 15-year-old cat. His appetite had declined. In all other regards, he seemed fine. Examination confirmed a 10% weight loss. Once I got over my guilt (how could my own cat have lost a pound, I'm an internist?) I took him in to my hospital for testing. Lab testing, radiographs, and abdominal ultrasound were all normal. I performed an upper GI endoscopy the next day, and biopsies confirmed intestinal small cell lymphoma. Although I had seen this dozens of times before, my name never appeared as the client on those other biopsy reports. After crying, I initiated treatment with oral steroid and chemotherapy.

Shortly after this diagnosis, I lectured to a local veterinary association group of about 20 colleagues and presented Whitney as the case example. After providing the history and handing out copies of the normal database and ultrasound, I asked my colleagues how many of them would have advised Whitney's owner to pursue further testing or referral. No one raised their hand.

Why was no one in this group willing to advocate that a 10% loss of body weight warranted further testing or referral? At the end of the discussion, one colleague approached me privately and said, "Look, I mean, the cat is 15 years old, he's going to be dead soon. I'm glad your cat is well, but I'm not going to recommend a scope or surgery ... I mean, he could die, or at best, I'm gonna be the bearer of bad news." Whitney lived for 17 months after this diagnosis.

Case Study 4.3   A Geriatric Dog with Lethargy and Declining Appetite

Shelby, a 15-year-old Dachshund, was seen by a colleague for lethargy, declining appetite, and weight loss. Blood tests showed a microcytic anemia and elevated liver enzymes. Imaging was not advised or performed. The owners were instructed to administer iron suspension at home for the anemia. You see Shelby after the owners independently sought a second opinion. Ultrasound confirmed a large liver tumor. After considerable discussion of benefits, risks, and costs, hepatectomy was elected, as there were no effective medical treatments to reduce tumor size. Shelby subsequently gained weight and quality of life was reported to be much improved. The owners were very pleased with their decision and gave you a five-star rating on a social media website.

(and much more commonly), if the owner relates that quality of life was good and that "he/she was still really feisty for his/her age" prior to the onset of illness, the clinician should encourage owners to pursue definitive treatment if quality of life after intervention can be restored and the owner can accept the uncertainty of how long the patient will live.

Age is not a disease. Making clinical decisions for senior patients is a very difficult undertaking, exacerbated by the paucity of clinical data on effective treatments and harms. Risk aversion and ageism are likely as prevalent in veterinary medicine as in the human medical profession, if not more so due to the capacity to elect for euthanasia. Veterinary clinicians should not consign senior patients as being somehow less valuable than any other patient. As companion animals may have longer lifespans due to improved veterinary care, the need to help our clients manage risks and benefits from interventions in these patients will become more important than ever before.

References

1 Morgan, D.J., Scherer, L.D., and Korenstein, D. (2020). Improving physician communication about treatment decisions: reconsideration of "risks vs benefits.". *Journal of the American Medical Association* 324 (10): 937–938.

2 harm (n.d., 2008). *West's Encyclopedia of American Law*, 2e. https://legal-dictionary.thefree dictionary.com/harm (accessed February 27, 2023).

3 Korenstein, D., Harris, R., Elshaug, A.G. et al. (2021). To expand the evidence base about harms from tests and treatments. *Journal of General Internal Medicine* 36 (7): 2105–2110.

4 Monteiro, B. and Robertson, S. (2022). Animal pain. In: *Ethics in Veterinary Practice: Balancing Conflicting Interests*, ch. 19 (ed. B. Kipperman and B.E. Rollin). Hoboken, NJ: Wiley-Blackwell.

5 Tversky, A. and Kahneman, D. (1981). The framing of decisions and the psychology of choice. *Science* 211: 453–458.

6 Gurm, H.S. and Litaker, D.G. (2000). Framing procedural risks to patients: is 99% safe the same as a risk of 1 in 100? *Academic Medicine* 75 (8): 840–842.

7 Fridman, I., Fagerlin, A., Scherr, K.A. et al. (2021). Gain–loss framing and patients' decisions: a linguistic examination of information framing in physician–patient conversations. *Journal of Behavioral Medicine* 44 (1): 38–52.

8 Gong, J., Zhang, Y., Yang, Z. et al. (2013). The framing effect in medical decision-making: a review of the literature. *Psychology, Health and Medicine* 18 (6): 645–653.

9 Royal Veterinary College (n.d.). About VetCompass. www.rvc.ac.uk/vetcompass/about/overview (accessed February 27, 2023).

10 O'Neill, D.G., James, H., Brodbelt, D.C. et al. (2021). Prevalence of commonly diagnosed disorders in UK dogs under primary veterinary care: results and applications. *BMC Veterinary Research* 17 (1): 1–14.

11 Conroy, M., Brodbelt, D.C., O'Neill, D. et al. (2019). Chronic kidney disease in cats attending primary care practice in the UK: a VetCompassTM study. *Veterinary Record* 184 (17): 526.

12 Paynter, A.N., Dunbar, M.D., Creevy, K.E. et al. (2021). Veterinary big data: when data goes to the dogs. *Animals* 11 (7): 1872.

13 Pailler, S., Slater, M.R., Lesnikowski, S.M. et al. (2022). Findings and prognostic indicators of outcomes for bitches with pyometra treated surgically in a nonspecialized setting. *Journal of the American Veterinary Medical Association* 260 (S2): S49–S56.

14 Song, K.K., Goldsmid, S.E., Lee, J. et al. (2020). Retrospective analysis of 736 cases of canine gastric dilatation volvulus. *Australian Veterinary Journal* 98 (6): 232–238.

15 Gill, S.S., Buote, N.J., Peterson, N.W. et al. (2019). Factors associated with dehiscence and mortality rates following gastrointestinal surgery in dogs. *Journal of the American Veterinary Medical Association* 255 (5): 569–573.

16 Merlin, T. and Veres-Nyeki, K. (2019). Anaesthetic management and complications of canine adrenalectomies: 41 cases (2007–2017). *Acta Veterinaria Hungarica* 67 (2): 282–295.

17 Bille, C., Auvigne, V., Libermann, S. et al. (2012). Risk of anaesthetic mortality in dogs and cats: an observational cohort study of 3546 cases. *Veterinary Anaesthesia and Analgesia* 39 (1): 59–68.

18 Hoffmann, T.C. and Del Mar, C. (2017). Clinicians' expectations of the benefits and harms of treatments, screening, and tests: a systematic review. *JAMA Internal Medicine* 177 (3): 407–419. https://doi.org/10.1001/jamainternmed.2016.8254.

19 Treadwell, J.S., Wong, G., Milburn-Curtis, C. et al. (2020). GPs' understanding of the benefits and harms of treatments for long-term conditions: an online survey. *BJGP Open* 4 (1): bjgpopen20X101016.

20 Morgan, D.J., Pineles, L., Owczarzak, J. et al. (2021). Clinician conceptualization of the benefits of treatments for individual patients. *JAMA Network Open* 4 (7): e2119747–e2119747.

21 Fowler, F.J. Jr., McNaughton Collins, M., Albertsen, P.C. et al. (2000). Comparison of recommendations by urologists and radiation oncologists for treatment of clinically localized prostate cancer. *Journal of the American Medical Association* 283 (24): 3217–3222.

22 Thomas, K.B. (1978). The consultation and the therapeutic illusion. *BMJ* 1 (6123): 1327–1328.

23 Gilberg, K., Bergh, A., and Sternberg-Lewerin, S. (2021). A questionnaire study on the use of complementary and alternative veterinary medicine for horses in Sweden. *Animals* 11: 3113.

24 Oussedik, E., Anderson, M.S., and Feldman, S.R. (2017). Risk versus benefit or risk versus risk: risk aversion in the medical decision-making process. *Journal of Dermatological Treatment* 28 (1): 1–2.

25 Thomas, W.B. (2010). Idiopathic epilepsy in dogs and cats. *Veterinary Clinics: Small Animal Practice* 40 (1): 161–179.

26 Hawkins, R.B., Mehaffey, J.H., Chancellor, W.Z. et al. (2020). Risk aversion in cardiac surgery: 15-year trends in a statewide analysis. *Annals of Thoracic Surgery* 109 (5): 1401–1407.

27 Shahian, D.M., Jacobs, J.P., Badhwar, V. et al. (2017). Risk aversion and public reporting. Part 1: observations from cardiac surgery and interventional cardiology. *Annals of Thoracic Surgery* 104 (6): 2093–2101.

28 Codman, E.A. (1914). The product of a hospital. *Surgery, Gynecology & Obstetrics* 18: 491–496.

29 Ben-Harush, A., Shiovitz-Ezra, S., Doron, I. et al. (2017). Ageism among physicians, nurses, and social workers: findings from a qualitative study. *European Journal of Ageing* 14 (1): 39–48.

30 Shem, S. (1978). *The House of God*. New York: Richard Marek Publishers.

31 Peake, M.D., Thompson, S., Lowe, D. et al. (2003). Ageism in the management of lung cancer. *Age and Ageing* 32 (2): 171–177.

32 Ferreira, S.F.S., Pires, L., Castelo-Branco, M. et al. (2022). Initial validation of the Portuguese version of the EVE discrimination questionnaire (EVE-D): the level of perceived ageism by physicians in the Portuguese healthcare system. *Educational Gerontology* 48 (11): 549–563. https://doi.org/10.1080/03601277.2022.2052406.

33 Fialová, D., Kummer, I., Držaić, M. et al. (2018). Ageism in medication use in older patients. In: *Contemporary Perspectives on Ageism* (ed. L. Ayalon and C. Tesch-Romer), 213–240. Cham: Springer.

34 Sutherland, K.A., Coe, J.B., and O'Sullivan, T.L. (2023). Exploring veterinary professionals' perceptions of pet weight-related communication in companion animal veterinary practice. *Veterinary Record* 194 (4): e1973.

35 Sutherland, K.A., Coe, J.B., Janke, N. et al. (2022). Veterinary professionals' weight-related communication when discussing an overweight or obese pet with a client. *Journal of the American Veterinary Medical Association* 260 (9): 1076–1085.

5

Client Education Beyond Informed Consent: The Most Important Thing an Owner Needs to Know

Barry Kipperman

Abstract

This chapter considers why it is important for veterinarians to enhance client education beyond informed consent during consultations via patient discharge instructions, and provides a template for their utilization. Case examples are provided. Access to veterinary care is cited as the most prominent welfare concern of companion animals. The role of the veterinarian in mitigating economic limitations via client education and preparation before an animal is ill is discussed. Finally, The Most Important Thing an Animal Owner Needs to Know from their veterinarian is proposed.

Keywords: *discharge instructions, cost discussions, monitoring appetite, delayed veterinary visits, client education, access to care, referrals*

As discussed in Chapter 3, obtaining informed consent is fundamental to satisfying the Principle of Patient Advocacy. This is both a legal and an ethical obligation of veterinarians and is also an important expectation of animal owners. Veterinarians should provide enough information that owners understand the nature of what is wrong with their animal and the options, costs, and consequences for what can be done to address it. The best option for each individual patient should be advised along with its rationale. Secondary and tertiary options should also be offered. Both written and verbal communication optimize client understanding. Visit durations for sick patients should be at least 30 minutes to accommodate this communication and the informational tools discussed in this chapter. Clinicians should strive to ensure that any substantiated consent also signifies that of an informed client.

Informed consent during consultations with sick animals should be considered "a good start" to providing owners the information they need to know to make educated decisions. After the consultation, other opportunities arise where the veterinary clinician should supplement and update the information provided during the initial consultation. This includes client informational handouts relevant to the patient's medical or surgical problem. Examples of these may include "Giving NSAIDS safely," "Postoperative care for the TPLO patient," "Seizures," "Diabetes Mellitus," etc. The advantage of these handouts is they can be created for any common disease treated by

Decision-Making in Veterinary Practice, First Edition. Barry Kipperman.
© 2024 John Wiley & Sons, Inc. Published 2024 by John Wiley & Sons, Inc.

the practice and can be provided to clients at the time of patient discharge from the hospital. The drawback is that they are not tailored to individual patients, and there may be exceptions or modifications to these standard handouts based on species, breed, patient size, temperament, or age.

Patient Discharge Instructions

Each client you see should be given discharge instructions unique to that patient, whether the animal is an outpatient or is being discharged from the hospital. For outpatients, these instructions serve to reinforce and augment the verbal discussion during the consultation as well as any standard client handout that may be provided. For inpatients, discharge instructions update the animal's owner regarding any changes that have occurred between the original consultation and patient discharge from the hospital, and improve continuity in the transition from hospital to home-based care.

These instructions can be saved as generic "macros" in the practice's software and modified and individualized for your patient. This takes about five minutes or so to complete and is invaluable as a resource both for your client to refer to as well as for any colleagues entrusted with the care of the patient when you are not available, as some of this information may not be included in the patient's medical record. A template for the information that should be provided in these instructions is outlined in Table 5.1. As clients may be intimidated by or may choose not to read documents that are multiple pages long, discharge instructions should ideally be limited to a few paragraphs on one page. Case Studies 5.1–5.4 provide examples using this template.

Table 5.1 Template for patient discharge instructions.

Patient diagnosis
What was done
Timeframe for recovery if patient was sedated or anesthetized
Precautions if patient was sedated or anesthetized
What was found
Implications/consequences of what was done and found
Actions being taken (if any) and goals
Side effects/complications of actions
Lifestyle or dietary modifications
Prognosis/time frame for patient improvement and what this looks like
When next recheck or progress report is advised
Potential next steps if no patient improvement
Concerns that warrant patient visit right away
Call with any questions

Case Study 5.1   Discharge Instructions for a Dog with a Presumptive Urinary Tract Infection

Patient Name: Cozy
Diagnosis: Urinary tract infection.

Cozy was seen today for frequent urinations and blood in her urine. X-rays showed no evidence of stones in her urinary bladder. A urine sample was obtained and sent to the laboratory for analysis. A urinary tract infection is considered the most likely cause of her symptoms. These are usually benign and respond quickly to appropriate antibiotic treatment. Please give the pain medication and antibiotic as directed right away. Her symptoms should be resolved in 48–72 hours. Until then, Cozy may need to go outside more often than normal to urinate. Side effects of the medications can include loss of appetite, vomiting, or diarrhea. Please stop the medications if these are noted and call us right away.

   Please call us for a progress report on her condition in three days. If her symptoms are not significantly improved, we may need to perform an additional test (urine culture) to identify the appropriate antibiotic to resolve her symptoms. A full recovery is expected. Cozy was a very good patient. Call with any questions.

Case Study 5.2   Discharge Instructions for a Dog with a Wound and Bandage

Patient name: Buster
Diagnosis: Degloving wound

Buster sustained a significant wound on his right forelimb secondary to trauma. Lab tests showed he is in good health, and x-rays showed no evidence of fractures or internal injuries. He was sedated today for minor surgery to clean and debride the wound and to place a protective bandage. Do not give any food or water until he is fully recovered in 3–6 hours. Please limit his access to any dangers such as stairs until he is fully recovered from sedation.

   Please give the antibiotic and pain medication as directed starting tomorrow morning. He received these by injection today. Side effects of the medications can include loss of appetite, vomiting, or diarrhea. Please stop the medications if these are noted and call us right away.

   It is imperative that you inspect the bandage daily to ensure it remains clean and dry. Please refer to the handout on Bandage Care for details. If the bandage is damp or has an odor, please bring Buster in right away for evaluation. Activity must be limited to short leash walks outside; no running or jumping. He should not go outside without supervision.

   Please make an appointment in three days to recheck the wound and replace the bandage. Delays in changing the bandage may increase the risk of complications and negative outcomes. Because the wound is extensive, it will probably take a few weeks to heal and require multiple bandage changes and further debridement under sedation. Risks include infection and prolonged healing in some patients. If this occurs, additional surgery (which may include referral to a surgical specialist) may be needed to facilitate healing. Buster was a good patient. Call with any questions.

Case Study 5.3   Discharge Instructions for a Dog with Congestive Heart Failure

Patient name: Henry
Diagnosis: Congestive heart failure

Henry received intensive care including oxygen and diuretics for congestive heart failure. This is a common disease of the heart valves in older, small-breed dogs. He has recovered well from coughing and difficulty breathing. Initial x-rays confirmed fluid in his lungs and today's x-rays show resolution of the fluid. Lab work showed no other problems. While this condition cannot be cured, many dogs can do well for 1–3 years with lifelong medications to slow progression of the disease and control symptoms.

Please give the medications as directed. Henry may drink and urinate more often from the diuretic. Water should be available at all times. Other side effects are uncommon and can include dehydration and lethargy, loss of appetite, vomiting, or diarrhea. Call if these are noted.

Please make an appointment in one week for a blood test to ensure Henry is tolerating the medications. If he is doing well, serial rechecks every few months will be needed. Signs of progression of heart disease include coughing and labored breathing. Please bring him in right away if these are noted. When this occurs, we can often increase medication doses or add additional medications to control the disease.

Activity should be limited to leash walks and moderate exercise. Please transition Henry's diet over the next week to a low-salt diet (see the handout Ideal Diets for Heart Disease). If he won't eat the commercial diet, homemade foods are another option. He was a very good patient. Call with any questions.

Case Study 5.4   Discharge Instructions for a Cat with Chronic Intestinal Disease

Patient name: Fluffy
Diagnosis: Chronic intestinal disease

Fluffy is recovering well from today's endoscopy to obtain biopsies of her stomach and intestine. Abdominal ultrasound revealed no evidence of any masses. Don't give any food or water until tomorrow morning. She should be fully recovered from anesthesia in about 24 hours.

Please give the medication (steroid) as directed starting tomorrow once daily. If Fluffy does not tolerate the suspension, a pill form is available. See the handout How to Medicate Your Cat for tips and guidance. While this condition cannot be cured, many cats can do well for 1–3 years with lifelong medication to slow progression of the disease and control symptoms. I expect her appetite to be much improved in 3–4 days, and the vomiting to resolve in about a week.

Please call me in one week for a progress report and to discuss pathology results. These may find inflammation or low-grade cancer. This will determine if any other medications are needed to maximize her response and survival time. Serial rechecks will be advised to assess her progress and to consider modifying medication doses. Please make an appointment for this in four weeks. Based on Fluffy's fear of visiting the hospital, I advise purchasing a cat scale so you can weigh her at home, and we can perform rechecks via telemedicine if she is doing well.

If vomiting or declining appetite recurs, she should be seen right away. This may reflect progression of her intestinal disease or could be due to another problem. Fluffy was a very good patient. Call with any questions.

Discussing Costs

A ubiquitous reality facing veterinary clinicians during patient visits is the query: "What will the tests and treatments cost, doctor?" For most practitioners, the responsibility for discussing the costs of veterinary care is limited to providing an estimate for proposed patient care at the end of consultations. This needs to be reconsidered to address the issue of access to veterinary care, which is the greatest animal welfare concern affecting companion animals in the United States. Access to veterinary care is defined as "recognizing when a pet needs care, having a physically reachable veterinary service provider, and the ability to pay for the care" [1]. When access to veterinary care is limited, a sick animal may face prolonged illness, pain, or recovery time, or premature death, causing emotional distress for the family.

Having the knowledge and desire to provide care but being thwarted in doing so due to financial limitations is an ethical dilemma inherent in the practice of veterinary medicine. Repeated instances of this dilemma can lead to burnout and moral stress, made worse when the situation results in patient euthanasia despite a treatable problem [2]. Discussion of veterinary care costs is fundamental to patient care, client satisfaction, and practice success [3]. Who should conduct these conversations? Veterinarians have a substantial influence on owners' behaviors regarding their pets' care because of their perception by society as healers and as advocates for animals. Veterinarians should view the issue of economic limitations to care with the same degree of concern we would apply for a disease endangering animal health.

Veterinarians hold proprietary knowledge about the costs of veterinary care that is unavailable to pet owners. It is time for a new paradigm in which practitioners reliably provide their clients with information and options to help them prepare for the costs of veterinary care for their animal companions *before* they are ill. Efforts to alleviate clients' economic limitations would also be financially beneficial to veterinarians. More details regarding why and how veterinarians should address this issue are provided in Chapter 8.

The Most Important Thing an Animal Owner Needs to Know

Many of the patients I saw in my practice had reduced appetite for weeks and had lost 20–40% of their body weight. Almost regardless of the patient's diagnosis, these animals were usually lost causes; my role was that of a grief counselor and mortician rather than an internist. I'd explain to the owner why the patient was a poor risk for surviving anesthesia or invasive procedures, and the poor prognosis for a full recovery, as the disease conditions of these patients were often too far advanced to survive the 1–2 weeks needed for interventions to take effect. On rare occasions, I'd salvage a few of these patients with nutritional support and therapeutic trials. The fundamental question is: "Why are clinicians regularly seeing patients in such a debilitated condition?" If this problem can be "diagnosed," then perhaps we can see patients in an earlier stage of disease and treatment can be initiated sooner to remedy the problem.

For an animal's owner to make an appointment with their veterinarian, they must recognize that their animal companion is ill or behaving in an unusual manner. As our patients cannot directly communicate or complain of pain, headaches, nausea, or weakness, combined with our patients' adaptive abilities to mask signs of sickness, it seems reasonable that detection is apt to occur later in the course of an illness. A common emotional response on recognition of something wrong with a beloved animal companion is denial, not wanting to conceive there may be a serious problem. The costs related to a veterinary visit may also prompt further delay, with the owner hoping that the problem will resolve without the need for veterinary care. Finally, the animal owner must make an appointment with their veterinarian that suits their schedule and experience the inconvenience and stress of transporting their animal to the hospital. The result of all these factors when animals are ill is delayed recognition and action. Consequently, by the time an animal sees their primary care veterinarian, the duration of illness is often far longer than is acknowledged by the owner.

On numerous occasions when I'd call to update a referring veterinarian about a patient with advanced weight loss, they'd apologetically tell me, "I can't believe they [the owners] waited so long to bring him in. I understand why the prognosis is poor. Thanks for trying." In some of these situations I asked my colleagues, "Do you ever inform your clients that if their animal's appetite has changed they should see you right away?" The responses included silence or the protestation, "Why should I do that? They ought to know that!" No colleague ever confirmed taking the time to do this. Why would we blame animal owners for not knowing something we never informed them of?

Almost all clinicians have heard medically unsound client rationales for why their pet stopped eating: "I assumed he was just tired of that food" or "When he stopped eating, I offered him some chicken, and he ate some of that, so I thought he was OK." While we cannot control the emotional and financial decisions of our clients, we can and must educate them regarding The Most Important Thing an Animal Owner Needs to Know: "If your animal's appetite declines in any way this is often a sign of a serious illness, and they should be seen right away."

The common theme associated with all life-threatening illness is reduced appetite and anorexia. Informing our clients in writing of this foundational knowledge during wellness visits allows us to satisfy the Principle of Patient Advocacy and may mitigate regularly seeing patients who are too sick to save.

References

1 Blackwell, M.J. (2022). Companion animals: access to veterinary care. In: *Ethics in Veterinary Practice*, ch. 10 (ed. B. Kipperman and B.E. Rollin). Hoboken, NJ: Wiley-Blackwell.

2 Kipperman, B.S., Kass, P.H., and Rishniw, M. (2017). Factors that influence small animal veterinarians' opinions and actions regarding cost of care and effects of economic limitations on patient care and outcome and professional career satisfaction and burnout. *Journal of the American Veterinary Medical Association* 250 (7): 785–794.

3 Bonvicini, K.A. (2009). Talking to clients about money. *Trends Magazine* 3: 61–66.

6

Euthanasia

Barry Kipperman and Kathleen Cooney

Abstract

Euthanasia is a common procedure in veterinary practice. Veterinarians must determine if the request for euthanasia is warranted or if other factors exist making the decision to euthanize inappropriate or objectionable. This chapter addresses ethical and practical concerns associated with companion animal euthanasia, including defining euthanasia; why, when, and where euthanasia should be performed; applying euthanasia; contemporary methods; fees; and aftercare of deceased animals. We contend that an intention-based definition of euthanasia should be strictly applied in veterinary practice and that practitioners view euthanasia decisions as requests that can (and in some cases should) be declined, rather than as mandates.

Keywords: *euthanasia, convenience euthanasia, economic euthanasia, objectionable euthanasia, moral stress, ethical dilemmas, dysthanasia, animal hospice, fees*

What Is Euthanasia?

Veterinary practice is unique, as clinicians are expected to end the lives of their patients. In a study of the cause of death of over 29 000 dogs under primary care in the United Kingdom, 89% were euthanized [1]. Euthanasia derives from the Greek roots of "a good death" and in human semantics is restricted to circumstances of mercy killing, in which death is viewed as a respite from inevitable suffering that cannot be alleviated by reasonable means [2]. The expectation is that if life is to be taken, it is at the right time for the right reason.

The American Veterinary Medical Association (AVMA) Guidelines for the Euthanasia of Animals define the following co-dependent, necessary requirements for euthanasia:

- Method-based: "the use of humane techniques to induce the most rapid and painless and distress-free death possible."
- Intention-based: "to induce death in a manner that is in accord with an animal's interest and/or because it is a matter of welfare" [3].

Even if an animal's "best interest" paradigm is used to justify euthanasia, Quain notes difficulties applying this principle: "Different stakeholders (for example, the veterinarian and the owner of the animal, the veterinarian and colleagues, or two different owners of the same animal) may

Decision-Making in Veterinary Practice, First Edition. Barry Kipperman.
© 2024 John Wiley & Sons, Inc. Published 2024 by John Wiley & Sons, Inc.

have different views about an animal's quality of life, prognosis and interests" [4]. Rollin observed that euthanasia is a double-edged sword, referring to its benefit in ending terminal suffering, but also its being performed in circumstances that appear less compulsory and do not conform with serving an animal's best interest [5]. Tannenbaum refers to euthanasia that does not align with an animal's best interest as "medically unnecessary euthanasia" [6].

Convenience euthanasia refers to requests to end the life of an animal due to unexpected changes in the owner's life, or the owner having insufficient time, capability (emotional or physical), or motivation to care for the animal [7, 8]. With the potential for significant caregiver burden brought on by an animal's condition [9], veterinarians are regularly tasked with deciding whose suffering is worse, the client's or the animal's. Economic euthanasia is defined as a circumstance in which "euthanasia is elected based primarily ... or to a large degree on the cost of veterinary ... care; or a condition in which veterinary care is sought and minimal or no testing/treatment is elected based on the costs of care, resulting in eventual euthanasia" [10]. As advances in veterinary care improve (along with the associated costs), veterinarians may find that owner decisions to euthanize an animal become more difficult to justify. More cases of convenience or economic euthanasia may emerge.

Quain has defined ethically indicated euthanasia as "euthanasia performed in what are believed to be the animal's interests and which is not considered to be primarily motivated by convenience, economics, or reasons to which veterinary team members object" [4]. Euthanasia that does not meet this standard should be referred to in medical records as convenience, economic, or objectionable euthanasia. Utilization of the term euthanasia (without a preceding qualification) in settings in which veterinarians are asked to cause the intentional death of healthy animals that are unwanted or of sick animals that could be restored to health by routine veterinary interventions obfuscates its meaning and should be discouraged. Classifying euthanasia may help clinicians avoid "normalizing" medically unnecessary euthanasia and encourage the pursuit of alternatives.

Why Euthanasia Should Be Performed

There will be many instances when a veterinarian must determine if euthanasia is the best, or most reasonable, course of action based on limited information, such as a physical examination alone, without the benefit of a diagnosis or response to treatment. Veterinarians are frequently expected to predict the future outcomes of their patients' conditions or even when a patient's natural death would be expected to occur. These uncertainties often accompany a burden of doubt for veterinarians regarding whether euthanasia should be elected. While there are many contributing factors for why euthanasia is chosen (immobility, behavior changes, lethargy, etc.), there are few objective tools to determine exactly when euthanasia is needed.

Veterinarians may be familiar with quality of life (QOL) scales that attempt to objectively measure negative states that may warrant euthanasia, such as pain and physiologic and emotional distress [11]. Unfortunately, these are subjective to the point that one household may score their pet's QOL very differently than another household in a similar situation. All assessments using modern QOL scales are classified as observer-reported outcome measures (OROs) because animal patients cannot speak [12, 13]. This means that scoring is based solely on observations made by proxy, through veterinarians and owners. In human medicine, proxies such as caregivers consistently report poorer QOL than is reported by patients [14–17]. Therefore, OROs and traditional QOL scales may not accurately reflect an animal's QOL. Veterinarians may use QOL scales to open dialogue with owners about disease trajectories, but must still rely on their instinct and medical acumen to guide what's best for their patient.

One of the pivotal decisions veterinary clinicians face is to determine if euthanasia is appropriate or if life is still worth living for the patient even in the face of disease symptoms. The concept of "a life worth living" is more of an ethical consideration than a scientific one. Euthanasia should be performed when no other options exist to address significant and permanent suffering. Suffering may be physical, mental, or both, and not every manifestation of suffering warrants euthanasia. It will depend on the degree of distress the animal experiences and how it copes. For example, a cat or small dog unable to walk on its back legs may still have a satisfactory QOL with the help of its family, while a recumbent large dog with pressure sores and decubital ulcers may not.

A major driver of euthanasia decisions for owners is the perception that their animal companion is suffering [18]. Owners may define suffering based on psychosocial factors such as previous experiences and beliefs. Their determination is as relevant (if not more so) as that of the veterinarian. The difference rests in the veterinarian's knowledge of diseases, the impacts on animal welfare, and available treatments. If agreement cannot be reached, an animal may suffer or die prematurely through euthanasia because the owner feels no other options exist.

Application of Euthanasia

It is to be expected that a veterinary practitioner will encounter conflicts about the suitability of euthanasia requests. In a survey of North American veterinarians, 93% had received what they considered to be an inappropriate request for euthanasia [19]. Complicating euthanasia decisions is the fact that animals are legal property and, barring violations of animal cruelty laws, are subject to the owner's disposition. A veterinarian may choose to comply with a euthanasia request, dissuade the animal's owner, or decline such a request. Veterinarians have the right to choose which services they will provide, including euthanasia.

In a study of small animal veterinarians, 80% reported having declined a euthanasia request at some point in their career; of these, 52% reported that they decline euthanasia requests every few years [20]. The most common reasons acknowledged for why veterinarians are hesitant to decline euthanasia requests included concerns that the owner may pursue other alternatives that might worsen the welfare of the animal, difficulty declining such requests once an owner had reached this decision, and concern that declining euthanasia requests might jeopardize their relationship with the owner [20].

There are ethical concerns about ceding the decision of when euthanasia is necessary to owners (Case Studies 6.1 [21] and 6.2 [22]). The reality that euthanasia in veterinary practice can end animal suffering but can also be used in circumstances that do not serve an animal's interest, can be a benefit for animals and a burden for veterinary professionals, respectively. Acting in ways that one believes to be suspect or wrong (i.e. euthanasia), based on the belief that another person (the animal's owner) may do something that leads to a poorer outcome for the animal, is an inadequate supposition on which to base an ethical decision. We are not responsible for the choices and actions of others. Veterinarians must instead be accountable for the consequences of their own behaviors. We contend that avoiding difficult decisions or retaining a client is not worth the moral stress (see Chapter 1) that may occur because of performing convenience, economic, or objectionable euthanasia.

Case Study 6.1   Euthanasia Request for a Cat with Chronic Illness and Good Quality of Life

Mrs. A is a nurse and a new client at your veterinary hospital. She presents her 12-year-old cat Debra for euthanasia. Hospital regulations require a consultation and examination before this procedure can be performed. Mrs. A tells you that Debra drinks water all day, eats all the time, and is losing weight. She relates that she can't bear to see Debra waste away, and she is convinced that Debra has diabetes mellitus, although no testing has been performed. Mrs. A expresses that she has no interest in treating her cat for diabetes. Examination reveals that Debra is alert, thin, and walks around and jumps on the chair in the exam room. You do not perceive that the cat is suffering. There is no hospital policy regarding declining euthanasia requests.

What should you do?

Case Study 6.2   Euthanasia Request and an Overwhelmed Owner

Mr. D and his wife live with four Chihuahuas. You have been treating two of the dogs for chronic medical conditions and see them regularly for checkups. Both dogs are in clinical remission on lifelong medications. At the next recheck, you learn that Mr. D's wife passed away. Each time you see Mr. D and the dogs for subsequent visits, he appears more erratic, and it is becoming more difficult to achieve compliance with your patients' medications and rechecks. The next time you see Mr. D, he brings in all four dogs and seems upset. He confides that since his wife died, he has lost his job and can no longer properly care for all the dogs. He relates that of the two dogs you are not treating, one of them (12 years old) requires dental extractions that he cannot afford, and the other (13 years old) is aggressive to anyone except Mr. D. He doesn't want to consider these two dogs spending time in a shelter where they may experience fear after living their entire lives with him. He tells you how much he trusts you and asks that you euthanize both dogs who are not receiving treatment, so he knows that they will not suffer and that their last memory is of being with him.

What should you do?

The rationale "If I don't do it [euthanasia], somebody else will" is archaic and diminishes our ethical integrity by perpetuating the image that we are willing to kill our patients on demand [6]. While euthanasia is the most common cause of companion animal death due to a deliberate choice by owners [1], when euthanasia is not justified practitioners should propose reasonable alternatives that better meet the animal's needs while reducing their moral stress by knowing that they advocated for what was in the patient's best interest. However, because veterinarians have compassion for both animals and their owners, it is very difficult to tell an owner "I'm not comfortable complying with your request." An owner who has made up their mind to euthanize their pet may be disappointed when the clinician disagrees and attempts to convince them otherwise, especially after significant owner preplanning for the event. Ethical behavior requires courage. We propose that all practices have a policy or standard operating procedure (SOP) supporting the declining of euthanasia requests on moral grounds (see Box 6.1). An intention-based definition of euthanasia may provide clearer guidance to veterinarians as they confront euthanasia decisions.

Box 6.1   Hospital Policy: Declining Euthanasia on Moral Grounds

This hospital takes the decision to euthanize a patient very seriously. Our veterinarians seek to learn every detail about a patient's quality of life and consider all available resources to care for their physical and emotional needs. It is also important for us to learn how owners can tend to their own personal/family needs while providing for their pet during the end of life. If a veterinarian feels that euthanasia is not the right medical decision, they have a responsibility to the animal and themselves to offer alternatives. The mental health of our veterinarians is of paramount importance, and if an ethical conflict arises, we may refuse to perform euthanasia on moral grounds.

When Euthanasia Should Be Performed

Even if one can confidently justify on a moral basis why an animal should be euthanized, it can be very difficult to know when euthanasia should be performed. One factor relevant to the timing of euthanasia is the question of whether veterinarians should initiate this difficult topic or wait for owners to do so. We believe it is the responsibility of the compassionate veterinarian to raise the topic of euthanasia when indicated and that abdication of this duty is likely to prolong animal suffering.

Because the need for euthanasia may arise during any life stage, we suggest opening dialogue about end-of-life options before euthanasia is necessary, especially for patients with congenital diseases, relatively short lifespans, and when chronic disease is diagnosed. While broaching the subject of death and dying is challenging [23], veterinarians uncomfortable with such discussions are missing an important opportunity to educate owners on what to expect and what to prepare for as their animal reaches the end of life. Preplanning details around euthanasia is ranked among the top five components of a good death experience according to owners [24].

It is common after discussion of euthanasia for owners to elect to take the animal home to allow them time to accept the situation, and/or for other family members to say goodbye. In some cases, the timeline proposed by the animal's owner may be a few weeks, when the veterinarian believes that a more appropriate timetable for euthanasia should be measured in hours or days. This circumstance creates ethical challenges for the veterinarian, who wishes to advocate for the interests of the suffering patient who will benefit from death, yet also respect the difficulty for the owner of letting go of a beloved family member. We believe that veterinarians must advocate for the timely euthanasia of suffering patients, even when this conflicts with owner desires. None of us wants to part with a beloved animal companion. Animal owners rely on veterinarians to be a source of objectivity and to be the animal's advocate to guide them in this difficult decision.

Conversely, owners concerned about imminent crisis events may prefer to euthanize an animal sooner rather than later to spare themselves the distress of watching their companion decline and the emotions that occur from fear of the unknown. Veterinarians should educate owners about disease symptoms and trajectories, including the likelihood and nature of possible crisis events, and whether and how these can be addressed, including costs, which may avert a premature euthanasia decision.

Palliative medicine is medical care to reduce the unpleasant symptoms of disease and improve QOL. Hospice care is a specialized form of palliative care that focuses on alleviating suffering in patients during the end stages of an illness [25]. A comprehensive understanding of the full scope of hospice and palliative care options and how to apply them in practice reduces the likelihood of premature euthanasia. Providing owners with guidance regarding which symptoms can be managed by palliative medicine and criteria for when euthanasia is justified (i.e. not eating any food, vomiting daily) can be very helpful. If veterinarians are candid about projections around death and dying, owners can feel more empowered to make sensible decisions for their animal, themselves, and their family. This equates to a more controlled decision about timing of euthanasia for all stakeholders.

There may be instances when euthanasia is performed due to veterinarian availability. For example, we see this situation arise before the close of a shift, before a vacation, or perhaps when a preferred home euthanasia can be performed. Fear can be the primary factor: fear of what would happen to the animal if the veterinarian wasn't available to euthanize, and in the location desired by the owner. We challenge veterinarians to seek alternative solutions to euthanasia based on veterinarian convenience, such as delegating to an associate or licensed technician (where allowed), leveraging community veterinary services, and increasing use of hospice and palliative care until such time as euthanasia should be provided.

Where Euthanasia Should Be Performed

Euthanasia is unique among veterinary procedures in that clients are often present and observing what occurs. To deliver on the definition of "a good death," veterinarians must also consider where the euthanasia procedure should be performed, ideally guided by where the animal patient and loved ones will be most comfortable. When considering all stakeholders in the decision on where to gather, a "one size fits all" model does not exist.

Veterinary hospitals are the most common site for companion animal euthanasia [26], where veterinary teams have greater control over access to the necessary resources and supplies, and owners may be reassured by the presence of their family veterinarian. If the patient is already hospitalized, this may avert the need for transport to an alternate location. This setting may present challenges due to physical space limitations, noises, the need to hurry due to emergencies or other appointments, or discomfort with the emotional nature of the procedure or with payment. Clients may also develop a strong negative association between the hospital and their animal's death; some clients will request not to be placed in the same exam room where a euthanasia previously occurred.

As the number of practices devoted to exclusively performing euthanasia is expanding, we suggest that practitioners offer a variety of viable location options for euthanasia in keeping with obtaining informed consent (Table 6.1).

Table 6.1 Options for where euthanasia can be performed.

Regular veterinary hospital
Specialty/emergency hospital
Client/patient home
Park or public space
Animal shelter
Euthanasia center
Pet crematory facility

Pet owners have expressed their desire for the home as the preferred location for euthanasia [27]. Home euthanasia is also the most comfortable setting for the animal due to familiarity, avoidance of the stress associated with travel, and the presence of loved ones including other companion animals. The proliferation of dedicated veterinary mobile euthanasia practices is a result of the rising demand for at-home euthanasia. The International Association for Animal Hospice and Palliative Care (IAAHPC) [28] reports having over 1200 members, including veterinarians, technicians, social workers, and other support personnel. An online directory of mobile, home hospice providers has some 300 listings from all over the United States [29]. Veterinary teams should refer to such services if they are unable to travel to the home to accommodate client requests.

Clients may elect for euthanasia to be in a public place to avoid having to do it in the hospital or home, which poses unique challenges. One may assume that euthanasia can be facilitated wherever the client wishes to gather (i.e. park, beach, etc.); however, some communities require a license for the procedure to be performed where the public may witness it. Unpredictable disturbances such as people encroaching and obtrusive sounds may have negative impacts on the experience in a public setting. There is also the consideration of deceased pet handling. A living animal will enter the public space, but a dead one will depart. This creates the risk of innocent bystanders seeing a deceased animal. Covering the patient completely and moving them with respect becomes necessary and is a component of the preplanning process.

Animal shelters commonly provide owner-requested euthanasia for pets. Owners choose to bring their pet to the shelter due to lack of local veterinarian availability or high cost. Shelters receive these pets specifically for euthanasia, although they have the option to discuss behavior training, rehoming, or medical support. Shelters typically do not allow owners to be present for euthanasia. Animal shelter euthanasia therefore is a less suitable location for owners who wish to remain with their pet. The veterinary profession can actively seek to reduce the pressures of owner-requested euthanasia on animal shelters by identifying better ways to meet the demand for euthanasia in the private sector.

The first reported pet euthanasia center was part of a veterinary mobile end-of-life practice, Home to Heaven™. It was designed to be a neutral location or "home away from home" for clients, circumventing the emotional trauma associated with memories of death occurring in the home or the busy hospital setting. Euthanasia centers may serve an even larger purpose: to reduce the burden on veterinary hospitals, mobile services, and animal shelters. These pressures include appointment availability and staff concerns (i.e. emotional wellbeing, technical skills). Euthanasia centers may be the bridge to provide compassionate euthanasia for companion animals in a timely, economical manner. A euthanasia center may be built for this purpose or established locations like pet aftercare facilities (i.e. pet crematory) can meet this need.

Whichever location is chosen, veterinarians must be aware of the implications of the experience for loved ones and witnesses. Veterinary teams, including veterinary technicians, will need to adapt to new environments, requiring movement of veterinary supplies to the patient to ensure the procedure goes as smoothly as in a hospital exam room. Where euthanasia is performed matters and can make the difference between a good experience and a bad one.

How to Perform Euthanasia

Euthanasia methodology with attention to patient comfort has advanced significantly in the past decade with the intention of providing a better experience for animals, owners, veterinarians, and involved veterinary personnel. Past approaches emphasized the rapid and efficient administration of euthanasia solution in conscious, alert animals; while this was effective, animal welfare concerns included anxiety from being separated from the owner and pain from placement of an intravenous (IV) catheter and/or from the injection itself, such as inadvertent extravasation. Recently, the paradigm has shifted from the primary goal being a fast death to a more calm and controlled death with loved ones present.

When euthanasia is elected, veterinarians have an ethical responsibility to provide all patients a good death, especially because there is only one opportunity to get it right. Owners want the option of being with their animal for the entirety of the appointment (never separated), to be provided with details to help them prepare, and to see their animal companion sleeping with little to no experienced pain or anxiety throughout the procedure [24, 30]. Only 33% and 47% of veterinarians in New Zealand cited always using sedation for euthanasia of dogs and cats, respectively [31], and 57% of Australian practitioners did so for dogs [26].

The evolving status of animals as family members means that companion animal euthanasia is now more of an experience with multiple components rather than a singular medical act. A good death includes proper delivery of the medication. While the administration of a euthanasia solution has predominantly been carried out via an IV injection, other techniques exist [32] and it is a veterinarian's duty to understand what they are, their indications (such as when insertion of an IV catheter is untenable), and how to perform them.

Owners can become emotionally traumatized by negative experiences (such as atypical vocalizations, body twitching, patient tremors, and feeling rushed) associated with euthanasia or "dysthanasia." A "dysthanasia" may cause a reluctance by owners to elect euthanasia of other animals in the future and create a negative perception of the veterinary profession as uncaring or incompetent. Avoiding a bad death becomes as important as performing euthanasia well.

Consequently, preventing errors during the euthanasia procedure should be the foremost consideration of the veterinarian. The use of SOPs based on peer-reviewed clinical practice guidelines helps build consistency in the delivery of care. The AAHA/IAAHPC end-of-life care guidelines offer clear instruction on how to perform euthanasia in both the hospital and home settings [33]. The AVMA [3], Companion Animal Euthanasia Training Academy [34], American Association of Feline Practitioners [35], and others have also produced guidelines or recommended best practices for the euthanasia of animals. Many veterinarians rely on SOPs to ensure the consistency and quality of their services, and many hospitals are accustomed to their use for activities such as surgery and practice management [36]. Yet less than half of veterinarians in a recent study reported that their clinic had a standard protocol for euthanizing dogs and cats [31].

Veterinary appointments often range from 15 to 20 minutes [37]. A recent report found that most non-emergency euthanasia appointments for dogs were 20–30 minutes in duration [26]. Such short times limit the application of modern euthanasia methods, which include what the Companion Animal Euthanasia Training Academy refers to as the 14 essential components of a good death (Table 6.2) [38]. The components are a compilation of recommendations from various sources intended to benefit patients, owners, and the veterinary team.

Companion animal euthanasia has evolved to be a pseudo-funeral: a unique, emotional medical procedure in full view of owners unlike anything else undertaken in veterinary practice. Lengthening scheduled euthanasia appointments is warranted to accommodate all the necessary components of modern euthanasia. We propose that longer appointment times in the range of 45–60 minutes for all sick patients become the standard, as some of these appointments may result in a euthanasia decision; if not, this still improves the veterinarian's capacity to acquire informed consent, discuss prognosis, and achieve shared decisions [39].

Table 6.2 The 14 essential components of companion animal euthanasia.

G: Grief support materials provided
O: Outline caregiver and pet preferences
O: Offer privacy before and after death
D: Deliver proper technique
E: Establish rapport
U: Use of pre-euthanasia sedation or anesthesia
T: Thorough, complete consent
H: Helpful and compassionate personnel
A: Adequate time
N: Narrate the process
A: Avoid pain and anxiety
S: Safe space to gather
I: Inclusion of loved ones
A: Assistance with body care

Source: Adapted from [38].

Animal owners expect a death process for their companion that is free of pain and fear and define "a good death" beyond just the procedure itself [24]. When an animal is considered a member of the family, making the decision to end its life can be a very distressing and protracted process, often described by owners as the hardest thing they have ever had to do. Owners reasonably expect emotional support during this time, including validation of their decision (if this can be offered sincerely) that mitigates feelings of guilt [27].

Fees

Veterinary practices are businesses and must generate revenue. Fees are necessary to keep the business operational and are driven by overhead costs plus the desired profit. Euthanasia as a medical procedure means someone is paying to end the life of an animal companion, which is often accompanied by significant emotional trauma. Consequently, the question of what to charge clients for euthanasia is complicated.

In some cases, the practitioner may perceive a euthanasia decision to be a result of a failure of diagnosis, treatment, and/or communication, which engenders feelings of guilt and incompetence. In these circumstances, clinicians may consider bypassing euthanasia fees or providing significant discounts to assuage such feelings. Practitioners may provide complementary euthanasia services to demonstrate respect for the emotional loss of the client and/or in gratitude for years of paid veterinary care. A discounted or free service may also be provided for clients unable to afford euthanasia. Conversely, some practitioners may consider euthanasia as another veterinary service that should be structured to accrue a profit for the practice. Tannenbaum has noted that "veterinarians ... should not take advantage of situations in which clients have a restricted choice of whether to accept their fees" [6].

We can consider four different components associated with euthanasia. First, veterinarians should charge appropriate fees for their time spent counseling owners about end-of-life decisions, whether euthanasia is ultimately chosen or not. Second, the time associated with the euthanasia procedure itself should be accounted for. The third component is the medical supplies, grief support materials/memorialization items, complying with the necessary regulations to manage the controlled substances needed for the procedure, and the costs of the medications used, which often vary based on patient weight. While many practices have a tiered scale of charges for euthanasia based on patient weight to account for the increased volume of medications for larger patients, we advise a single euthanasia fee for all patients that accounts for all the steps associated with the procedure. A standard fee accounting for the median weight of patients in the practice is simpler and more readily facilitates providing an accurate estimate for the procedure to clients. Finally, there are fees associated with patient aftercare. We suggest that while it is quite reasonable to incorporate a profit based on the clinician's time and medications, aftercare (i.e. cremation) fees should not constitute a profit center for the practice, unless the practice itself performs the aftercare.

When euthanasia is the purpose of the appointment, collecting fees can be done before the appointment starts. When a euthanasia decision is the outcome of an appointment for a sick patient, costs and payment will need to be handled gently. In these situations, many practitioners prefer to collect payment before the procedure begins to spare emotionally upset clients from having to make payment. Alternatively, the practice could bill the client, which may raise the concern of non-payment.

Just because a client is willing to pay for euthanasia should not compel the veterinarian to perform it. It is common for euthanasia appointments to be scheduled for both established and new patients, leading to questions of suitability for new patients that the veterinarian has never seen before. A client may feel the time is right for euthanasia and request it be scheduled, placing the practice in a tricky spot. One way around this is to inform clients that new patients, those not familiar to the attending veterinarian, and those who have not been seen for a year require a physical exam and consultation before euthanasia will be considered. These are commonly referred to as end-of-life consultations and veterinarians use them to open dialogue around what the patient and the client are experiencing. End-of-life consultations determine what's best without the expectation of euthanasia. They can be priced the same as for euthanasia, with the understanding that if the veterinarian feels euthanasia is an acceptable path forward, they may do so during the same appointment at no extra charge.

Pet Aftercare

How the deceased animal's body is handled while in the care of the veterinarian also deserves attention. Clients have voiced their preference for body handling/storage that chooses more respectful containers (e.g. specially designed transport bags) over the commonly used plastic refuse bags [40], yet these bags are still regularly used in practice. Hospitals typically use freezers to hold client-owned animals until the crematory service can pick them up, a less than ideal system for those who would prefer the body to arrive expeditiously at its destination. In our experience, veterinarians shield owners from witnessing how the deceased's body is contained and stored until crematory pickup, perhaps due to their own disapproval of current norms. When we know better, we do better, and veterinarians have an opportunity to elevate ethical behaviors related to the aftercare of deceased patients, treating the body as if it were their own pet.

Use of deceased animals for teaching and training purposes should be limited to those in which informed consent is acquired from the owner. It may once have been considered acceptable to routinely practice learning exercises on cadavers to advance medical knowledge without the owner's awareness, but professional ethics prompts reconsideration of this behavior. In our experience, owners have been receptive to donating their pet's body for select teaching purposes and have signed agreements indicating such consent. For all approaches to aftercare, veterinarians should ask themselves: "Would I be willing to inform my clients or my colleagues of these practices?"

Conclusion

Companion animal euthanasia is fraught with ethical challenges and emotions and can lead to moral and traumatic stress for veterinary professionals and clients, respectively. We define euthanasia as the intentional ending of life primarily to benefit the animal's interest only when suffering is imminent or permanent and cannot be alleviated. While making the decision to euthanize an animal companion may be difficult due to limited information and uncertainty about the patient's condition, veterinarians should ensure a peaceful death, establish an ethical approach to aftercare, and demonstrate compassion to grieving animal owners, the veterinary team, and themselves.

References

1 Pegram, C., Gray, C., Packer, R. et al. (2021). Proportion and risk factors for death by euthanasia in dogs in the UK. *Scientific Reports* 11: 9145.

2 Dyck, A. (1975). Beneficent euthanasia and benemortasia: alternative views of mercy. In: *Beneficent Euthanasia* (ed. M. Kohl), 117–129. Buffalo, NY: Prometheus Books.

3 Leary, S., Underwood, W., Anthony, R. et al. (2020). *AVMA Guidelines for the Euthanasia of Animals*. Schaumburg, IL: American Veterinary Medical Association. https://www.avma.org/sites/default/files/2020-02/Guidelines-on-Euthanasia-2020.pdf (accessed December 18, 2022).

4 Quain, A. (2021). The gift: ethically indicated euthanasia in companion animal practice. *Veterinary Sciences* 8 (8): 141. https://doi.org/10.3390/vetsci8080141.

5 Rollin, B.E. (2011). Euthanasia, moral stress and chronic illness in veterinary medicine. *Veterinary Clinics Small Animal* 41 (3): 651–659.

6 Tannenbaum, J. (1995). *Veterinary Ethics: Animal Welfare, Client Relations, Competition and Collegiality*, 2e. St. Louis, MO: Mosby.

7 Batchelor, C.E.M. and McKeegan, D.E. (2012). Survey of the frequency and perceived stressfulness of ethical dilemmas encountered in UK veterinary practice. *Veterinary Record* 170 (1): 19.

8 Rathwell-Deault, D., Godard, B., Frank, D. et al. (2017). Conceptualization of convenience euthanasia as an ethical dilemma for veterinarians in Quebec. *Canadian Veterinary Journal* 58 (3): 255–260.

9 Spitznagel, M.B., Patrick, K., Gober, M.W. et al. (2022). Relationships among owner consideration of euthanasia, caregiver burden, and treatment satisfaction in canine osteoarthritis. *Veterinary Journal* 286: 105868.

10 Kipperman, B. (2010). Economic euthanasia: a disease in need of prevention. Davis, CA: Humane Society Veterinary Medical Association. https://www.hsvma.org/economic_euthanasia_disease_in_need_of_prevention#.Y1mdNC-B30o (accessed June 12, 2023).

11 Villalobos, A.E. (2011). Quality-of-life assessment techniques for veterinarians. *Veterinary Clinics North America. Small Animal Practice* 41 (3): 519–529.

12 Fulmer, A.E., Laven, L.J., and Hill, K.E. (2022). Quality of life measurement in dogs and cats: a scoping review of generic tools. *Animals* 12 (3): 400.

13 McMillan, F.D. (2003). Maximizing quality of life in ill animals. *Journal of the American Animal Hospital Association* 39 (3): 227–235.

14 Schulz, R., Cook, T.B., Beach, S.R. et al. (2013). Magnitude and causes of bias among family caregivers rating Alzheimer disease patients. *American Journal of Geriatric Psychiatry* 21 (1): 14–25.

15 Janssen, D.J., Spruit, M.A., Wouters, E.F. et al. (2012). Symptom distress in advanced chronic organ failure: disagreement among patients and family caregivers. *Journal of Palliative Medicine* 15 (4): 447–456.

16 Hsu, T., Loscalzo, M., Ramani, R. et al. (2017). Are disagreements in caregiver and patient assessment of patient health associated with increased caregiver burden in caregivers of older adults with cancer? *Oncologist* 22 (11): 1383–1391.

17 Oechsle, K., Goerth, K., Bokemeyer, C. et al. (2013). Symptom burden in palliative care patients: perspectives of patients, their family caregivers, and their attending physicians. *Support Care Cancer* 21 (7): 1955–1962. https://doi.org/10.1007/s00520-013-1747-1.

18 Marchitelli, B., Shearer, T., and Cook, N. (2020). Factors contributing to the decision to euthanize: diagnosis, clinical signs, and triggers. *Veterinary Clinics: Small Animal Practice* 50 (3): 573–589.

19 Moses, L., Malowney, M.J., and Boyd, J.W. (2018). Ethical conflict and moral distress in veterinary practice: a survey of North American veterinarians. *Journal of Veterinary Internal Medicine* 32 (6): 2115–2122.

20 Kipperman, B., Morris, P., and Rollin, B. (2018). Ethical dilemmas encountered by small animal veterinarians: characterization, responses, consequences and beliefs regarding euthanasia. *Veterinary Record* 182 (19): 548. https://doi.org/10.1136/vr.104619.

21 Kipperman, B. (2022). Veterinary advocacies and ethical dilemmas. In: *Ethics in Veterinary Practice*, ch. 7 (ed. B. Kipperman and B.E. Rollin). Hoboken, NJ: Wiley-Blackwell.

22 Jurney, C. and Kipperman, B. (2022). Moral stress. In: *Ethics in Veterinary Practice*, ch. 22 (ed. B. Kipperman and B.E. Rollin). Hoboken, NJ: Wiley-Blackwell.

23 Shaw, J.R. and Lagoni, L. (2007). End-of-life communication in veterinary medicine: delivering bad news and euthanasia decision making. *Veterinary Clinics North America Small Animal Practice* 37 (1): 95–108.

24 Cooney, K. and Kogan, L. (2022). How pet owners define a "good death": new study reveals some surprising facts. *DVM360 Magazine* 53 (8): 12.

25 Monteiro, B. and Robertson, S. (2022). Animal pain. In: *Ethics in Veterinary Practice: Balancing Conflicting Interests*, ch. 19 (ed. B. Kipperman and B.E. Rollin). Hoboken, NJ: Wiley-Blackwell.

26 Pepper, B.M., Chan, H., Ward, M.P. et al. (2023). Euthanasia of dogs by Australian veterinarians: a survey of current practices. *Veterinary Sciences* 10 (5): 317. https://doi.org/10.3390/vetsci10050317.

27 Matte, A.R., Khosa, D.K., Coe, J.B. et al. (2020). Exploring pet owners' experiences and self-reported satisfaction and grief following companion animal euthanasia. *Veterinary Record* 187: e122.

28 International Association for Animal Hospice and Palliative Care (IAAHPC). https://iaahpc.org (accessed June 7, 2023).

29 In-Home Pet Directory. www.inhomepeteuthanasia.com (accessed June 7, 2023).

30 Kogan, L. and Cooney, K. (2023). Defining a "good death": exploring veterinarians' perceptions of companion animal euthanasia. *Animals* 13 (13): 2117.

31 Gates, M.C., Kells, N.J., Kongara, K.K. et al. (2023). Euthanasia of dogs and cats by veterinarians in New Zealand: protocols, procedures and experiences. *New Zealand Veterinary Journal* 71 (4): 172–185. https://doi.org/10.1080/00480169.2023.2194687.

32 Cooney, K. (2020). Common and alternative routes of euthanasia solution administration. *Veterinary Clinics North America Small Animal Practice* 50 (3): 545–560.

33 Bishop, G., Cooney, K., Cox, S. et al. (2016). AAHA/IAAHPC end-of-life care guidelines. *Journal of the American Animal Hospital Association* 52 (6): 341–356.

34 Companion Animal Euthanasia Training Academy. https://caetainternational.com (accessed June 12, 2023).

35 American Association of Feline Practitioners (n.d.). End of life educational toolkit. https://catvets.com/public/PDFs/Toolkit/EOL/EOL-TK-Euthansia-Process.pdf (accessed June 12, 2023).

36 Freeman, K.P., Cook, J.T., and Hooijberg, E.H. (2021). Standard operating procedures. *Journal of the American Veterinary Medical Association* 258 (5): 477–481.

37 Corah, L., Lambert, A., Cobb, K. et al. (2019). Appointment scheduling and cost in first opinion small animal practice. *Heliyon* 5 (10): e02567.

38 Companion Animal Euthanasia Training Academy (2019). What's behind a good pet euthanasia? https://caetainternational.com/whats-behind-a-good-pet-euthanasia (accessed November 23, 2022).

39 Janke, N., Coe, J.B., Bernardo, T.M. et al. (2021). Pet owners' and veterinarians' perceptions of information exchange and clinical decision-making in companion animal practice. *PLoS One* 16 (2): e0245632.

40 Cooney, K., Kogan, L., Brooks, S. et al. (2021). Pet owners' expectations for pet end-of-life support and after-death body care: exploration and practical applications. *Topics Companion Animal Medicine* 43: 100503.

7

Referrals

Barry Kipperman

Abstract

This chapter discusses the growth of veterinary specialization and the goals of patient referrals. Barriers to referral are considered, including emotional concerns and costs. Guidance is provided regarding when and how to refer and receive patients, including the obligations of the referring veterinarian and specialist in this process. Practices to foster trust and collaboration between referring veterinarians and specialists are outlined. Whether specialists should educate and report referring veterinarians is considered. Because they see patients in advanced stages of illness who are sometimes referred too late to be helped, veterinary specialists are at high risk of moral stress.

Keywords: *specialist, referring veterinarian, referrals, barriers, communication, collaboration, educating, reporting, moral stress*

To meet societal demand that medical care for animals rival that of humans, specialization in veterinary medicine has expanded. The number of referral and emergency practices offering specialized care in the United States has increased dramatically in the last three decades. Of the estimated 124 000 veterinarians in America [1], 11% are board-certified specialists [2]. This figure has increased by 23% since 2012 [3]. Veterinary specialists have the same diverse obligations as referring veterinarians (RDVMs), but in addition must satisfy the perceived or real demands of RDVMs. The questions of whether, when, and how to refer a patient to a specialist, and the obligations of the specialist to the RDVM, have important ethical dimensions.

There should be little debate about the duty of *whether* to refer a patient. Rollin [4] asserts that "If the animal will benefit ... the veterinarian has a moral duty to refer and defer to greater expertise." The American Veterinary Medical Association (AVMA) Principles of Veterinary Medical Ethics state: "When appropriate ... veterinarians are encouraged to seek assistance in the form of ... referrals" [5].

Goals of Referrals

Over a century ago, Codman noted in human medicine that desperate measures are often necessary to treat critical illnesses, particularly when the alternative is death [6]. He suggested that the most knowledgeable and capable medical professionals (i.e. those with specialized training) should perform such procedures: "Who should attempt these desperate operations—the man anxious to make a reputation, or the man who has made one?" Stoewen et al. nicely summarize the goal of referrals in veterinary practice: "The provision of the best possible medical care to veterinary patients may be envisioned as a collegial partnership between general practitioners (GPs) and board-certified specialists, with specialty care as a direct extension of primary care service" [7].

The ideal benefits of referral include providing your patient with access to equipment your practice does not have (i.e. ultrasound or CT scanner) and/or to someone with more knowledge in managing the patient's condition. A report of the beliefs of human GPs aligns with these motives, finding that the main driver for the choice to refer was the perception that the specialist knows more about the problem and/or can do more to address it [8]. In a report of equine RDVMs, the top two factors associated with the decision to refer were quality of care and clinician expertise [9].

Barriers to Referrals

By their choice to limit their expertise to one field, I believe that veterinary specialists are more apt to appreciate their respective strengths and limitations than are GPs. As an internist, I would never conceive of performing a major surgery on a patient. Although many of my clients asked me to do so, it was easy to inform them that I wasn't qualified for the job. I had no reservations or shame in acknowledging the boundaries of my expertise. Yet, the GP is considered a jack of all trades, with a social license to perform virtually any procedure they wish. Consequently, the onus to acknowledge and respect one's limitations is greater on the part of the GP. This task is made even more difficult because an objective evaluation of one's professional capabilities is intrinsically difficult, if not impossible to assess [10].

Bergman et al. [11] observe that dental practice and veterinary practice are similar in that few patients have insurance, but suggest that clients are more likely to expect a referral from their dentist: "patients are likely to expect a referral to a specialist for non-routine dental services, including periodontics and orthodontics. Few expect their general dentist to have the expertise needed ... to meet the patient's needs. As a result, there is no loss of 'image' or confidence when a general dentist refers patients to a specialist." I recall my dentist telling me: "While I can perform a root canal, I just don't do them anymore, so I'll refer you to someone who does them every day." In contrast to the acceptance of referrals in dentistry, a report found that human GPs often "struggle to decide whether or not they should refer patients to specialists" [8]. This sentiment may be even more problematic in veterinary practice given the lack of societal awareness of veterinary specialists, the property status of animals, and the reality that veterinary clinicians have virtually no malpractice concerns or economic liability for failing to refer.

In a rare survey of veterinary specialists, 78% of small animal internal medicine specialists believed that RDVMs keep cases that a specialist in their field should be seeing [12]. My own experience parallels these concerns: based on seeing thousands of patients that were transferred from the emergency service to my internal medicine service (so these patients had not been referred and whose owners consented to my consultation), many patients in need of referral are not being referred.

Multiple studies have documented the perceived high costs of referral care by RDVMs as the major barrier regarding the decision to refer [9, 12–14]. It's important to recognize that the RDVM's assumptions about an animal owner's financial capacity and their willingness to spend money on their animal companion may be inaccurate [11]. RDVMs should never assume that a client cannot afford to see a specialist. Main has observed: "it is ... simply impossible to predict how much an owner is prepared to spend on an animal. I would contend that attempting to do so would also be to conflict with the owners 'right' to make an autonomous decision on how to spend his or her own money" [15]. A recent report on human GPs also discovered concern over the financial and/or psychological "cost" for patients as undesirable consequences of referral [8].

These beliefs may discourage or prevent appropriate referrals. My experience has been that attempting to judge which clients will spend considerable resources on their animal companions is a fool's errand. Rollin has argued that it is ethically justifiable for an RDVM to discourage referral if they believe that this may cause the client to exhaust their financial or emotional capacity [4]. This raises the question of whether it is appropriate for the RDVM to be the "guardian of their client's pocketbook" or whether animal welfare considerations should be prioritized.

Another obstacle to referral is perceived loss of income of the RDVM, with the specialist seen as competition for finite revenues associated with each patient. In one investigation, equine RDVMs reported that their greatest source of dissatisfaction was the competition the referral hospital posed to their practice, including concerns of client solicitation [9]. Main notes regarding referral that "If the goal ... is to advocate the best treatment option, then the loss of clinical income for the practitioner should not be a relevant factor" [15]. Surely a live patient cared for by a colleague is more valuable to the practice than one that is deceased! Specialist availability regarding appointment dates and times as well as proximity can also be limiting factors to referral.

It is common for RDVMs to call specialists requesting advice about a patient. As the premise for such queries, the RDVM may tell the specialist that the client either cannot afford or will not accept referral. Many of these phone consults last 5–15 minutes and guidance is often provided that helps the RDVM to order additional tests or treatments, for which they are compensated by their client. In some cases, the RDVM will also request that the specialist help them interpret the results of the new tests. During my career, I tried to provide the best advice I could in this setting, but I sometimes felt that my knowledge had been taken advantage of to bypass a formal referral. As most specialists don't charge fees for time spent on the phone supporting RDVMs and their patients, referring veterinarians should offer to compensate the specialist for these informal consultations to demonstrate respect for their time and expertise. If after the phone discussion the case is referred, the specialist can then choose to waive the fee as a courtesy.

One's perceived lack of autonomy within a practice can also limit referrals. I've taken numerous calls from associate colleagues inquiring whether a patient they are caring for should be referred. If I believed that the patient should be referred, they would sometimes whisper into the phone, "I can't refer the patient today because my boss is here. I'll send him [the patient] tomorrow when he [my employer] is not here." Such intimidation by employers influences referral patterns. Finally, poor communication between the RDVM and the specialist has also been noted as an important hindrance to referrals [9].

Emotions and Referrals

Physicians' decisions to refer are influenced by emotions, including experiencing stress and challenges to their self-esteem [8]. Because of these emotional factors, "Referral is a sensitive topic for general practitioners, involving ... relationships with patients, colleagues, specialists and supervisors. The decision to refer ... is influenced by multiple contextual, personal and clinical factors that dynamically interact and shape the decision-making process" [8]. Consequently, another impediment to referral may be ego and pride; for some practitioners, acknowledging (to themselves and to clients) that a colleague is better suited to care for a patient is difficult. This emotional component of decision-making about referrals is important for veterinary specialists to appreciate and may require an emotionally intelligent skill set to navigate successfully. It also suggests that validation of a timely and appropriate referral by the specialist may ease this uncertainty, as we do to support clients who have made difficult euthanasia decisions.

When to Refer

There is little information available regarding *when* to refer. Block et al. [16] suggest that "any animal that has not received a definitive diagnosis or fails to improve despite medical treatment should be considered a candidate for a second opinion." Reasons to refer veterinary patients are summarized in Table 7.1.

An unnecessary referral is a waste of client and specialist time and resources; these can easily be diminished via a screening phone call to the specialist. A suitably timed referral is most likely to achieve the ideal goals. Delayed referrals often have devastating consequences, including poor patient prognosis and suffering, increased client costs, loss of faith in the value of specialists by clients and GPs, the perception by the specialist that the GP did not prioritize the patient's welfare, and demoralization for the specialist, who feels they cannot disclose to the client or the GP that an earlier referral would have achieved a better patient outcome or allowed the patient to survive.

Making the Decision to Refer and Expectations of the Referral Process

As most pet owners are not aware of the existence of specialists [12], the RDVM is considered the gatekeeper to the referral process. Consequently, they *in conjunction with the client* should consider if the potential benefits of referral outweigh the cost, inconvenience, and necessity of trusting a clinician with whom the client often has no previous relationship. Multiple studies have confirmed that RDVMs expect to be involved in decisions regarding the patients they refer, including frequent communication and collaboration [9, 18]. At the time of referral, the referring veterinarian assigns

Table 7.1 Reasons to refer veterinary patients.

Inability to make a diagnosis

A patient has lost 10% or more of their body weight

Patient survival is more likely

Patient condition is progressing

Less invasive diagnostic or treatment options

The patient would benefit from 24-hour monitoring

The client is dissatisfied

The client requests a second opinion

The client is considering a euthanasia decision

Source: Adapted from [16, 17].

case management and responsibilities to the specialist. An excellent set of guidelines regarding referrals in veterinary medicine is available [17].

How to Refer

When an RDVM advises referral to a client, they should address the purpose or rationale of the referral, express confidence in the specialist, and assure the client that they will be communicating with the specialist. Clients should be informed of possible diagnoses that may be discovered and tests that may be performed, without committing the specialist to a specific expectation. Ensuring that the specialist receives all pertinent and up-to-date medical records and test results at least 12 hours prior to the patient's appointment (for non-emergency cases) maximizes the value of the consultation by avoiding potential delays that could compromise patient care or redundant diagnostic tests being performed [16]. All medical records should be typed; it is difficult to justify handwritten (and often illegible) medical records when even our most inane tweets and texts are typed. Clarifying the clinical issue that the specialist is expected to address in the medical record or on a referral form (i.e. "Referred for evaluation of icterus") is also very important.

RDVMs should counsel their clients on the anticipated costs associated with referral. Meeting this duty is challenging; informing a client that the bill is likely to be hundreds to thousands of dollars when the patient may only require a consultation may overestimate the fees involved. Conversely, quoting only the consultation fee and then having the specialist advise extensive tests or treatments misleads clients by underestimating the costs. If an RDVM is uncertain as to the outcome of the referral, it may be best to tell the client: "The consultation fee with the specialist is approximately 'x' dollars. If additional tests or treatments are needed, this may cost hundreds to thousands of dollars. The specialist will provide you with choices and estimates."

A screening call to the specialist may allow for a more accurate estimation of costs when the result of the referral is predictable (such as repair of cruciate ligament disruption or intensive care for a sick patient with diabetic ketoacidosis), and in some cases may determine that referral is inappropriate. Kipperman et al. note:

> Too often, pets are presented only for the owner to find out that needed care is prohibitively expensive. Referring a patient only to have it end up getting care that could have been provided by their family veterinarian, or worse, one who is euthanized immediately after the initial evaluation at the referral hospital, represents a failure of communication between all involved. [19]

How to Receive Referrals

To address RDVMs' concerns about competition and to foster mutually trusting relationships, specialists should limit the scope of care to the problem for which the animal is referred. If an alternate problem that requires attention is discovered, communication to update the RDVM is essential. Specialists must avoid any perceived attempts to encourage clients to seek primary care at their practice. Failure to communicate effectively and cultivate trust can result in poor patient outcomes and client dissatisfaction, and can have an adverse effect on the partnership between the RDVM and the referral hospital. Emphasizing the importance of communication associated with referrals, veterinarians have reported timeliness of communication as a recommended improvement to the referral process [20].

The specialist has a responsibility to communicate with the RDVM to summarize the nature of the consultation, including patient condition, diagnoses, and options offered to the client. Ideally, this should include at least one phone call within 24 hours of presentation to facilitate any input from the RDVM and to express appreciation for the referral. It's important to send all medical records and treatments provided, daily progress reports for hospitalized patients, and discharge instructions. These should be received no later than the day of discharge from the hospital and should clarify if follow-up is warranted, when this is necessary, and who should supervise it. As these documents can in some cases run to dozens of pages, a one-page referral letter summarizing the case is more likely to be read in its entirety. The referral letter should be received within seven days of patient discharge.

By virtue of the client's long-standing relationship with the GP, they may be in a better position to help guide the animal owner faced with difficult decisions. The trust that has been built over years with the GP cannot be rivaled by the specialist, where the duration of interaction with one client is often brief. Consequently, clients should be expected to confer with their GP regarding decisions about their animal companions. This reinforces the need for the specialist to contact the GP quickly after the initial consultation, especially if the client cannot make a decision.

In some cases, reaching out to the RDVM can help the specialist provide proper guidance to clients. I recall seeing Dusty, a black Labrador, for acute onset of vomiting. While the number of episodes reported was concerning, he seemed happy and alert. As a result, I was conflicted as to whether to treat Dusty as an inpatient or an outpatient (see Chapter 21). To help me make a good decision, I called the RDVM, who asked me, "Is Dusty jumping in your face and kissing you?" When I reported that he was not conducting this amorous behavior he said, "He's sick. Better be aggressive."

It has been suggested that "Specialists should always encourage referred clients to follow up with the referring veterinarian if the specialist and referring veterinarian believe that the referring veterinarian is capable of performing follow-up diagnostic testing and care" [16]. Adhering to this advice in practice is more challenging than it appears due to the difficulties in objectively assessing one's competence. As an example, I have seen numerous patients referred in very poor condition due to RDVM incapacity to recognize hypoadrenocorticism as the cause of illness. Yet, after patient stabilization when I inquired regarding monitoring, many of these RDVMs assured me they could manage the treatment going forward. Is this a reasonable expectation when they had not considered this diagnosis? Should I assure the client that all will be well by transferring care back to the RDVM? If there is any doubt about the RDVM's capacity to provide follow-up care, the specialist can suggest that they perform the first one or two rechecks to ensure the patient is stable and then transfer the case back. I have found that many RDVMs prefer this gradual hand-off of difficult cases. This also reduces the likelihood that the patient must be referred again for a relapse.

Finally, it is imperative that referral hospitals immediately inform the RDVM if a patient has died, to avoid a call to the client from the RDVM for a progress report, and to ensure that the RDVM can express condolences and provide support to the client.

Educating Referring Veterinarians

Do veterinary specialists have a duty to educate RDVMs? Block et al. support this role:

> Specialists have a responsibility to educate referring veterinarians ... when they believe animals ... should have been managed differently. Referring veterinarians should not be

defensive or confrontational when specialists attempt to ... suggest other ways they may have managed patients, nor should specialists discourage referring veterinarians from providing suggestions or advice regarding case management. Referring veterinarians should not respond by withholding future referrals. [16]

In my experience this seldom occurs; just as general practitioners are careful not to offend animal owners since they are economically dependent on them, specialists feel the same way toward referring veterinarians out of concern of losing referrals and their associated income. Unfortunately, also in my experience, attempts to constructively discuss what could have been done better with referring colleagues sometimes results in a punitive loss of future referrals. Professionally crafted referral letters are an opportunity to educate the RDVM in a less confrontational format. Specialists are more comfortable fulfilling this duty by providing continuing education on topics relevant to their expertise via lectures and case presentations.

Reporting Referring Veterinarians

Whether specialists are obligated to report RDVMs has been addressed: "Veterinarians have an ethical obligation to report what they believe to be patterns of professional negligence or malpractice to the appropriate authority" [16]. The AVMA Principles of Veterinary Medical Ethics state: "If there is evidence that the actions of the former attending veterinarian have clearly and significantly endangered the health or safety of the patient, the new attending veterinarian has a responsibility to report the matter to the appropriate authorities" [5].

I have never seen or heard of a practitioner reporting a colleague. I have recognized negligence (Case Studies 7.1 and 7.2) and been told by GPs of financial motivations to perform costly, invasive procedures on patients, and for failure to refer. I seldom have confronted these actions and have never witnessed one of my colleagues doing so. When I addressed a delayed referral that resulted in prolonged illness with a colleague, I was thanked for my candor and told that future referrals would be sent elsewhere. A utilitarian calculation may conclude that the risks of

---

Case Study 7.1   A Labrador with Vomiting and Anorexia

Shane, a four-year-old male Labrador retriever, is seen by an RDVM for lethargy, vomiting, and declining appetite for five days. He is sent home on an antiemetic and bland diet without any testing being offered. Numerous progress reports via telephone are noted in the medical record for the next five days, suggesting that the owner perceives appetite may be improving, but vomiting persisted. Abdominal radiographs, lab tests, and hospitalization are advised and approved, and supportive care with intravenous fluids and an antiemetic is initiated for a tentative diagnosis of pancreatitis. Shane is transferred for four consecutive days and nights between the RDVM and a local emergency clinic to receive supportive care with no improvement. On Friday afternoon (two weeks after the initial symptoms), Shane is referred to your internal medicine practice for evaluation. The previous radiographs reveal an intestinal foreign body. Surgery is advised with a guarded prognosis based on the two-week duration of illness. The owner approves all necessary care for Shane. An intestinal resection and anastomosis are required to remove a corn cob from his small intestine. Shane develops hemolytic anemia and severe thrombocytopenia and is euthanized days after surgery.

Case Study 7.2   A Dog with Weight Loss and Lymphadenopathy

Clancy, a 13-year-old male Golden retriever, has seen his RDVM his whole life. Clancy weighed 94 lb in June. In December, his weight was 88 lb and lab work was unremarkable. In February, Clancy is brought in for a lump on the left side of his neck. Weight is now 83 lb. The RDVM notes confirm slight lymph node enlargement. The medical record states: "Discussed possible lymphoma. Advise antibiotic trial × 1 week. If lymphoma, nodes will continue to enlarge."

One week later, Clancy's owner calls and reports that his gland is still enlarged. Recheck at that time revealed that Clancy's weight was 78 lb and another week of antibiotic was dispensed. The medical record documents: "Advise ultrasound and lymph node biopsy if continues to lose weight. Recheck 1 week." Clancy is referred to you one week later (21 days after initial presentation), due to persistent vomiting. Weight is now 76 lb.

Testing reveals an irregular spleen, abdominal lymph node enlargement, azotemia, dilute urine, hypoalbuminemia, and anemia. Lymph node aspirates confirm lymphoma. You discuss a guarded–poor prognosis for recovery given his debilitated condition and kidney failure. The owners tell you that Clancy is a member of the family, and they wish to be as aggressive as possible. They elect to pursue supportive care for the kidney failure via diuresis and to start chemotherapy injections. Despite four days in the hospital receiving intensive care, Clancy becomes weaker and is unable to stand. You inform the owners that Clancy is not likely to respond because of declining condition and euthanasia is elected.

---

speaking up in these circumstances outweigh the benefits: the perceived harm has already occurred, and loss of future referrals may harm the financial viability of the practice and limit the potential number of referred patients that could be helped in the future. Moreover, divulging such concerns to a colleague within your practice could be viewed as jeopardizing one's career, employment, and financial security. But there is a compelling reason to consider "speaking up" in these circumstances.

Moral Stress

Moral stress (or moral distress) has been defined as "The experience of psychological distress that results from engaging in, or failing to prevent, decisions or behaviors that transgress ... personally held moral or ethical beliefs" [21]. Moral stress is therefore recognized as a consequence of conflicts experienced involving work-related obligations or expectations that do not coincide with one's values [22]. Contributing factors to moral stress related to the killing or euthanasia of animals include a reverence for animals by those within the veterinary profession, the perception that one must suppress one's moral outrage at those responsible for creating the ethical conflict, and a disinclination to discuss the problem with friends or family [23].

I sought professional counseling to help me cope with the moral stress that developed from regularly seeing patients whose care I believed to be unacceptable, while feeling that I could not disclose my concerns to the RDVM or the client to adhere to standards of professionalism, resulting in feelings of guilt, anger, and discouragement. Veterinary specialists should be considered at high risk for moral stress and efforts to provide them with resources for mitigating moral stress and enhancing resilience during residency training are warranted [24].

A virtuous profession would seek a way forward for the problem of failure of self-regulation. Improved policing of our profession could reduce client complaints, mitigate moral stress, and enhance public trust. Such conversations should elevate the standards of care of the profession.

Conclusion

A recent report on human GPs' beliefs about the referral process found that they wanted improved relationships with specialists [8]. Forging trusting and mutually respectful relationships is a common outcome when specialists and RDVMs adhere to the recommendations in this chapter. When the RDVM and the specialist appreciate the boundaries of their respective areas of expertise, communicate well, and work as a team on behalf of the best interests of the animal, the wellbeing of our patients and the reputation of the profession are best served.

References

1 American Veterinary Medical Association (AVMA). US veterinarians 2022. https://www.avma.org/resources-tools/reports-statistics/market-research-statistics-us-veterinarians (accessed March 3, 2023).

2 American Veterinary Medical Association (AVMA). Veterinary specialists 2020. https://www.avma.org/resources-tools/reports-statistics/veterinary-specialists-2020 (accessed March 3, 2023).

3 American Veterinary Medical Association (AVMA). Market research statistics: veterinary specialists 2012. https://www.avma.org/resources/reports-statistics/market-research-statistics-veterinary-specialists-2012 (accessed March 3, 2023).

4 Rollin, B. (2006). The ethics of referral. *Canadian Veterinary Journal* 47 (7): 717.

5 American Veterinary Medical Association (AVMA). Principles of veterinary medical ethics of the AVMA. https://www.avma.org/KB/Policies/Pages/Principles-of-Veterinary-Medical-Ethics-of-the-AVMA.aspx (accessed March 3, 2023).

6 Codman, E.A. (1914). The product of a hospital. *Surgery, Gynecology and Obstetrics* 18: 491–496.

7 Stoewen, D.L., Coe, J.B., MacMartin, C. et al. (2013). Factors influencing veterinarian referral to oncology specialists for treatment of dogs with lymphoma and osteosarcoma in Ontario, Canada. *Journal of the American Veterinary Medical Association* 243 (10): 1415–1425.

8 Tzartzas, K., Oberhauser, P.N., Marion-Veyron, R. et al. (2019). General practitioners referring patients to specialists in tertiary healthcare: a qualitative study. *BMC Family Practice* 20 (1): 1–9.

9 Best, C., Coe, J.B., Hewson, J. et al. (2018). Survey of equine referring veterinarians' satisfaction with their most recent equine referral experience. *Journal of Veterinary Internal Medicine* 32 (2): 822–831.

10 Carter, T.J. and Dunning, D. (2008). Faulty self-assessment: why evaluating one's own competence is an intrinsically difficult task. *Social and Personality Psychology Compass* 2 (1): 346–360.

11 Bergman, P., Brogdon, R., Coates, J.R. et al. (2015). Specialist referrals among companion animal veterinary practices. Collaborative Care Coalition. https://collaborativecarecoalition.org/wp-content/uploads/2020/02/VetSOAP_Phase-1-Research-Full-Report-Jan2016.pdf (accessed March 3, 2023).

12 Buechner-Maxwell, V. and Byers, C. (2013). ACVIM member engagement and brand assessment survey Corona Insights survey results summary. *Journal of Veterinary Internal Medicine* 27 (5): 1287. doi: 10.1111/jvim.12171.

13 Alvarez, L.X., Fox, P.R., Van Dyke, J.B. et al. (2016). Survey of referring veterinarians' perceptions of and reasons for referring patients to rehabilitation facilities. *Journal of the American Veterinary Medical Association* 249 (7): 807–813.

14 Magalhães-Sant'Ana, M., More, S.J., Morton, D.B. et al. (2017). Challenges facing the veterinary profession in Ireland: 1. Clinical veterinary services. *Irish Veterinary Journal* 70 (1): 1–8.

15 Main, D. (2006). Offering the best to patients: ethical issues associated with the provision of veterinary services. *Veterinary Record* 158 (2): 62–66.

16 Block, G., Ross, J., and Northeast Veterinary Liaison Committee (2006). The relationship between general practitioners and board-certified specialists in veterinary medicine. *Journal of the American Veterinary Medical Association* 228 (8): 1188–1191.

17 American Animal Hospital Association (AAHA) (2013). Referral and consultation guidelines. https://www.aaha.org/globalassets/02-guidelines/referral/aaha-referral-guidelines-2013 (accessed March 3, 2023)

18 Burrows, C.F. (2008). Meeting the expectations of referring veterinarians. *Journal of Veterinary Medical Education* 35 (1): 20–25.

19 Kipperman, B., Block, G., and Forsgren, B. (2022). Economic issues. In: *Ethics in Veterinary Practice*, ch. 8 (ed. B. Kipperman and B.E. Rollin). Hoboken, NJ: Wiley-Blackwell.

20 Jakobek, B.T., Stull, J.W., Munguia, G. et al. (2023). Veterinarians' self-reported needs and attitudes on the Atlantic Canada Veterinary College and associated teaching hospital in relation to continuing education, research, and clinical referrals. *Journal of Veterinary Medical Education* 50 (2): 243–250.

21 Crane, M.F., Bayl-Smith, P., and Cartmill, J. (2013). A recommendation for expanding the definition of moral distress experienced in the workplace. *Australasian Journal of Organisational Psychology* 6: e1. https://doi.org/10.1017/orp.2013.1.

22 Fawcett, A. and Mullan, S. (2018). Managing moral distress in practice. *In Practice* 40 (1): 34–36.

23 Rollin, B.E. (2011). Euthanasia, moral stress, and chronic illness in veterinary medicine. *Veterinary Clinics of North America-Small Animal Practice* 41 (3): 651–659.

24 Jurney, C. and Kipperman, B. (2022). Moral stress. In: *Ethics in Veterinary Practice*, ch. 22 (ed. B. Kipperman and B.E. Rollin). Hoboken, NJ: Wiley-Blackwell.

8

The Influence of Economics on Decision-Making

Barry Kipperman

Abstract

This chapter examines the implications of economics in veterinary practice. The frequency with which veterinarians encounter economic limitations to care, their consequences, and actions practitioners can take to mitigate them are discussed. Practitioners should prepare their clients for the costs of veterinary care before patients are ill. All practices should have a protocol for dealing with financially limited clients to mitigate negative repercussions to patient care. The chapter considers whether veterinarians should work to preserve client resources or modify their recommendations based on presumed client capacity to pay, and what veterinarians should do when clients acknowledge incapacity to afford veterinary care.

Keywords: *business, economic limitations, costs of care, pet insurance, economics, paying, education, responsibility, money*

The origins of small animal practice in the United States were associated with efforts to help animal owners who could not afford veterinary services [1]. Over a century later, economic limitations still have a pervasive influence on access to veterinary care.

Veterinary Medicine as a Business

Most human patients have health insurance that insulates them from the costs of medical care. Veterinarians in practice utilize a fee-for-service model of income. The practices are businesses, and clients of companion animals are typically expected to leave a deposit prior to their animal receiving care and pay the balance of the fees when the patient leaves the hospital.

The repercussions of this model are summarized by Rosoff et al.:

> Unlike human medicine, veterinary medicine has no safety net that ensures that patients receive needed care, and thus the role of money ... very much dictates the treatment received. Since only a small ... minority of owners purchase health insurance for their animals, veterinary medicine's payment structure leaves owners liable for the full cost of veterinary care. Thus, the ability to receive treatment is intimately tied to both the ability and the willingness of the owner to pay for it. Some owners can't afford to get the care they believe their pet needs. [2]

A report assessing the implications of this economic model discovered that 28% of pet-owning households indicated they were unable to access veterinary care for one or more of their pets at least once in the past two years [3]. Studies have concluded that cost is the largest barrier to veterinary care [4, 5]. Substantiating this concern, 72% of veterinarians agreed that the for-profit business model is not meeting the needs of all pets [3] (Case Study 8.1).

Case Study 8.1   Economic Limitations to Life-saving Surgery

You see Molly, a six-month-old dog, for vomiting for three days, progressive lethargy, and declining appetite. You advise blood testing and radiographs to discern the cause and provide an estimate of $500 including your consultation. Molly's owners request that you perform testing in an incremental fashion. You start with abdominal radiographs, which reveal segmental dilation of small intestinal bowel loops, consistent with intestinal obstruction, most likely from ingestion of a foreign object. You discuss this finding with the owners and inform them that surgery will be necessary to resolve this problem. Without surgery, there will be a progressive decline in Molly's condition and then death. The estimated cost for surgery and postoperative care is $5000. You provide an 85% chance of complete recovery and a 15% chance of perioperative complications. The owners respond that if you cannot make Molly well for less than $1000, "We will have to put her down." You offer a financial line of credit program per hospital protocol: the owner's application is declined. The hospital has no other policies regarding addressing clients and pets with financial limitations.

What should you do?

How Often Do Veterinarians Encounter Economic Limitations to Care?

Client financial limitations compromising patient care have been documented as the most common ethical dilemma encountered by small animal veterinarians [6, 7]. In a study of small animal veterinarians, 57% reported that economic limitations of clients adversely affected their ability to provide the quality of care they would like at least once or multiple times per day [8]. In another report, many veterinarians cited financial limitations as the most common barrier to doing what they felt was right [9]. In another study of small animal veterinarians, euthanasia requests perceived to be based on a lack of financial means occurred with a median frequency of once a month, and euthanasia requests where the practitioner believed this decision was due to client unwillingness to pay for treatment occurred with a median frequency of a few times a year [6].

Consequences of Economic Limitations

The consequences of economic limitations for animals and veterinary professionals include a decrease in the number of visits to the veterinarian, delayed presentation to the veterinarian so the animal is seen when illness is more advanced, compromised patient care, economic euthanasia (where the cause of the animal's death is owner inability or unwillingness to afford care rather than a poor prognosis), and professional income limitations. Veterinarians have the desire and capacity to heal their patients, and to have that capability be repeatedly denied because of economic limitations is inevitably disheartening; 77% of small animal veterinarians reported that the economic limitations of clients were either a moderate or primary contributor to their burnout [8]. For caring practitioners, the moral stress (see Chapter 7) incurred by economic constraints may have debilitating consequences such as career disenchantment and premature transition out of clinical practice, demoralization, feelings of guilt, or desensitization to the plight of patients and blaming clients as an adaptive mechanism.

Morris [10] observed that small animal veterinarians negotiate with clients to evaluate their inclination to pay for needed care, and to avert economic euthanasia veterinarians bargain with animal owners for less costly treatment options. These types of discussions place the clinician in the role of financier rather than healer, a position that many are unprepared and disinclined to assume: "Negotiations that involve bargaining with owners over treatment costs to avoid euthanasia are particularly unsavory for most veterinarians" [10].

In veterinary practice, money is a common cause for client complaints [11, 12]. Frequent criticisms on websites that review hospitals include spending money on diagnostic testing when results are inconclusive or normal, or on treatments that are not successful. Veterinarians may feel the greatest burden when clients "invest" in animals that die. Some clients accuse the veterinarian of exploiting the patient for income, knowing the outcome would be poor. This can have a profoundly detrimental effect on a veterinarian's willingness to recommend costly and risky procedures that may benefit patients.

Another consequence of economic limitations is reluctance to refer patients based on perceived loss of income, with the specialist seen as competition for the finite revenues associated with each patient.

From a client's perspective, being denied access to the best care available for their animal over money may elicit feelings of guilt, resentment, and a negative perception of the veterinary profession as placing profits over patients. The reason most frequently cited among pet owners for leaving a practice was cost of care [13].

Despite many advances in the veterinary profession in the past few decades, on the issue of economic limitations little progress has been made. If no action is taken by the profession to change this, veterinarians are likely to hear the following statements from clients over the course of their careers:

- "If you only cared enough, you would do the work without profit" [14].
- "You're a veterinarian; you're supposed to love animals" [14].
- "You're going to let him die over $1000?"

Options for Addressing Economic Limitations

Most veterinarians report using the following methods to address economic limitations [3]:

- Offering a variety of treatment options.
- Payment options such as installment plans and credit services.
- Providing services for reduced fees or no charge.
- Other financial resources such as pet health insurance.

Veterinarians have always offered clients multiple options for care. Veterinarians must be aware of less expensive alternatives that are suitable for the patient even if they are not the ideal method of care. Some of the increasingly utilized financing options include independent credit services such as CareCredit® (http://CareCredit.com) or ScratchPay (http://scratchpay.com), hospital-administered extended payment plans, and accepting postdated checks [15].

The veterinary profession must consider difficult questions regarding its role in providing care for animals whose owners are in economic need. Should veterinarians be expected to offer discounted or free services? One report revealed that 59% of practitioners discounted services and products; most veterinarians who offered discounts did so from several times a month to several times a year [16]. The most common reason cited for discounting was to provide the best possible care for the animal. Veterinarians are not expected to be charitable, and practitioners deserve a reasonable income for their knowledge and services. Practice owners also have an interest in being profitable to ensure that their hospital can afford the equipment and trained staff to properly care for its patients; therefore, the practice is not obligated to divert its own resources at a financial loss to save patients.

When presented with an estimate for care many clients say "I can't afford that." Seldom do clients relate "I won't spend this much money on this animal." Should a veterinarian distinguish a client who is unwilling to pay from one who is unable to pay, and if so, how? Tannenbaum expands on this dilemma:

> Many people purchase goods and services for which they cannot pay in full at the time of purchase. Many clients who say ... that they "cannot afford" an alternative to euthanasia can afford it in the sense in which they would literally be able to pay for it if they made financial arrangements to do so. What they really mean is that they do not regard saving the animal to be worth the economic burden. [17]

Most veterinarians in one report agreed that pet owners should be required to supply verification of income before receiving veterinary care at a reduced fee or at no cost [3].

Offering for the hospital to subsidize patient care provides many benefits, including knowing that this aligns with our role as caretakers, improves the morale of the professional team, and should result in a high level of client satisfaction, with positive public relations for the practice. But this is not a viable long-term business strategy, as the need for economic relief for all patients far surpasses any hospital's capacity to perform pro bono work. What if the word gets out that your practice is the "place to go" for those who can't afford veterinary care? The ethical principle of justice suggests that if the hospital is willing to intervene in this way for one patient, then the hospital should do so for all patients who meet similar criteria. Is this expectation reasonable? If so, is this strategy sustainable? This option also does not address recurrence of vulnerability due to economic limitations for a future illness that the patient may incur.

As of 2022, almost 4.4 million pets in North America were insured [18]. Based on a conservative estimate of 145 million companion animals in the United States [19], the prevalence of insurance is about 3%. A study substantiates this, as 76% of small animal veterinarians estimated that less than 5% of their clients had pet health insurance [8].

Rollin asserts that compromising veterinary care due to economic limitations or performing economic euthanasia violates our social contract with companion animals and suggests that prospective pet owners be subject to screening: "The only solution to our ... moral irresponsibility toward animals is to regulate ... the acquisition ... of companion animals. They [potential animal owners] should demonstrate that they have the ... ability to care for an animal in a responsible fashion" [20]. Such regulations could mandate the acquisition of pet insurance or proof of economic means as a prerequisite for ownership. Most small animal veterinarians in one study opposed such measures [8].

Effects of Client Awareness of Veterinary Care Costs and Pet Health Insurance on Patient Care

Before a recommendation can be made regarding what veterinarians should do to mitigate economic limitations, the potential benefits associated with improved client education regarding future veterinary care costs and pet health insurance must be known. In a report examining these issues, most small animal veterinarians felt that increased client awareness of potential future veterinary care costs would have a positive effect on financial stress and money-saving behavior of clients, the veterinary–client relationship, and professional stress and job satisfaction [8]. Approximately three-quarters of practitioners believed that an increase in client awareness of potential future veterinary care costs would have a positive effect on their ability to provide the medical care they feel is in the best interest of their patients.

In the same study, most small animal veterinarians also believed that increased adoption of pet health insurance would have a positive effect on financial stress for clients, the veterinary–client relationship, economic euthanasia, professional stress and job satisfaction, and their ability to provide the desired medical care for their patients [8]. A recent study concluded that dog owners with pet health insurance spent significantly more money on veterinary visits [21]. A retrospective study of dogs with gastric dilatation-volvulus presenting to emergency clinics found that euthanasia decisions were primarily due to costs: only 10% of insured dogs were euthanized before surgery and non-insured dogs were seven times more likely to be euthanized [22].

These studies suggest significant benefits to all parties involved in the practice of veterinary medicine from greater awareness among owners of the costs of veterinary care and pet health insurance.

Discussion of Veterinary Care Costs and Pet Health Insurance

Discussion of veterinary care costs is fundamental to patient care, client satisfaction, and practice success [14]. Animal owners may be distrustful because of the tension they perceive between veterinary medicine as a healing profession as opposed to veterinary medicine as a business [23]; i.e. whether profitability is viewed as being ancillary to caring for animals or whether patients are viewed primarily as a means to being profitable. Communicating about the costs of veterinary care with emotional clients in a manner that will be perceived as caring can be challenging and is a source of anxiety for many veterinary professionals [23]. Morris concluded that veterinarians experience guilt regarding the costs of care and that "veterinarians often hate talking with clients about money" [10].

Results of a focus group indicated that pet owners are generally not satisfied with the extent of discussions regarding costs provided by small animal veterinarians [23]. Moreover, costs were discussed in only 42% of visits in which diagnostic testing was recommended. A more recent report found that only 23% of recorded veterinary visits included cost discussions [24]. Almost 75% of such discussions related to services being advised that day; only 14% of cost discussions related to future health concerns.

In accord with these findings, in another study only 31% and 23% of small animal veterinarians discussed potential future veterinary care costs and pet health insurance, respectively, with over half of their clients [8]. Reasons most frequently cited for not discussing these topics were lack of time and the belief that it would not change client behavior or financial preparation. Yet, most of these veterinarians believed that there should be an increase in efforts to improve client awareness and adoption of pet health insurance. In fact, a recent report concluded that providing pet owners information about the costs of disease can increase their willingness to purchase pet insurance [25].

It is difficult to reconcile the documented benefits associated with improved client education regarding potential future veterinary care costs and pet health insurance with the small proportion of veterinarians who routinely discuss these topics with their clients.

An Ethical Argument for Discussing Costs of Care with Clients

Neutering of small animal patients is customary in the United States and virtually all general practitioners address this topic with most of their clients [8], despite a recent report documenting that gonadal retention is associated with fewer health and behavioral problems and enhanced lifespan in dogs [26]. I will now offer an ethical argument for routinely discussing costs of care with clients.

Hypothetically, if veterinarians did not routinely perform gonadectomy in dogs and cats, it is estimated that 20–60% of these animals would develop mammary cancer or become ill from pyometra [27, 28]. These diseases typically affect older animals, and may be reversible with treatment or may be fatal. Based on the evidence presented in this chapter, it is reasonable to assume that at least 20% of all owned companion animals are subject to economic limitations to veterinary care. But unlike mammary cancer and pyometra, susceptibility to economic limitations is lifelong, affecting both young and old animals. Economic limitations to care may be reversible or may have fatal outcomes. While a strong case can be made that these two issues have comparable welfare impacts on companion animals, at this time veterinarians uniformly discuss neutering with clients and do not discuss economic preparation.

Who should conduct these conversations (see Case Study 8.2)? Veterinarians have a substantial influence on owners' decisions regarding their pets' care. In one study, the veterinarian was identified as the most vital source of knowledge regarding pet care by 70% of pet owners [29], and another report found that 65% of consumers purchased pet health insurance because a veterinarian advised it [30]. Rollin also contends that this task is uniquely suited to veterinarians:

> No animal should be denied life and health because of the owner's ... unwillingness to pay. The veterinarian should not be forced to bear the financial burden either. They [veterinarians] ought to be educating their clients and the ... public regarding ... pet ownership. If anyone can speak knowledgeably for the rights of pet animals, it is veterinarians. [20]

Case Study 8.2   Cost of Care Discussion

"Winston is a cute little guy, and I'm honored to be on your and Winston's healthcare team. We've discussed several important measures for ensuring that Winston lives a long, happy, and healthy life, including regular veterinary visits and vaccinations. If Winston gets sick, our profession can provide care comparable to human medicine, including access to specialists and 24-hour monitoring. A serious illness can cost thousands of dollars, whether at this hospital or another I may refer you to. I want to help you prepare for an illness or injury while Winston is young and healthy, by giving you some resources including information about health insurance (which I recommend), so that our decisions about Winston's medical care can be based primarily on what is best for Winston, and not so much on what things cost. Do you have any questions?"

Potential drawbacks of addressing this issue are that clients may perceive the veterinarian as mercenary; clients may be dissatisfied with insurance company policies over which the practitioner has little control; or the client may not comply or prepare.

If veterinarians believe in the value of neutering to prevent reproductive diseases and vaccinations to prevent infectious diseases, why would we not prioritize preventing the harmful impacts of economic limitations? If there was an infectious disease afflicting millions of our patients, there would be clamor within the profession for a vaccine. Veterinarians should view the issue of economic limitations to care with the same degree of concern as we would for a disease endangering animal health. Veterinarians hold proprietary knowledge about the costs of veterinary care that is unavailable to pet owners. It is time for a new paradigm in which general practitioners reliably provide their clients with information and options to help them prepare for the costs of veterinary care for their animal companions *before* they are ill. The potential benefits to animals, clients, and the profession outweigh an individual veterinarian's interest in avoiding difficult discussions. Efforts to alleviate client economic limitations would also be financially beneficial to veterinarians.

Establishing a Financial Assistance Policy

Despite a practitioner's best efforts to prevent economic limitations, they are still inevitable. Therefore, it is critical that all hospitals have a well-articulated, easily accessible financial assistance policy that everyone from the receptionists to the doctors understands and finds acceptable. A clear sequence of steps should be consistently followed to ensure that the funds are equitably and impartially administered based on previously identified criteria [15]. Having a policy in place is a better way of ensuring a consistent approach to financially limited clients, thereby averting the potential for unfairness in distributing limited economic resources [17]. Such policies make it clear that the practice acknowledges the importance of this problem, encourage management to be aware of available resources including rescue groups, and reduce the emotional burden on the veterinarian to decide who should receive assistance and via which sources.

Should Veterinarians Be the "Guardian of Their Client's Pocketbook"?

Given how often veterinarians encounter clients with economic limitations, it's reasonable to consider whether we should routinely endeavor to save our clients as much money as possible. One means of safeguarding client resources is by using a conservative diagnostic and treatment strategy. This can be accomplished by offering tests in an incremental fashion ("Let's start with a blood test today and go from there"), or via bypassing tests completely and conducting a therapeutic trial (see Chapter 22) in the hope that this will improve the animal's condition. Patients who would be best served by hospitalization may instead be treated as outpatients.

While one may contend that such a perspective is intended to benefit animal owners, these actions often are detrimental to positive outcomes for patients. By the time a veterinarian sees a patient, the extent of illness is frequently advanced due to delays in the client recognizing the signs of illness and because many clients hope that the identified problem will resolve without the need to see the veterinarian. Consequently, a tentative approach by the practitioner often delays diagnoses, prolongs patient suffering, and worsens patient prognosis. I have witnessed this countless times in my career. On some of these occasions, a colleague was quite surprised to find that a client assumed to be financially limited had spent thousands of dollars at my practice. This may reflect that the veterinarian's efforts to spare their client were unnecessary or that the decision to spend was due to the need for emergency care due to the decline in patient condition that occurred because of the conservative posture.

I experienced numerous examples of "financial protectionism," including a colleague who performed a splenectomy on a 14-year-old dog and kept the dog in their hospital overnight unobserved. No other options for postoperative care were noted in the medical record. In another case, a veterinarian dispensed steroid for a dog with a diagnosis of lymphoma without offering the client chemotherapy. The clients discovered that chemotherapy offered a better prognosis and independently pursued this at my practice. I recall seeing a febrile, painful small-breed dog referred at 7 p.m., who I diagnosed with bile peritonitis from a ruptured gall bladder mucocele. When I called the referring veterinarian to discuss the diagnosis and advise immediate surgery by a specialist surgeon at our 24-hour hospital, he replied, "Just send the dog back to me and I'll do the surgery here." When I noted that their hospital had already closed, he replied, "I'll have someone stay here all night to monitor."

In all these cases, these actions were defended by the veterinarian, citing saving the client money. Additionally, colleagues justified these actions because the patients did not die. Patients may survive *despite* rather than *because* of our efforts; survival is not synonymous with quality care.

Veterinarians are hired by humans, not by animals. Therefore, the veterinarian is dependent on the animal owner who pays for veterinary services. Consequently, a common practice philosophy is that profitability is commensurate with client satisfaction. In an ethnographic study of small animal veterinarians, Morris concluded that "Because animals are legally considered property and veterinarians depend on clients for income, veterinary medicine is more client oriented than patient oriented" [10]. Rather than attributing efforts to save clients money as being considerate of the supposed needs of animal owners, I believe a contributing factor to this behavior is the desire to be viewed favorably by clients, which is self-serving. Most practitioners understand there is often an inverse association between the cost of veterinary bills and client satisfaction. The Veterinarian's Oath does not instruct clinicians to conserve client resources. Instead, the Oath calls for "the protection of animal health and welfare" [31], which is frequently at odds with a practice philosophy emphasizing preservation of client monies.

Should Veterinarians' Recommendations Change Based on Presumed Client Capacity to Pay?

Veterinarians in practice are commonly compensated based on a proportion of their revenues [32]. Although such systems are purportedly intended to reward those who see many patients, they also create an incentive for veterinarians to advise costly testing, procedures, hospitalization, and surgery. Consequently, an implicit conflict of interest exists that may influence veterinary recommendations, contributing to unnecessary treatment [2]. It can be argued that because of the economic burdens faced by veterinarians, and since they are profoundly underpaid relative to physicians (simply compare the fees charged to human insurance companies by physicians), they are justified in exploiting clients with economic resources. For example, a veterinarian's awareness that a patient has insurance could lead to overuse of diagnostic tests or overtreatment [33]. Such behavior challenges the perception and role of the veterinarian as an animal advocate compared to a salesperson and abuses the trust that animal owners place in their veterinarian.

After sociological research in veterinary practices in the Netherlands, Swabe asserts: "The notion that profit may possibly influence veterinary decision-making ... conflicts strongly with the collective image of the ... animal doctor that we hold. In deciding the course of action to take, practical and financial considerations may well often outweigh sentiment and idealism" [34]. This conflict of interest is also perceived by clients, as 30% of pet owners agreed that veterinarians advise additional services to make money [13].

Veterinarians were found to routinely make judgments about their clients, including categorizing them as "good" or "bad" in terms of inclination to pursue treatments or pay the fees [35]. Therefore, if a veterinarian assumed that a client could not afford diagnostic testing or would not pay for it, testing may not be offered. A study corroborates this, finding that approximately a third of small animal veterinarians indicated that they do not offer ideal diagnostic or treatment options in the list of alternatives provided to all clients [8] (Case Study 8.3).

I worked with clinicians whose recommendations were strongly influenced by their presumption of the client's capacity to pay or by the client's previous patterns of spending. Clients driving expensive cars were more likely to be offered diagnostic evaluations, while those in budget brands were offered therapeutic trials. Clients with a track record of spending were often sent home with multiple medications, while those who declined counsel in the past were often given an inexpensive placebo. During my career I have been told by numerous colleagues that the justification for their medical recommendations included "I've got a house to pay for" and "I've got kids to send to college."

Main advocates for a consistent approach regardless of assumed client capacity to pay:

> Do veterinary surgeons need to worry about causing distress (in this case, guilt) to clients concerning the cost of treatments? Provide the information in such a way as to clearly explain the best option for the animal without coercing an approval from the client. The profession need not be reticent (or even embarrassed) in advocating expensive treatments provided they are truly in the best interests of the animal. Even if the best option happens to be the most profitable for the practice, and provided the client is not coerced into a decision, advocating the best is not abusing the trust that clients place in their veterinary surgeon. [36]

Case Study 8.3   Employer Request Not to Discuss MRI Scans

Mandy, a 12-year-old schnauzer, is presented to you for evaluation of recent onset grand mal seizures. The owner also reports that Mandy seems more disoriented and less alert. Physical examination is unremarkable. You discuss your concern and share that the most likely causes include metabolic diseases or a brain tumor. You advise lab work as an initial screen and discuss that if this is inconclusive, a brain tumor would be the most likely diagnosis and two options could be considered. An MRI scan of the brain is the best means to confirm a brain tumor. You inform the owner of the cost of the scan and the need for anesthesia, and that rationales for the MRI include that knowing the cause of the seizures may assist decision-making if Mandy's condition declines, and it facilitates surgery or radiation as definitive treatments if these are viable options, which may provide a longer lifespan compared to medications alone. Alternatively, symptomatic treatment for a presumed tumor can often be helpful without the MRI with a possibly shorter lifespan.

The next day your employer, Dr. B, calls you into his office. He relates that he received a call from Mandy's owner expressing concern that she cannot afford the MRI scan. He tells you that it is important to him that "our clients feel good when they leave our practice," and that as very few clients can afford an MRI scan, he prefers that you not offer this procedure to clients to mitigate any feelings of guilt or inadequacy.

Clients often complain about the costs of good veterinary care, and veterinarians are frequently put in a position of providing a lower level of care than they would prefer the animal to receive. In addition, clients sometimes do not take responsibility for their own financial decisions and criticize us for our inability to have achieved a positive outcome for the patient. Although these realities are frustrating, veterinarians cannot become so disheartened and "beaten down" that they no longer offer the best care to every client and patient. Attempting to judge a client's ability to pay veterinary fees is notoriously unreliable and discriminatory. Veterinarians should not attempt to presume a client's capacity to pay. While it can be uncomfortable to offer services and have clients decline them, this is a part of fulfilling our obligation to obtain informed consent (see Chapter 3). It is equally ethically problematic for veterinarians to take advantage of clients believed to have resources by advising unnecessary care. How should veterinarians find a balance between being sensitive to the fact that many clients may have trouble affording needed care for their animals, while simultaneously advocating for the best care for the animal?

What Should Veterinarians Do When a Client Acknowledges Inability to Pay?

It is common in veterinary practice for clients to express that they cannot afford the recommended care. Financial limits that pet owners place on veterinary care reflect their perception of the value of animals and economic realities. While most clients do not distinguish whether this represents an inability or an unwillingness to spend, the result is the same. Practitioners often either modify the plan for patient care if this is feasible or guide the client toward resources to assist, or to a euthanasia decision if the animal is suffering and no other recourse is viable.

Should veterinarians expect owners to provide veterinary care for their animals when they are ill? Burgess-Jackson contends that they should:

> human beings have special responsibilities to the animals they voluntarily bring into their lives – precisely because they bring them into their lives and create a dependent relationship. The act of bringing an animal into one's life ... generates a responsibility to care for its needs. If you believe that a parent is responsible for his or her children, then ... you should believe that humans are responsible for the animals they bring into their lives. [37]

But Coghlan notes differing societal expectations regarding the financial obligations of animal owners compared to human parents:

> it remains true that pediatricians enjoy *comparatively* more power over good patient health outcomes than do veterinarians ... this difference in authority is partly connected to the ... moral point: that society holds parental responsibilities to surpass client responsibilities to animal companions. For example, we might well expect parents to risk serious financial hardship ... to help their very ill children. [38]

If we look to the legal system, we find no clear answers. Not all state laws require that owners provide their animals with veterinary care. Even when they do, it is not clear what level of care is required. The duty to provide veterinary care, to the extent that it exists, can only be found in animal cruelty statutes [39]. The California Veterinary Medical Association's Eight Principles of Animal Welfare, Care, and Use address this responsibility, noting that "owners are responsible for ... timely and appropriate veterinary care" [40].

To pay for veterinary care, should clients be expected to forgo their own interests [41]? Patient advocacy may be less ethically justifiable to pursue when a client expresses that they are unable to pay or if it is determined that such costs would be detrimental to them or their families [38]. Do veterinarians as animal advocates have a duty to inform their clients in these situations that an integral responsibility of caring for their animals includes providing veterinary care? Tannenbaum [17] believes that the best way of challenging the attitude that a companion animal is not worth the economic sacrifice is to promote the view of the animal as a member of the family.

When encountering clients with acknowledged economic limitations, a clinician adhering to the Principle of Patient Advocacy should provide them with all available resources (referring to the practice's financial assistance policy) to avoid compromising patient care and economic euthanasia. Unfortunately, some clients may perceive this as coercive, confrontational, devoid of empathy, and inducing guilt. These circumstances can be challenging, requiring a resolute awareness of one's professional identity and excellent communication skills.

Rather than address the moral dimensions of a veterinarian's or client's duty to animals when faced with a client's acknowledged incapacity to afford care, spectrum of care adherents suggest that a veterinarian should simply accept these limitations and offer care that may reduce the likelihood of a favorable outcome within the sphere of informed consent: "A continuum of ... care that considers ... evidence-based medicine while remaining responsive to client expectations and financial limitations" [42]. I am very concerned that the spectrum of care philosophy may result in veterinarians feeling more at ease providing care that is not conducive to optimizing patient outcomes, thereby abandoning patient advocacy in lieu of client satisfaction and lowering acceptable standards of care.

Conclusion

Because money has a ubiquitous influence on access to veterinary care, practitioners should take the time to prepare their clients for the costs of veterinary care before patients are ill. All practices should have a protocol for dealing with financially limited clients (including multiple resources) that attempts to mitigate negative repercussions on patient care. Veterinarians are instructed by their oath to protect animal welfare, not client resources. This mandate does not include exploiting veterinary clients who are able to spend money. Clinicians should utilize a consistent approach to all clients and patients and should not attempt to presume client capacity to pay. When clients acknowledge financial limitations, veterinarians, as animal advocates, should work with clients to find a way to provide care without compromising patient outcomes prior to considering less optimal choices or euthanasia.

References

1 Animal Medical Center (n.d.). About us. https://www.amcny.org/meet-amc/about-us (accessed August 20, 2022).

2 Rosoff, P.M., Moga, J., Keene, B. et al. (2018). Resolving ethical dilemmas in a tertiary care veterinary specialty hospital: adaptation of the human clinical consultation committee model. *American Journal of Bioethics* 18 (2): 41–53.

3 Access to Veterinary Care Coalition and the Center for Applied Research and Evaluation (2018). *Access to Veterinary Care: Barriers, Current Practices, and Public Policy*. Knoxville: University of Tennessee https://pphe.utk.edu/wp-content/uploads/2020/09/avcc-report.pdf (accessed August 16, 2022).

4 American Animal Hospital Association (AAHA) (2017). New research from AAHA reveals changing pet owner perceptions of veterinary hospitals. https://www.aaha.org/publications/newstat/articles/2017-03/new-research-from-aaha-reveals-changing-pet-owner-perceptions-of-veterinary-hospitals (accessed August 16, 2022).

5 Park, R.M., Gruen, M.E., and Royal, K. (2021). Association between dog owner demographics and decision to seek veterinary care. *Veterinary Sciences* 8 (1): 7. https://doi.org/10.3390/vetsci8010007.

6 Kipperman, B., Morris, P., and Rollin, B. (2018). Ethical dilemmas encountered by small animal veterinarians: characterisation, responses, consequences and beliefs regarding euthanasia. *Veterinary Record* 182 (19): 548. https://doi.org/10.1136/vr.104619.

7 Quain, A., Mullan, S., McGreevy, P.D. et al. (2021). Frequency, stressfulness and type of ethically challenging situations encountered by veterinary team members during the COVID-19 pandemic. *Frontiers in Veterinary Science* 8: 647108. https://doi.org/10.3389/fvets.2021.647108.

8 Kipperman, B.S., Kass, P.H., and Rishniw, M. (2017). Factors that influence small animal veterinarians' opinions and actions regarding cost of care and effects of economic limitations on patient care and outcome and professional career satisfaction and burnout. *Journal of the American Veterinary Medical Association* 250 (7): 785–794.

9 Moses, L., Malowney, M.J., and Boyd, J.W. (2018). Ethical conflict and moral distress in veterinary practice: a survey of North American veterinarians. *Journal of Veterinary Internal Medicine* 32 (6): 2115–2122.

10 Morris, P. (2012). *Blue Juice: Euthanasia in Veterinary Medicine*. Philadelphia, PA: Temple University Press.

11 Bryce, A.R., Rossi, T.A., Tansey, C. et al. (2019). Effect of client complaints on small animal veterinary internists. *Journal of Small Animal Practice* 60 (3): 167–172.

12 Gordon, S.J.G., Gardner, D.H., Weston, J.F. et al. (2019). Quantitative and thematic analysis of complaints by clients against clinical veterinary practitioners in New Zealand. *New Zealand Veterinary Journal* 67 (3): 117–125.

13 Brown, B.R. (2018). The dimensions of pet-owner loyalty and the relationship with communication, trust, commitment and perceived value. *Veterinary Sciences* 5 (4): 95.

14 Bonvicini, K.A. (2009). Talking to clients about money. *Trends Magazine* 3: 61–66.

15 Kipperman, B., Block, G., and Forsgren, B. (2022). Economic issues. In: *Ethics in Veterinary Practice*, ch. 8 (ed. B. Kipperman and B.E. Rollin). Hoboken, NJ: Wiley-Blackwell.

16 Kogan, L.R., Stewart, S.M., Dowers, K.L. et al. (2015). Practices and beliefs of private practitioners surrounding discounted veterinary services and products. *Open Veterinary Science Journal* 9 (1): 1–9.

17 Tannenbaum, J. (1995). *Veterinary Ethics: Animal Welfare, Client Relations, Competition and Collegiality*, 2e. St. Louis, MO: Mosby Year Book.

18 North American Pet Health Insurance Association (NAPHIA) (2022). NAPHIA: State of the pet insurance industry in North America. https://naphia.org/about-the-industry (accessed August 16, 2022).

19 American Veterinary Medical Association (AVMA) (2017–2018). U.S. pet ownership and demographics sourcebook. https://www.avma.org/resources-tools/reports-statistics/us-pet-ownership-statistics (accessed August 16, 2022).

20 Rollin, B.E. (2006). *Animal Rights and Human Morality*, 3e. Amherst, NY: Prometheus Books.

21 Williams, A., Williams, B., Hansen, C.R. et al. (2020). The impact of pet health insurance on dog owners' spending for veterinary services. *Animals* 10 (7): 1162.

22 Boller, M., Nemanic, T.S., Anthonisz, J.D. et al. (2020). The effect of pet insurance on presurgical euthanasia of dogs with gastric dilatation-volvulus: a novel approach to quantifying economic euthanasia in veterinary emergency medicine. *Frontiers in Veterinary Science* 7: 590615. https://doi.org/10.3389/fvets.2020.590615.

23 Coe, J.B., Adams, C.L., and Bonnett, B.N. (2007). A focus group study of veterinarians' and pet owners' perceptions of the monetary aspects of veterinary care. *Journal of the American Veterinary Medical Association* 231 (10): 1510–1518.

24 Groves, C.N., Janke, N., Stroyev, A. et al. (2022). Discussion of cost continues to be uncommon in companion animal veterinary practice. *Journal of the American Veterinary Medical Association* 260 (14): 1844–1852.

25 Verteramo Chiu, L.J., Li, J., Lhermie, G. et al. (2021). Analysis of the demand for pet insurance among uninsured pet owners in the United States. *Veterinary Record* 189 (1): e243. https://doi.org/10.1002/vetr.243.

26 Zink, C., Delgado, M.M., and Stella, J.L. (2023). Vasectomy and ovary-sparing spay in dogs: comparison of health and behavior outcomes with gonadectomized and sexually intact dogs. *Journal of the American Veterinary Medical Association* 261 (3): 366–374.

27 Kustritz, M.V.R. (2007). Determining the optimal age for gonadectomy of dogs and cats. *Journal of the American Veterinary Medical Association* 231 (11): 1665–1675.

28 Howe, L.M. (2015). Current perspectives on the optimal age to spay/castrate dogs and cats. *Veterinary Medicine: Research and Reports* 6: 171–180.

29 Sprinkle, D. (2019). Competing in the omnichannel era: A customer perspective on veterinary services. United Veterinary Services Association Member Webinar, Abingdon, MD, June 12.

30 Williams, A., Coble, K.H., Williams, B. et al. (2016). Consumer preferences for pet health insurance. *2016 Annual Meeting, Southern Agricultural Economics Association*, San Antonio, TX, February 6–9. https://doi.org/10.22004/ag.econ.230144.

31 American Veterinary Medical Association (n.d.). Veterinarian's Oath. https://www.avma.org/KB/Policies/Pages/veterinarians-oath.aspx (accessed May 18, 2023).

32 Opperman, M. (2019). Pro on ProSal. *Today's Veterinary Business*, February/March. https://todaysveterinarybusiness.com/pro-on-prosal (accessed August 16, 2022).

33 Springer, S., Lund, T.B., Grimm, H. et al. (2022). Comparing veterinarians' attitudes to and the potential influence of pet health insurance in Austria, Denmark and the UK. *Veterinary Record* 190 (10): e1266. https://doi.org/10.1002/vetr.1266.

34 Swabe, J. (2000). Veterinary dilemmas: ambiguity and ambivalence in human–animal interaction. In: *Companion Animals and Us: Exploring the Relationships between People and Pets* (ed. A.L. Podberscek, E.S. Paul, and J.A. Serpell), 292–312. Cambridge: Cambridge University Press.

35 Morgan, C.A. (2009). Stepping up to the plate: animal welfare, veterinarians and ethical conflicts. PhD thesis, University of British Columbia, Vancouver, BC, Canada.

36 Main, D. (2006). Offering the best to patients: ethical issues associated with the provision of veterinary services. *Veterinary Record* 158 (2): 62–66.

37 Burgess-Jackson, K. (1998). Doing right by our animal companions. *Journal of Ethics* 2 (2): 159–185.

38 Coghlan, S. (2018). Strong patient advocacy and the fundamental ethical role of veterinarians. *Journal of Agricultural and Environmental Ethics* 31 (3): 349–367.

39 Hankin, S.J. (2005). What is the scope of the duty to provide medical care? Baltimore, MD: University of Maryland School of Law. https://digitalcommons.law.umaryland.edu/fac_pubs/920 (accessed August 11, 2023).

40 California Veterinary Medical Association (2023). The California Veterinary Medical Association's eight principles of animal welfare, care, and use. https://cvma.net/about-us/policies/the-california-veterinary-medical-associations-eight-principles-of-animal-care-use-and-welfare (accessed May 18, 2023).

41 Morgan, C.A. and McDonald, D. (2007). Ethical dilemmas in veterinary medicine. *Veterinary Clinics Small Animal* 37 (1): 165–179.

42 Fingland, R.B., Stone, L.R., Read, E.K. et al. (2021). Preparing veterinary students for excellence in general practice: building confidence and competence by focusing on spectrum of care. *Journal of the American Veterinary Medical Association* 259 (5): 463–470.

9

How to Optimize Patient Outcomes

Barry Kipperman

Abstract

This chapter introduces the Principle of Optimizing Patient Outcomes as the primary goal of the veterinary clinician in satisfying their role as patient advocate. The indications for when this principle should be applied are discussed. The nine rights for optimizing patient outcomes are introduced and considered using case examples. These include right client, right budget, right patient, right doctor competence, right doctor state of mind, right staff, right time of day and duration allotted for procedures, right equipment, and having a backup plan or Plan B.

Keywords: *optimizing patient outcomes, client, budget, competence, state of mind, staff, timing, equipment, nine rights, Plan B*

In Chapter 1, the Principle of Patient Advocacy was introduced as a philosophy of clinical practice as well as the ideal benchmark for assessing your success as a clinician. The main goal of the Principle of Patient Advocacy is to optimize patient outcomes. While veterinary clinicians can't control whether their patients live or die or flourish or fail to meet predetermined goals of therapeutic success, we can play a significant and influential role in ensuring we give our patients their best opportunity to succeed.

This chapter introduces the Principle of Optimizing Patient Outcomes, which should ideally be applied to all our patients. Let's consider when it's most imperative to do so. When I was an intern, I knew that I had little interest in performing surgery and even less aptitude. As a result, I requested that I not be placed on surgical rotations. My request was declined with little debate, as the opinions of interns don't carry much credibility, perhaps rightfully so. My memories of performing surgery during my internship are both amusing and painful. While on surgery service my peers were aware of my limited skills, so I usually drew the patient in need of the easiest procedure.

One day our service was very busy, and I was slated to perform a splenectomy on a stable, asymptomatic dog with a splenic mass. Having never done this, I was quite anxious. My supervising resident reassured me as he left to assist someone else, "Kippy, just ligate all the vessels, get that sucker out, and yell if you need me." I did as he requested, and within 40 minutes the spleen and the tumor attached to it were removed. While I likely took twice as long to do this as the resident (and lost buckets of sweat from nerves), the patient survived, and his outcome and postop pain levels were likely minimally different than had a more experienced surgeon performed the procedure.

The message is that applying the Principle of Optimizing Patient Outcomes is least imperative when the patient's condition is not serious and the consequences of being less competent or making errors are minimal. Most young dogs and cats undergoing routine gonadectomy don't require the best surgeon available, nor would inappropriate treatment of a urinary tract infection (UTI) likely result in a catastrophic patient outcome. While one could argue that an inexperienced surgeon may cause more tissue trauma or create a larger incision resulting in enhanced patient pain, or that delayed resolution of a UTI may cause prolonged pain and stress, these problems likely don't affect life and death or success or failure for patients. In fact, at some point we all must perform our first procedure on a patient to gain experience. Such experience ideally is gained under the supervision of a mentor with vast proficiency to ensure that the potential detrimental consequences of our inexperience are minimized.

Yet, for many new veterinarians such guidance is unavailable. This may be because no one else in the practice has the necessary experience to train you, the person with the knowledge is unwilling or unable to teach you, or the person with the expertise doesn't work on days you are at the practice. For all these reasons, less experienced veterinarians may feel compelled to perform procedures without the requisite knowledge or training. This is exacerbated if the veterinarian works in a practice where referrals to those with more experience are discouraged within the culture of the practice (see Chapter 7).

Consequently, I'm aware of novice veterinarians who taped the instructions for how to perform a hepatectomy (a high-risk surgery with bleeding as a prominent complication) from a textbook to the operating room wall, or who requested their technicians read them the instructions for the surgical procedure in the operating room. Such behavior clearly is not in accord with the Principle of Optimizing Patient Outcomes and we must therefore consider when such actions are inappropriate. Indications for applying the Principle of Optimizing Patient Outcomes are given in Table 9.1.

The Nine Rights for Optimizing Patient Outcomes

There are nine different factors clinicians should consider when applying the Principle of Optimizing Patient Outcomes. These nine "rights" are outlined in Table 9.2 and will be discussed individually with case examples.

Right Client

Virtually all patients recovering from procedures or receiving treatment require their caretakers to either observe for side effects or complications, modify the animal's activity and appetite, and/or administer medication(s). For example, the caregiver of a canine patient recovering from

Table 9.1 Indications for applying the Principle of Optimizing Patient Outcomes.

Consequences of poor decision may cause patient death

Consequences of poor decision may cause prolonged patient pain or suffering

Consequences of poor decision may cause client distress or increased costs

Consequences of poor decision may cause client complaint or malpractice claim

Consequences of poor decision may cause moral stress or burnout for team or clinician

Consequences of poor decision may cause disrepute for the profession

Table 9.2 The nine rights for optimizing patient outcomes.

Right client

Right budget

Right patient

Right doctor competence

Right doctor state of mind

Right staff

Right time of day and duration allotted for procedures

Right equipment

Right Plan B or backup plan

orthopedic surgery may be instructed not to allow their dog to walk up or down stairs or to run, as this may create complications such as fractured implants. Many prescriptions have contingencies in the instructions for when the medication should be discontinued. Some practitioners do not consider the importance of the capacity of the client (physical, emotional, and time) in optimizing patient outcomes (see Case Studies 9.1–9.2).

Case Study 9.1 Treating a Dog with Hyperadrenocorticism

You see Max, a geriatric male dachshund, for polyuria and polydipsia, polyphagia, and excessive panting. Lab testing reveals hyposthenuria and elevated alkaline phosphatase (ALP). You suspect hyperadrenocorticism and inform the client that another blood test is needed to confirm your suspicion of the cause. You impart an optimistic prognosis for resolution of Max's symptoms, noting that lifelong medication and serial monitoring will be necessary. Additional testing including an adrenocorticotropic hormone (ACTH) stimulation test and abdominal ultrasound confirm pituitary-dependent hyperadrenocorticism. You dispense mitotane and your written discharge instructions to the client are to stop medication immediately if Max's appetite declines or if he seems lethargic. Six days into treatment, a neighbor who was asked to walk Max at lunchtime brings him in in a collapsed state. Testing confirms iatrogenic hypoadrenocorticism from medication overdose. Max recovers after a brief hospital stay to receive intravenous (IV) fluids and steroid.

After this episode, you ask the client if she understood your instructions to closely monitor Max for reduced appetite. The client tells you that she works 12 hours a day at an office and there is no one to observe Max until she gets home at 8 p.m. She seems frustrated and tells you if she had known this might be a problem, she would have declined induction therapy with medication-induced risks.

Despite your best intentions, all clients may not remember your verbal instructions for care or may not read or understand your written instructions. While it's easy to blame the client in this circumstance, it was the veterinarian's obligation to evaluate the client's capacity to closely observe this patient prior to dispensing the medication. In fact, such a conversation should ideally have occurred *before* the second tier of diagnostics was performed. At that point, the client could have declined treatment as the disease is not fatal, planned for assistance in monitoring Max's appetite, or been informed of a treatment alternative that reduced this risk.

Case Study 9.2   Treating a Cat with Chronic Kidney Failure

You see Buster, a 12-year-old cat, for poor appetite, lethargy, and weight loss. Lab testing confirms moderate azotemia and dilute urine, consistent with a diagnosis of chronic kidney failure. You inform the client that Buster will need to be hospitalized for a few days to receive IV fluids to improve his condition. The client approves, and Buster begins eating as the azotemia subsides with treatment. On the day of discharge from the hospital, you inform the client that Buster will require lifelong, daily fluid administration under the skin to maintain a good quality of life. The client informs you that she is afraid of needles and will be unable to provide the recommended care. You are surprised by this and tell the client that she can arrange for a technician to come to her home, but this will incur an additional cost. The client now seems upset, telling you, "If I had known about this *before* the hospital stay was advised, I would have declined the hospitalization and its associated costs and requested euthanasia."

Based on your veterinary school training, the patients in Case Studies 9.1 and 9.2 had problems that were relatively easy to diagnose with reasonable prognoses with treatment. Consequently, as a patient advocate, you were eager to initiate testing and advise the client to pursue treatment. Yet, in both cases good intentions ended up with undesirable patient outcomes and unhappy clients. The concept of client caregiver burden associated with providing care for companion animals with protracted illness has been acknowledged [1] and can correlate with client euthanasia decisions [2] (Case Study 9.3). Explicitly assessing the client's capacity to provide appropriate care for your patients is imperative to satisfying the Principle of Optimizing Patient Outcomes. Ideally this should entail a dialogue directly with the client before any risky or costly intervention occurs.

Case Study 9.3   A Dog with Recurrent Seizures

You are seeing Lucy, a two-year-old border collie with recurrent, cluster seizures. The client and Lucy have incurred two hospitalizations for rescue treatment to abort seizures. You are treating Lucy with phenobarbital as an anticonvulsant. Your instructions to the client outline the common side effects of the medication and the need to seek emergency care if Lucy has three or more seizures in a 24-hour period. The instructions also suggest that the client bring Lucy to you for evaluation if any single seizure occurs. Two months later, Lucy is again brought into an emergency hospital for cluster seizures and the client requests euthanasia.

In this common example, the reason for Lucy's death was client emotional and financial exhaustion, rather than the seizures. The supervising veterinarian's treatment plan was too conservative and assumed that the client could tolerate the consequences of Lucy's recurrent seizures. Instead, the veterinarian should have taken a more aggressive posture that included therapeutic drug monitoring of blood levels of the phenobarbital every 2–4 weeks regardless of reported seizure activity, increasing the drug dose as needed to attain levels of $25-30\,\mu g/$ ml as rapidly as possible to reduce the probability of recurrent seizures. The veterinarian should have also evaluated the client's capacity to endure another hospitalization for Lucy. If this query suggested otherwise, then combination therapy with two medications might have been more likely to control the seizures and prevent Lucy's death.

Right Budget

In addition to selecting the right client, client budgets have a dramatic impact on patient outcomes and client satisfaction, as only about 2–3% of small animal patients in the United States are covered by health insurance [3]. Veterinarians in practice utilize a fee-for-service model of income. The practices are businesses, and clients of companion animals are typically expected to pay the balance of the fees when the patient leaves the hospital. When the costs of care are not accurately communicated to or understood by clients, problems may arise (Case Study 9.4).

It is an unfortunate reality that our clients' inability to afford the increasingly complex levels of veterinary care available profoundly limits viable options to help our patients [4]. While many veterinarians are aware of the costs of diagnostic tests and hospitalization, as these are expected to be accounted for in client estimates and consent forms, the cost of medications, especially those prescribed for outpatients, are more likely not to be included in the initial financial estimates given to clients by the veterinary team. Ideally, in Case Study 9.4 the cost of the mineralocorticoid monthly injection would have been included in the original estimate before hospitalization. This would have been more honest and transparent, reflecting the actual costs incurred by the client for Fifi's full recovery. In a recent report, 58% of owners of dogs with hypoadrenocorticism were worried about costs [5]. Fortunately, studies have documented efficacy of desoxycorticosterone pivalate at doses well below those recommended by the manufacturer, which can mitigate the costs of treating this disease [6].

When new medications are available to improve patient outcomes, these can often be quite expensive, as no generic form is available for years after the new drug comes to market. Even when the cost of medications is accounted for by clinicians, it may increase significantly due to supply chain disruptions, resulting in the need for unanticipated and unpleasant discussions with clients. Ensuring that your client can afford all the anticipated tests or treatments needed by providing comprehensive estimates and transparent communication is an imperative right to satisfy the Principle of Optimizing Patient Outcomes. Such conversations may then prompt the provision of resources for clients (see Chapter 8) or a change in plan, such as bypassing tests and emphasizing treatment, utilizing less expensive medications, or referral to a veterinarian who provides more economical services.

Case Study 9.4 Treating a Dog with Hypoadrenocorticism

You see Fifi, a young female Rottweiler, for progressive lethargy and vomiting. Lab testing reveals azotemia, hyponatremia, and hyperkalemia. You suspect hypoadrenocorticism and inform the client that another blood test is needed to confirm your suspicion of the cause of her symptoms. You impart a very optimistic prognosis for resolution of Fifi's illness, noting that lifelong medication and serial monitoring will be necessary. An ACTH stimulation test confirms hypoadrenocorticism. You advise hospitalization for treatment with IV fluids and steroid and inform the client that Fifi should feel dramatically better in about 36 hours. The client approves the estimate and Fifi improves and is ready to go home.

Your written discharge instructions to the client are to administer an oral steroid daily and to bring Fifi in tomorrow for a monthly injection that she will need for the rest of her life to have a normal quality of life and lifespan. At that time, Fifi receives the recommended dose of 2 mg/kg of desoxycorticosterone pivalate and the bill is $300. The client asks to speak to you and tells you she can't afford to spend almost $4000 annually for the rest of Fifi's life just on this medication. The client becomes emotional and requests euthanasia.

Right Patient

Perhaps the most obvious right to satisfy the Principle of Optimizing Patient Outcomes is selecting the right patient for the proposed treatment or intervention. Patient characteristics such as species, breed, size, condition, and age are most commonly considered by veterinary clinicians. For example, we wouldn't suggest high-dose aspirin in a cat, we would reduce the dose of vincristine in dog breeds with the *MDR1* mutation, we may discourage amputation to treat osteosarcoma in a giant-breed dog who is obese and therefore may have trouble ambulating on three limbs, we may bypass anesthetic hepatic biopsies in patients deemed unlikely to survive or live long enough to justify the procedure, and we may discourage pancreatectomy and choose medical management to treat insulinoma in a 15-year-old dog. In my experience, however, patient temperament (stress, fear, aggression) is too often overlooked in clinical decisions, with potentially detrimental outcomes for the quality of life of the patient and the owner (Case Studies 9.5–9.7).

Investigations have documented what common sense would indicate: that many (if not all) animals visiting veterinary hospitals experience stress [7, 8]. Recent awareness within the profession of this reality (prompted by a study documenting that cat owners were reluctant to bring their cats to veterinarians due to perceived stress [9]) has prompted multifaceted methods and approaches to address this problem [10]. Recognition of patient temperament by the clinician is as important to achieving optimized outcomes, as are more common concerns such as species, breed, and age.

Case Study 9.5   Giving Subcutaneous Fluids to a Cat with Chronic Kidney Failure

You see Buster, a 12-year-old cat, for poor appetite, lethargy, and weight loss. Lab testing confirms moderate azotemia and dilute urine, consistent with a diagnosis of chronic kidney failure. You inform the client that Buster will need to be hospitalized for a few days to receive IV fluids to improve his condition. The client approves, and Buster begins eating as the azotemia subsides with treatment. On the day of discharge from the hospital, you inform the client that Buster will require lifelong, daily fluid administration under the skin to maintain a good quality of life. The client informs you that Buster will likely not tolerate this, as he has tried to bite her when she attempted to trim his nails in the past. The client now seems upset, telling you, "If I had known about this before the hospital stay was advised, I would have declined the hospitalization and its associated costs."

Case Study 9.6   A Fearful Dog Needing Chemotherapy for Lymphoma

Yoda is a five-year-old female Yorkshire terrier diagnosed with high-grade lymphoma. You discuss the nature of this diagnosis and offer combination chemotherapy as the best means to achieve remission and prolong survival times. You have been taught that a multi-drug protocol requiring weekly visits to the hospital for chemotherapy injections for eight weeks, then tapering to every other week, provides the best outcome for patients with this type of cancer. The suggested protocol is approved.

Your technician observes that Yoda is hiding in the back of the cage and shivering prior to being handled to receive her first treatment. After the treatment, the technician informs you that it was difficult to administer the IV chemotherapy injection safely because Yoda was struggling. You are reluctant to address this with the client due to concern that this might reflect negatively on you or the practice, or they may stop the treatments, and this may lead to premature death for Yoda. After the third week of treatment, your technician calls and asks the client how Yoda is doing and is told that she wishes to stop chemotherapy, because Yoda has diarrhea for days after coming home from treatments and hides under the bed.

Yoda's temperament for tolerating frequent visits to the hospital should have been considered *before* a chemotherapy option was elected. Once Yoda's fearful nature was acknowledged by the owner and the clinician, alternate options could have been offered, including utilization of a chemotherapy protocol that minimizes trips to the hospital, and/or the administration of anxiolytics given at home prior to bringing Yoda to the hospital.

Case Study 9.7   Monitoring a Fearful Cat with Low-Grade Gastrointestinal Lymphoma

You see Theo, a 13-year-old female cat, who presented for chronic vomiting and weight loss, and who is diagnosed with low-grade lymphoma based on endoscopic biopsy results. The prognosis is good with lifelong medications and serial monitoring of body weight, appetite, and vomiting. Rechecks have been advised every four weeks for the first few months, to be tapered to every six weeks thereafter. During the first two rechecks, you are pleased to see that vomiting has resolved and Theo is gaining weight. You also notice that Theo struggles to escape when handled, but this is common in your feline patients. You congratulate the client for doing a great job administering the medications and observe that Theo is in clinical remission. After the first two rechecks, the client no longer keeps her scheduled appointments. Your technician calls and is told that the rechecks are too stressful for Theo, especially when the client perceives that she's doing so well.

Ideally, once the clinician recognized signs of Theo's stress during the rechecks, options to mitigate this should have been offered, including anxiolytic medications prior to visits or the use of telemedicine to perform the rechecks from home. The author has commonly utilized telephone rechecks in these cases: owners are requested to purchase a cat scale, so they are empowered to weigh their cats regularly and report body weights. These owners are also informed to schedule an in-person visit any time weight loss is documented.

Right Doctor Competence

As discussed in the introduction to this chapter, self-evaluation of clinician competence should be commensurate with the factors outlined in Table 9.1. That is, the more serious the patient's condition or the consequences of an error or inexperience in conducting an intervention, the more imperative it is to ensure proficiency in the required procedure before it is performed. In these patients, the question that should be asked is not "Can I probably do this?" but "Am I the most qualified person available to do this?" (see Chapter 7 on referrals).

Numerous considerations may influence such decisions:

- Objectively evaluating our own competence may be intrinsically difficult, if not impossible [11], and may be affected by other factors such as ego and financial gain from doing the procedure.
- The fact that the likelihood of an animal owner discovering that another colleague was better suited to perform the procedure is small given that most animal owners are not aware of the existence of veterinary specialists.

- More qualified colleagues may be unavailable in the time frame needed or may be inaccessible due to distance.
- As animals are legal property and fair market value for most animals is negligible, and non-economic damages for injuries or malpractice are not recognized by the US legal system, veterinarians have minimal legal or economic concerns regarding negative patient outcomes due to incompetence.
- Veterinarians are loath to report a colleague for malpractice or negligence. While the American Veterinary Medical Association Principles of Veterinary Medical Ethics provide a framework for self-regulation, the translation of this principle into a meaningful vehicle for professional accountability leaves much to be desired.

While all these factors might lead a clinician to overestimate their competence and subsequently violate the Principle of Optimizing Patient Outcomes, let's look at considerations that might prevent you from misjudging your ability and "getting in over your head." First, if an anesthetic, painful, or costly procedure is being contemplated, clients are understandably reluctant to repeat such procedures on their animals. It's one thing to ask a client to return a patient for a repeat blood draw because the complete blood count could not be run due to a blood clot; it's quite another to request a second spinal tap or surgery or explain to clients why a repeat ultrasound procedure by a radiologist is necessary after their primary care veterinarian performed one. Second, adverse patient outcomes have been reported to affect clinicians emotionally [12].

Self-evaluation of one's competence is a critical right to satisfy the Principle of Optimizing Patient Outcomes.

Right Doctor State of Mind

While one may have determined that the right client, budget, patient, and professional competence have been established, another important consideration is clinician state of mind. For example, you may receive emotionally upsetting news such as a phone call regarding the death or critical condition of a family member. You may be distraught after recognizing an error has occurred that caused harm to your patient (see Chapter 10), or you may have euthanized a beloved animal companion earlier that day.

Performing procedures on one's own animal is also a likely recipe for a distracted clinician. I recall performing a rhinoscopy on my dog and forgetting to remove the gauze sponges I placed in the back of his throat to reduce the inhalation of water. Fortunately, my technician reminded me before recovery from anesthesia. It seems logical to presume that when working on your own animal, you would be so concerned with survival-related factors such as anesthesia and vital signs that this would distract you from performing the procedure correctly. In the legal profession, this analogy is reflected by the common motto that "A person who is their own lawyer has a fool for a client."

Another common cause of clinician distraction is work-related stress. Several studies have evaluated the prevalence of occupational stress among veterinarians. A recent investigation noted that 50% of veterinarians had high burnout scores [13]. A study of small animal veterinarians found that 49% reported a moderate to substantial level of burnout [4]. Another report found that when North American veterinarians were asked "How often have you felt distressed or anxious about your work?" 52% responded "often" or "always" [14].

One of the most common stressors is perceiving there is too much to do and too little time to do it [15]. This often relates to having too many procedures scheduled on the same day, or because emergencies added procedures to the schedule. Feeling stressed and perceiving that you need to rush through procedures to get them all done is likely a common cause of procedural error and negative patient outcomes [16]. In my experience, trying to rush through diagnostic endoscopy procedures resulted in iatrogenic intestinal perforations in patients on more than one occasion. Of course, dealing with rectifying and communicating about these negative outcomes only worsened my stressed state.

Another cause of clinician impairment is sleep deprivation. For much of my career I was on call for emergency endoscopies and ultrasounds, and surgeons are commonly on call and are expected to come in after hours to perform select procedures. I can attest that despite downing numerous chocolate Frappuccinos to allay my weary state, inadequate sleep affected my capacity to provide optimal care. A recent study of house officers at nine veterinary teaching hospitals discovered that most of them worked 11–13 hours on a typical day and work hours were inversely related to sleep quantity [17]. The majority of house officers felt that fatigue negatively affected their technical skills and clinical judgment. The authors concluded that most house officers failed to obtain sufficient sleep for optimal cognitive function and physical and mental health. Many colleagues view working through sleep deprivation as a source of pride or as something to boast about, as if this demonstrates an extraordinary commitment to patients. In fact, this is a risk factor for our patients. This archaic perspective should end.

Ideally, a clinician would recognize when their state of mind is not conducive to adequately performing a scheduled procedure and, if possible, either delegate it to a colleague or postpone it to later in the day or to an alternate day. Unfortunately, there are strong forces that will be discussed later in this chapter that render this a difficult, and therefore uncommon, posture.

Right Staff

Clinicians should recognize the importance of collaborating with the right paraprofessional staff to optimize patient outcomes. Paraprofessionals in many practices are responsible for performing most of the diagnostic and some therapeutic patient procedures. For many routine practices such as obtaining blood or urine, the level of expertise required is low, and patient care is unlikely to be compromised based on who is performing the procedure. Placement of IV catheters and taking radiographs require more experience, and the selection of which team members complete these tasks could influence patient outcomes, especially if the patient's condition is critical and time sensitive (shock, dyspnea). In many practices, proficiency in performance of advanced procedures such as chemotherapy injections, CT scans, endoscopy, etc. is often limited to one to two highly trained team members. In addition to individual capabilities, most procedures performed on animals require more than one technician for a portion of or the entire procedure, due to the need to properly restrain the patient, monitor them, or assist.

What happens, then, when one of these procedures is necessary for a patient, and the proficient team member(s) or enough technicians are unavailable, either because they are out sick, it's their scheduled day off from work, they are on vacation, or the practice is understaffed relative to patient needs? I can recall a Saturday when I diagnosed a patient with lymphoma and the degree of lymph node enlargement was so severe that the dog had marked stridor and trouble breathing. The weekend team were not trained in safely administering IV chemotherapy injections. I considered the available options, including postponing chemotherapy until Monday (understanding the patient may die or be euthanized if breathing difficulties worsened), referring the patient elsewhere (I surmised that other referral practices probably did not routinely perform chemotherapy on weekends), calling in the experienced technician (and interrupting their personal time and paying overtime costs), or proceed with the treatment and increase the risk of local extravasation or drug error.

I decided to proceed with treatment and took extra time to provide written and verbal resources to my lead shift technician on duty, who volunteered to assist even though she was inexperienced with this task. Despite these measures and double-checking the dose before treatment, the patient jumped during the injection and extravasation of a caustic medication occurred. This was the only time in my career that one of my patients with cancer suffered significant local trauma from an extravasation. I still regret that decision to this day.

While cross-training of team members is ideal to mitigate being put in the position of performing a procedure with inadequately trained staff, such issues arise in practice more often than is documented or discussed. Consideration of the nature of the anticipated procedure, the availability of qualified personnel in proper numbers to assist you with the procedure, and the potential risks of proceeding with less qualified or insufficient staff are pivotal to satisfying the Principle of Optimizing Patient Outcomes.

Right Time of Day and Duration Allotted for Procedures

At most veterinary practices scheduled appointments are seen in the morning, patients are admitted to the hospital as warranted, and diagnostic and therapeutic procedures and surgeries are performed in the afternoon. In general practices that close at 6 p.m., there is an expectation among clients as well as within the culture of most practices that these patients will be sent home prior to closing time. This reality must be accounted for by veterinary clinicians as they plan the sequence of afternoon procedures to optimize patient outcomes.

It seems logical that patients that will need longer times to recover from anesthesia (i.e. older or debilitated patients) or high-risk patients (thoracotomy) would be scheduled earlier in the day compared with younger patients recovering from sedation or anesthesia. Another argument for proceeding with the most difficult procedures or high-risk patients first is that the clinician's state of mind may be poorer the later in the day a procedure is begun due to exhaustion. Patients who do not need to recover from anesthesia or a painful event might be scheduled last.

In my experience, scheduling of procedures is often influenced by many other factors, including client demands and expectations, clinician preferences, and staff schedules. In many cases, it's difficult to understand the rationale for the sequence of scheduled procedures. While clinicians working in 24-hour practices have the capacity to keep patients in the hospital overnight or until later in the evening, they are still subject to satisfying client expectations (Case Study 9.8).

Case Study 9.8   To Proceed with or Postpone an Elective Endoscopy

You are an internist working in a 24-hour referral practice. You have multiple procedures to perform this afternoon, and you considered all the factors noted in this chapter in ensuring the right sequence has been chosen. You are scheduled to begin a brief, elective, diagnostic endoscopy procedure with biopsies on a stable patient at 4 p.m. An emergency arises that you must attend to, and it is now 5 p.m. before you are able to consider starting the procedure. While you are willing to do this, there are numerous consequences to this decision: (i) your endoscopy technician leaves work at 6 p.m. or will incur overtime costs; (ii) you need to be available at 6 p.m. for patient rounds, where your patients are transferred to the overnight doctor; (iii) you promised the client that the patient would be sent home between 6 and 7 p.m., which would not be feasible if you proceed; and (iv) the prospect of these concerns may cause you to experience stress, which may increase patient risk from the procedure. What should you do?

In addition to selecting the proper time of day to begin patient procedures, an equally important component of optimizing patient outcomes relates to anticipating the right duration for each procedure to be performed (Case Studies 9.9 and 9.10). While scheduling ample time by, for instance, adding 30 minutes beyond the anticipated duration for each procedure would be ideal, this luxury often cannot be afforded in clinical practice, as it reduces the number of procedures that can be performed. In fact, the number of patient procedures is far more likely to increase at the last minute on a given day due to unexpected arrivals, emergencies, etc. When this happens, the clinician must make difficult decisions, including:

- Do I cancel less urgent procedures and postpone them to another day?
- Can I fit all the procedures in by working more quickly?
- If I work more quickly, am I able to complete the procedures properly?

In Case Studies 9.9 and 9.10, the surgeon should never have begun an elective major surgery so near to closing time without calling the client beforehand to discuss the potential ramifications, and should have understood that there would be client- and patient-related problems from the decision to proceed without informed consent.

Case Study 9.9   Postoperative Referral after Elective Nephrectomy

You are a general practitioner in a busy practice that closes at 6 p.m. You have multiple procedures to perform in the afternoon, including two gonadectomies of healthy animals, two ultrasounds, a splenectomy, and a nephrectomy for a stable dog with a unilateral renal mass. You begin the last procedure, the nephrectomy, at 4:45 p.m., and you and your team stay late to complete the surgery, which ends at 6:30 p.m. You inform the pet owner that the surgery went well and that you and your team stayed late to complete the procedure. You refer the patient to a local 24-hour emergency practice for overnight care and monitoring (see Case Study 9.10) without discussing the need for additional costs for this service. What were your alternatives to proceeding with the procedure? Can this decision be justified?

Case Study 9.10   Postoperative Care for a Nephrectomy Patient

You are an intern working at a 24-hour emergency practice. At 6:45 p.m., Holly, a 12-year-old Boston terrier, arrives on a gurney after a nephrectomy procedure. She is intubated with an endotracheal tube and is unconscious. You determine that vital signs are stable and instruct your team to closely monitor Holly while you talk with the client. The client asks when Holly can come home, as their regular veterinarian promised she'd be discharged shortly after the surgery. You feel "caught in the middle" and refer to Holly's medical record for guidance regarding client postoperative expectations. None is documented. You inform the client that Holly is unconscious and will need time to safely recover from anesthesia, and that you cannot promise what time frame this may require. The client seems displeased, and their demeanor worsens after you provide a $500 estimate for postoperative care and analgesics.

Should the surgeon have called the emergency practice to alert them to the transfer of care? Was this all that was needed, or was a discussion with the emergency doctor warranted to discuss client expectations? Should the surgeon or the client be expected to incur the unforeseen costs for ongoing monitoring? How should the intern navigate these concerns?

Allotting the proper duration for a procedure must incorporate not only the clinician's expertise (it's difficult to assess the right duration when you are inexperienced or rarely perform the task), but potentially unanticipated patient-related factors (i.e. not complying with handling or IV catheter placement, aggressive behaviors requiring sedation), emergencies, and staff-related factors (scheduled lunch hours and breaks, need to train staff that prolongs procedure time).

Scheduling procedures for the right patient, with the right doctor and staff, at the right time and having allotted the right duration are pivotal to satisfying the Principle of Optimizing Patient Outcomes.

Right Equipment

When scheduling patient procedures, it is inevitable that you may discover while your patient is in the hospital that the equipment you rely on to complete the procedure is not or may not be available or is not functioning properly. In some situations, such as learning that all the suitable surgical packs were not sterilized and cannot be used, or a certain type of collection tube or medication is not available, you may be able to readily solve these problems with the cooperation of a local colleague who can loan you the materials. What if your technician who screens equipment function before all procedures are started informs you that the x-ray machine or light source for the endoscope is working intermittently, and therefore may not work reliably when your patient is under anesthesia? In other cases, you may discover that the x-ray machine fails only after your patient is anesthetized. This is, of course, the worst-case scenario for the clinician and the patient.

When clinician concerns about satisfying rights five to eight (right doctor state of mind, right staff, right time of day and duration allotted, and right equipment) arise, two options are available:

- *Proceed and hope that the impacts on your patient and client will be minimal.*
  The advantages of continuing with the proposed plan are that you may be able to successfully accomplish the task and not have to confront and disappoint a client. Potential problems with forging ahead could include patient morbidity or mortality, inadequate diagnosis or treatment, need to repeat the procedure, moral stress for clinician and staff, client complaints or increased costs, and loss of respect by team members. I have seen many incomplete upper gastrointestinal (GI) series and nasal radiographs that were non-diagnostic and quite costly for clients, and numerous other poorly performed procedures that compromised patient outcomes and client emotional states because of "forging ahead."
- *Postpone or reschedule the procedure.*
  The advantages of delaying or rescheduling select procedures are peace of mind that you are optimizing patient outcomes and reduced stress levels for you and your staff. Drawbacks are primarily related to client communication and potential embarrassment at disclosing the truth. Having been in this position many times in my career, I can attest that clients are apt to express their disappointment. While honesty is an inherent aspect of ethical behavior, it is not necessary to tell your client that "I forgot today is Susan's day off" or "We forgot to sterilize the pack." While honesty is usually laudable, in these circumstances overt honesty is not apt to change the plan, is likely to discredit you, your practice, and the profession, and will probably exacerbate the client's unhappiness with the decision to postpone or reschedule.

In these situations, I suggest calling the client and explain that unanticipated circumstances arose that were beyond your control, and that you believe that delaying the procedure is in their animal's best interest. While clients often complain that they are being inconvenienced and that their companion missed a meal while fasting, remind them that "Unlike a blood test, we only want to do this procedure once and I want to ensure that (animal name) has the best chance of a successful outcome." Most clients will understand if the cause of the postponement is related to patient emergencies that disrupted your schedule, and many have told me, "Of course, if my animal had an emergency, I'd want her care to be prioritized."

In summary, postponing select procedures is sometimes required to fulfill your role as patient advocate by following the Principle of Optimizing Patient Outcomes.

Right Plan B or Backup Plan

Another fundamental requirement to optimize patient outcomes is always to have a Plan B or a backup plan. This means planning for the potential outcomes of any procedure *before* it is begun and preparing to institute measures to address each outcome. Instituting a Plan B is relevant in the exam room when we discuss medical issues and provide estimates to clients, as well in the treatment or operating room. Let's examine the concept of having a Plan B in Case Studies 9.11–9.13.

Case Study 9.11 Exploratory Surgery for a Vomiting Dog

You see Bella, a two-year-old Labrador retriever, for vomiting and weight loss of three weeks' duration. Based on testing completed, you are highly suspicious of an intestinal foreign body as the cause. You advise exploratory abdominal surgery, which is approved. During the laparotomy, you find no evidence of a foreign object and end the procedure. A few days later, you call the local internal medicine specialist requesting that Bella have an endoscopy to obtain intestinal biopsies.

Had you planned for the contingency that a foreign body might not be discovered before the surgery was begun and used your differential diagnosis list as a guide, you could then have discussed with the client, received approval for, and instituted Plan B, which would have included obtaining intestinal biopsies during the surgery to diagnose inflammatory bowel disease. The consequences for not planning included increased costs for Bella's owner, another anesthetic procedure for Bella, further delay in attaining a diagnosis and beginning a treatment plan, and possibly a poorer prognosis if Bella loses more weight. Finally, if the client somehow becomes aware that the endoscopy could have been averted with proper planning, there could be consequences for the primary clinician.

Case Study 9.12 A Cat with Chronic Vomiting (No Plan B)

You see Blackie, a 12-year-old cat, for chronic vomiting and significant weight loss. Lab testing and radiographs are inconclusive. You advise an abdominal ultrasound to help determine the cause. An intestinal mass is discovered, at which time you call the client to inform them and to request ultrasound-guided aspirates to identify the tumor type. You provide an estimate for the fees for this procedure. The client becomes very upset with the news that Blackie has cancer and is unable to approve the unexpected procedure due to her emotional state and need to discern if she can afford the costs for sedation, the aspirates, and the pathology report. She asks if she can call you back in a few hours, which postpones the procedure for at least another day.

While the veterinarian in this case pursued the proper means for diagnosis and provided the correct advice considering the ultrasound results, the client was unprepared for the news, and this resulted in the need to postpone the aspirate procedure, resulting in frustration for the veterinarian, significant distress for the client, and delay in diagnosis for the patient.

The veterinarian should have discussed with the client before the ultrasound that based on the differential diagnosis list, the two most likely findings would be intestinal cancer or intestinal inflammation. Discussion regarding the most suitable plan for each outcome and their associated costs and prognoses should have been provided (see Figure 3.1). This advanced notice and estimates for the care would have improved the chances that the owner approved the aspirates and would have mitigated the need to call after the ultrasound study.

Case Study 9.13   A Cat with Chronic Vomiting (Including Plan B)

You see Blackie, a 12-year-old cat, for chronic vomiting and significant weight loss. Lab testing and radiographs were inconclusive. In the exam room, you discuss that the two most likely causes for these symptoms are intestinal cancer or intestinal inflammation. You suggest an abdominal ultrasound to help determine the cause. If a mass is discovered, you advise sedation and ultrasound-guided aspirates to determine the tumor type and prognosis. If no mass is discovered, you advise anesthesia for endoscopic biopsies and placement of a short-term feeding tube for nutritional support, with a good prognosis with lifelong medication and serial evaluations. You provide two separate estimates for these potential outcomes, and the client approves both. Blackie is admitted to the hospital.

In this scenario, the clinician adhered to the concept of having a Plan B, which facilitated client understanding and approval, and expedited the medical care needed. In addition, planning reminded the clinician that nutritional support would also be beneficial as a bridge between recovery from anesthesia for the endoscopy and onset of action of the prescribed medication. This planning created a win–win–win scenario for clinician, client, and patient.

Learning and applying the nine rights for satisfying the Principle of Optimizing Patient Outcomes are pivotal to guide the veterinary clinician in satisfying their role as patient advocate.

References

1 Spitznagel, M.B., Jacobson, D.M., Cox, M.D. et al. (2017). Caregiver burden in owners of a sick companion animal: a cross-sectional observational study. *Veterinary Record* 181 (12): 321.

2 Spitznagel, M.B., Marchitelli, B., Gardner, M. et al. (2020). Euthanasia from the veterinary client's perspective. *Veterinary Clinics Small Animal Practice* 50 (3): 591–605.

3 North American Pet Health Insurance Association (NAPHIA) (2022). State of the pet insurance industry in North America. https://naphia.org/about-the-industry (accessed August 16, 2022)

4 Kipperman, B.S., Kass, P.H., and Rishniw, M. (2017). Factors that influence small animal veterinarians' opinions and actions regarding cost of care and effects of economic limitations on patient care and outcome and professional career satisfaction and burnout. *Journal of the American Veterinary Medical Association* 250 (7): 785–794.

5 Hupfeld, J., Dölle, M., Volk, H. et al. (2022). Effect of long-term management of hypoadrenocorticism on the quality of life of affected dogs and their owners. *Veterinary Record* 191 (1): e1977.

6 Sieber-Ruckstuhl, N.S., Reusch, C.E., Hofer-Inteeworn, N. et al. (2019). Evaluation of a low-dose desoxycorticosterone pivalate treatment protocol for long-term management of dogs with primary hypoadrenocorticism. *Journal of Veterinary Internal Medicine* 33 (3): 1266–1271.

7 Quimby, J.M., Smith, M.L., and Lunn, K.F. (2011). Evaluation of the effects of hospital visit stress on physiologic parameters in the cat. *Journal of Feline Medicine and Surgery* 13 (10): 733–737.

8 Bragg, R.F., Bennett, J.S., Cummings, A. et al. (2015). Evaluation of the effects of hospital visit stress on physiologic variables in dogs. *Journal of the American Veterinary Medical Association* 246 (2): 212–215.

9 Volk, J.O., Felsted, K.E., Thomas, J.G. et al. (2011). Executive summary of the Bayer veterinary care usage study. *Journal of the American Veterinary Medical Association* 238 (10): 1275–1282.

10 Riemer, S., Heritier, C., Windschnurer, I. et al. (2021). A review on mitigating fear and aggression in dogs and cats in a veterinary setting. *Animals* 11 (1): 158.

11 Carter, T.J. and Dunning, D. (2008). Faulty self-assessment: why evaluating one's own competence is an intrinsically difficult task. *Social and Personality Psychology Compass* 2 (1): 346–360.

12 Kogan, L.R., Rishniw, M., Hellyer, P.W. et al. (2018). Veterinarians' experiences with near misses and adverse events. *Journal of the American Veterinary Medical Association* 252 (5): 586–595.

13 Ouedraogo, F.B., Lefebvre, S.L., Hansen, C.R. et al. (2021). Compassion satisfaction, burnout, and secondary traumatic stress among full-time veterinarians in the United States (2016–2018). *Journal of the American Veterinary Medical Association* 258 (11): 1259–1270.

14 Moses, L., Malowney, M.J., and Boyd, J.W. (2018). Ethical conflict and moral distress in veterinary practice: a survey of North American veterinarians. *Journal of Veterinary Internal Medicine* 32 (6): 2115–2122.

15 Ashton-James, C.E. and McNeilage, A.G. (2022). A mixed methods investigation of stress and wellbeing factors contributing to burnout and job satisfaction in a specialist small animal hospital. *Frontiers in Veterinary Science* 9: 942778. https://doi.org/10.3389/fvets.2022.942778.

16 Oxtoby, C., Ferguson, E., White, K. et al. (2015). We need to talk about error: causes and types of error in veterinary practice. *Veterinary Record* 177 (17): 438.

17 Scharf, V.F., McPhetridge, J.B., and Dickson, R. (2022). Sleep patterns, fatigue, and working hours among veterinary house officers: a cross-sectional survey study. *Journal of the American Veterinary Medical Association* 260 (11): 1377–1385.

10

Medical Errors

Barry Kipperman and Jim Clark

Abstract

Human beings are imperfect, so medical errors in veterinary practice are inevitable. This chapter discusses the different types of events related to patient safety, the challenges distinguishing a medical error from an adverse event or complication, the frequency, most common causes, and consequences of errors, and how a practice should respond to errors. It also provides discrete strategies for mitigating errors and disclosing errors and bad news to clients. Ethical concerns regarding disclosure are addressed. Every veterinary practice should develop policies and procedures for responding to medical errors that can guide decision-making in the face of these unfortunate events.

Keywords: *medical error, error, adverse event, complication, ethics, communication, reporting, lying*

While the dictum "first, do no harm" is commonly attributed to the Hippocratic Oath, literal translations find no statement to this effect. As virtually every intervention proposed by veterinarians – be this a medication, procedure, anesthetic event, or surgery – carries risk, if veterinarians were to abide by such a statement, we could only help our patients by offering their owners emotional support, hope, and consolation. Shmerling proposes a more realistic interpretation: "Doctors should help their patients as much as they can by recommending tests or treatments for which the potential benefits outweigh the risks of harm" [1]. These principles were discussed in the chapters on informed consent (Chapter 3) and managing risks (Chapter 4). Another interpretation of this saying could be to mitigate *preventable harms* that are within the control of the clinician, staff, or practice (some are discussed in Chapter 9). Despite good intentions, human beings are imperfect, therefore every person who works in veterinary practice will occasionally make mistakes. Unfortunately, some of these mistakes can and do harm our patients.

Definitions

Several terms have been used to describe conditions related to patient safety, which are summarized in Tables 10.1 and 10.2.

Table 10.1 Definitions of types of events related to patient safety.

Term	Definition
Near miss	An incident that could have had adverse consequences but did not reach the patient
Harmless hit	An error that reached the patient but did not cause harm
Medical complication	An unfavorable evolution of a disease, condition, or therapy
Adverse event/ outcome	Unanticipated harm caused by the medical treatment rather than the disease process itself
Medical error	An action or omission with potentially negative consequences for the patient that would have been judged wrong by peers at the time it occurred, independent of whether there were negative consequences [2]

Source: Adapted from [3].

Table 10.2 Circumstances associated with different types of events related to patient safety.

Term	Reached patient?	Harmed patient?	Team member(s) and/or system at fault?
Near miss	No	No	Yes
Harmless hit	Yes	No	Yes
Medical complication	Yes	Yes	Yes or no
Adverse event/outcome	Yes	Yes	Yes or no
Medical error	Yes	Yes or no	Yes

Case Study 10.1 demonstrates different types of patient safety events.

Case Study 10.1   Patient Safety Events in a German Shepherd with Osteosarcoma

After developing lameness in his right front limb, Prince, a nine-year-old neutered male German shepherd dog, was diagnosed via radiographs and a bone biopsy with osteosarcoma, an aggressive and painful bone cancer. After consulting with their veterinarian, the clients elected amputation of Prince's diseased limb followed by chemotherapy. The following are patient safety events that might have occurred in this case.

- *Near miss*: Not realizing that two German shepherd dogs with similar appearances were in the hospital, and failing to check the cage card, a technician anesthetized Champ rather than Prince for surgery. She clipped the hair from the right front leg and prepared the limb for surgical removal. Before Champ was transferred into the operating room, a kennel worker noticed the error and the procedure was aborted.
- *Harmless hit*: Prior to his surgery, Prince was scheduled to receive an analgesic injection. Due to a miscalculation, he received a 1.5 times overdose of the medication. The error was quickly recognized and reported to the veterinarian, who determined that this was not a safety concern for Prince and did not require any change in his treatment plan.
- *Medical complication*: After being hospitalized on the morning of his scheduled surgical procedure, Prince became acutely painful on his right forelimb and could no longer bear any weight. Recheck radiographs showed that the bone, weakened by the cancer, had fractured.

> This event, termed a "pathologic fracture," is a recognized complication associated with osteosarcoma. In this case, there was no error on the part of the staff or hospital. In other situations, complications may be due to errors, and/or may be due to the medical intervention itself.
>
> - *Adverse event/outcome*: Near the end of the surgical procedure, Prince abruptly went into cardiopulmonary arrest. Cardiopulmonary cerebral resuscitation was unsuccessful. A detailed analysis of his medical care revealed no known cause for his sudden death. In this case, there was no error on the part of the staff or hospital. In other types of adverse events, there is an error. Note that although adverse events are caused by a medical intervention, this does not necessarily mean that an error occurred.
> - *Medical error*: Near the end of the surgical procedure, Prince abruptly went into cardiopulmonary arrest. Cardiopulmonary cerebral resuscitation was unsuccessful. A detailed analysis of his medical care revealed that the pop-off valve in the anesthetic circuit had been left fully closed, which resulted in excessive pressure causing respiratory arrest, which then led to cardiac arrest. The error was the fault of an inexperienced technician, who had taken over because her colleague called in sick that day. The system and equipment were also at fault.

Distinguishing a Medical Error from an Adverse Event or Complication

When something bad happens to our patients after an intervention, distinguishing a medical error (which creates a professional liability) from an adverse event (AE) or complication (where responsibility is less certain) can be challenging. As an example, we have been associated with numerous patients who developed peritonitis after an enterotomy or intestinal resection and anastomosis. This is a serious outcome requiring a second surgery and significant expense. We've never seen a surgeon ascribe these events to a medical error. Since most surgeons likely mention peritonitis as a risk of intestinal surgery, these instances are attributed to an AE or complication related to the patient's condition.

When administering intravenous chemotherapy using a vesicant drug such as vincristine, drug extravasation is a risk usually mentioned to clients. This may occur when the oncology team ensures that proper injection technique was followed but the patient moved or jumped unexpectedly, causing the injection to leak out of the vein. In other cases, the patient may not move at all and the extravasation is due to clinician or technician error. As the person injecting the medication is concentrating on this task only, it can be difficult to know which of these patient safety events caused this undesirable outcome.

Looking back, we are certain there were instances in our careers where a procedural error by one of us or a technical error by the team was inadvertently conveyed to clients as an AE or complication. The point is that when patient safety events occur in real time, it can be challenging to discern whether a team member is at fault, because efforts at that point are usually directed toward the patient's needs and such investigations require time, which is often in short supply in busy practices. In addition, if the clinician involved in an undesirable patient outcome does not consider an error as the cause, other team members are very unlikely to come forward to discuss such a sensitive subject.

Prevalence of Medical Errors

Studies in the past few years have examined the prevalence of medical errors in veterinary practice. A survey of 606 veterinarians showed that 74% indicated being involved with at least one AE or near miss (NM) in the preceding 12 months [4]. In a study from three companion animal teaching/

multi-specialty private practice hospitals using a voluntary reporting system, approximately five medical errors occurred per 1000 patient visits (0.5%) [3]. Most veterinary students (86%) reported being present during a medical error, and 60% reported causing a medical error [5]. As these results were based on self-reporting, they likely underestimate the actual prevalence of errors. Medical errors are probably far more common and consequential than is acknowledged within the veterinary profession.

Causes of Medical Errors

The primary reasons to determine the causes of veterinary team errors should be to comprehend what happened, learn from the mistake, and make changes to diminish the likelihood of repeating errors, rather than to ascribe blame. The terms *error reduction* or *error mitigation* best characterize the rationale behind these efforts, rather than the idea that errors can be prevented. Broadly, errors may be due to individual factors and/or environmental factors. Individual errors by healthcare team members may include those of commission (wrong action) or omission (failure to act). As an example, if a clinician adds a new medication but inserts this into the wrong patient's treatment sheet, that's an error of commission, whereas if they forget to add the new medication, that's an error of omission. Factors contributing to errors associated with a practice's systems and culture include inadequate staff training or numbers, poor communication systems, and staff members not feeling safe enough to speak up when they recognize that something may cause harm or has gone wrong.

Few investigations have been performed in veterinary medicine examining causes of errors. In a multi-center study conducted in the United States, drug errors were the most frequently reported error type, accounting for 55–69% of all errors [3]. Drug errors were categorized as wrong patient, wrong drug, wrong route, wrong time, or wrong dose. Giving the wrong dose was the most common form of medication error. Communication errors were the second most common (30%) error type. Communication errors were classified as a failure of transmission (illegible handwriting, poor medium for transmitting information), a failure of the source (missing or incomplete information), or receiver failure (information forgotten or incorrectly interpreted). This study revealed that 39% of communication errors were transmission errors, 35% were source errors, and 21% were receiver errors.

In a study of voluntary incident reports submitted by 130 small animal practices in Europe [6], medication-related incidents were the most frequent type recorded (40%). In another investigation evaluating over 1000 medication errors, errors were most frequent during the drug administration phase accounting for 51% of cases, of which 68% were due to the wrong dose, frequency, or duration [7].

Veterinarians often have arduous work schedules. One of us (BK) was on call for much of my career and can personally attest that I was tired when working with less than seven hours of sleep. I also often did not take a lunch break nor eat lunch, proclaiming that I was too busy caring for patients. Basic self-care strategies such as maintaining reasonable work hours, exercise, sleep, and hydration have benefits to cognition and wellbeing [8]. In many cases, deficiencies in these basic aspects of self-care have been directly linked to impaired cognitive abilities in healthcare workers [9].

While personal responsibility for self-care is important, we should also consider the cultural and workplace norms that enable deficiencies of self-care among veterinary professionals. In a recent study, veterinary house officers reported working 11–13 hours a day and 32% reported clinical duties 7 days a week. Working hours were negatively related to sleep quantity. Most of these veterinarians felt that fatigue had negative impacts on their technical skills and clinical judgment [10]. In developing healthy work environments, organizations must create plans conducive to the self-care of their employees [11]. Simply put, sleep deprivation, dehydration, and hunger do not promote one's capacity to navigate the mental and physical requirements needed to ensure patient safety.

Stress has also been recognized as a cause of errors affecting patient safety in veterinary practice [12]. In our experience, stress associated with the perception of having too many procedures to perform and not enough time to complete them properly was commonly associated with AEs or errors.

Consequences of Errors

It is difficult to overstate the importance of medical errors given their potentially devastating impacts on patients, family members, and veterinary team members. A study in the human medical field found that more than 250 000 patient deaths per year in US hospitals are attributable to medical errors, making medical errors the third leading cause of death [13]. In one veterinary study, 15% of errors resulted in harm [3]. The frequency of errors causing permanent harm or death was less than 2% of reported incidents. Following an AE, more than 82% of patients had temporary harm, and 8% of patients harmed suffered permanent morbidity or death. In another investigation, 30% of medication errors were associated with mild harm, 3% with moderate harm, and 0.2% caused severe harm [7]. In a European study [6], incidents caused harm in 42% of voluntary reports. Treatment-related incidents were the most common type of incident causing patient harm (55%). Anesthesia-related incidents were the most severe type, resulting in patient death in 18% of these reports.

Most veterinary clients consider their animals to be members of the family, so the consequences of serious AEs can be emotionally devastating. Despite efforts by members of the veterinary healthcare team to explain potential risks in advance (as required to obtain informed consent), many owners are not emotionally prepared for something bad to happen to their beloved animal companion. This is understandable and requires that the disclosure and handling of these events be conducted with compassion, empathy, and respect. Even when AEs are handled in this fashion, many clients will experience a range of emotions that can include denial, anger, guilt, and profound grief.

Following the occurrence of a medical error or perceived medical error, hurt and disgruntled clients have at least three responses that strike fear into every veterinarian: (i) file a lawsuit; (ii) file a veterinary medical board complaint; and/or (iii) broadcast accusations (whether founded or not) on social media. Thus, the consequences of making an error could be financial loss, loss of the ability to continue to practice, and/or widespread public humiliation, in addition to the emotional pain of the initial event. Litigation also occurs in the veterinary field and defending oneself can be a daunting and expensive process. Every practicing veterinarian should obtain good-quality professional liability protection insurance and license defense insurance. Several large veterinary organizations offer this coverage and working with agents with veterinary-specific experience may have advantages. As this coverage is often arranged and paid for by employers, it is important for veterinary associates to understand that they are *not* protected when performing veterinary work that is not associated with their place of employment. When reviewing policies, veterinarians should ensure that they retain control of whether a case will be settled or not.

Medical errors can also cause mental and emotional harm to members of the medical team, who should be considered as secondary victims of these events. If a clinician fails to disclose an error to a client yet still charges a fee, they may not legally or morally deserve this payment [14]. A survey of US veterinarians indicated that following an AE, 78% experienced a short-term negative impact on their personal life and 51% had a long-term negative impact [4]. Detrimental effects reported included diminished confidence in their abilities, reduced job satisfaction, increased feelings of burnout, reduced happiness, feeling persistently guilty, and having difficulty sleeping. Many veterinary students also report experiencing anxiety or distress in relation to medical errors [5]. Medical errors and their disclosure can worsen occupational stress and exacerbate poor mental health in veterinarians.

This evidence clearly highlights the importance of providing care, kindness, and support not just for animal patients and their families affected by AEs, but also for members of the veterinary healthcare team. Though research is lacking on the impact of errors on members of the veterinary team beyond veterinarians, there is little doubt that they are also significantly affected and deserve equal compassion and support.

Responding to Errors

When an error occurs, the initial focus is understandably and appropriately on efforts to mitigate harm to the patient and their family. Except in the case of fatal errors, immediate medical steps to care for affected patients should be prioritized. Once the immediate patient care has been initiated, the following steps are often helpful:

- If the animal owner is present and witnessed the event, you should immediately communicate with them.
- If the owner is not present, pause and take a deep breath. If you are directly involved in a serious error, it's normal and understandable that emotions may arise that could make it difficult for you to function normally. If possible, discuss the situation with a colleague and ask for their support. This might include their taking over care of the patient so you can focus on other things and/or offering advice on how to proceed with the patient and client.
- Unless you own the practice, immediately notify the owner and/or hospital administrator and seek their advice.
- Make some quick notes. This is not the time for a detailed analysis; instead, capture the initial facts of the event, including the time frame and names of any individuals who were involved in any way, even as just witnesses to the event. When time permits (but relatively soon after the event) it is essential to record detailed notes in the patient medical record, including communications with the client.
- It may be appropriate to contact your professional liability insurance carrier. Some agents have extensive experience with these situations and can offer helpful advice. Remember, however, that *you* need to feel comfortable with how the situation is handled.
- Take a little time to review and mentally rehearse how you will communicate with the client.
- Share the news with the client following the guidelines discussed later in this chapter. This should be a two-way conversation and include suggestions for a plan forward.
- For all AEs, complete a structured investigation.
- Implement changes to reduce the risk of the event occurring again.
- Consulting with trusted professional colleagues, friends, and family can be helpful following the decision to acknowledge and address errors.

After communicating with the client, the next step is often investigating the AE, error, or NM. The veterinary profession is well behind the human medical profession in establishing systems to track, report, and productively address medical errors [3]. Use of a structured investigation process is helpful. A root cause analysis is a technique seeking to identify underlying causes or contributory factors that led to an unfortunate outcome. A simple and helpful approach is referred to as the "5 whys." The investigator begins by describing the most obvious cause for the AE and then repeatedly asks why that, and additional contributing events, occurred.

For example: A patient received a medication overdose. *Why?* Beth gave the wrong dose. *Why?* The dose was incorrect on the treatment sheet. *Why?* When Larry created the treatment sheet, he wrote the wrong dose. Beth is not familiar with this drug, so did not realize the error. *Why?* Larry was distracted when he created the treatment sheet and had trouble remembering the doctor's verbal dosing instructions. *Why?* The hospital was understaffed as two team members were out sick. Larry is not trained on creating treatment sheets nor Beth on use of this drug as our training program does not include these tasks. We also do not have a call-in list to fill shift vacancies.

Once the investigation of the AE, error, or NM has been completed, it's important to share and learn from this information. The goal should not be to assign blame, though in the case of repeated errors of the same type by the same individual, action must be taken to protect the safety of patients. This might include additional coaching, greater supervision, a change in position or responsibilities, or termination of employment. Far more often, the appropriate action is to support those individuals who were involved and collectively agree on changes in protocols indicated by the analysis, with the goal of improving patient safety in the future. In other words, the focus shifts from looking backward to looking forward. Unfortunately, only 50% of veterinarians in one study reported that their disclosure resulted in a system change [4].

Creating standard operating procedures (SOPs) can be another helpful approach to reducing errors. An SOP for a condition or procedure should include (i) name of condition/procedure; (ii) which team members are qualified to provide care; (iii) helpful definitions; (iv) specific steps for testing and/or treatment; and (v) known risks or hazards to mitigate. Clearly defining important specific steps can be facilitated using checklists.

As medication administration errors are among the most common types of errors in practice, particular attention should be paid to reducing the likelihood of these events. A tried-and-true reminder for anyone administering medications is to review the "Five Rights of Medication Administration" [15]:

- Right patient
- Right time and frequency
- Right dose
- Right route
- Right drug

Another approach is to require that doses of high-risk medications such as chemotherapy agents are double checked by a second team member before administration.

Handwritten medical records are often indecipherable by other people. Countless times we were unable to interpret some of the contents of a referring veterinarian's handwritten record. Fortunately, this is changing due to the availability of software that facilitates typed records. In an era in which we type our most inconsequential thoughts in tweets and texts, all medical records and treatment sheets should be digital. The practice of "closed-loop communication," where the receiver restates the message (for example, a medication dose or treatment plan) to ensure clarity and understanding, can reduce miscommunication and errors. Another simple intervention is the requirement that all medication orders from doctors be typed rather than delivered verbally.

Choosing to disclose medical errors can be scary. A tension exists between the moral duty to acknowledge a mistake with the resulting harm and the desire to protect oneself from the potentially serious repercussions of admitting errors. In our experience, reporting allows caregivers to honor their values and ethical beliefs, has the potential to rebuild trust and retain clients, and may reduce the likelihood of legal action or veterinary medical board complaints.

Unfortunately, a study in veterinary medicine indicates there is underreporting of NMs, AEs, and errors. A survey of veterinarians explored reporting of AEs and NMs [4]. When asked if they had disclosed an AE to a client within the last 12 months, 77% reported doing so. The majority of those who reported an AE to their client reported feeling satisfied with the result. Of veterinarians who experienced one or more AEs in the prior 12 months, 29% failed to disclose it to their client, with 79% failing to report one or more NMs. The most common reasons cited for not disclosing an AE were wanting to avoid needlessly upsetting the client, being afraid of damaging their relationship with the client, and being afraid the client would be angry or upset.

Given this evidence of underreporting of errors, AEs, and NMs, it's clear there are powerful impediments. A multi-pronged approach will be most effective in overcoming these barriers and must be supported by the leaders of the practice through both words and actions. Reporting will improve when there is a culture of support, opportunities for anonymous disclosure, and response is focused on learning rather than assignment of blame.

Improving the culture within a practice is another worthwhile strategy to reduce the incidence of medical errors. If non-doctors on the team do not feel empowered or welcomed to raise potential concerns related to patient safety, more errors are likely to occur. Conversely, when doctors treat other members of the healthcare team as respected colleagues, team members are more likely to feel comfortable asking questions and raising concerns. Every veterinary practice would be wise to proactively develop policies and procedures for responding to medical errors that can guide decision-making in the face of these unfortunate events. Although members of the medical team will always feel badly about AEs, it will help if they can feel good about how these incidents are handled by their employer (Case Study 10.2).

Case Study 10.2   A Medical Error Causing Death in a Young Dog

You are the owner of a 24-hour small animal practice. Brandy, a six-month-old female shih tzu, is seen during the night because she ingested a few Hershey's Kisses chocolate candies. She is healthy and asymptomatic. As chocolate ingestion can potentially be toxic, your associate, Dr. A, advises the routine protocol including induction of vomiting and administration of activated charcoal, which is approved. Brandy is transferred to your care the following day because of progressive decline in alertness after receiving the narcotic to cause vomiting. You perform blood testing, which reveals severe hypernatremia. Shortly after you receive approval to treat Brandy for this unexpected complication, she arrests and expires. You call the owners to inform them of her death.

You are aware that hypernatremia can be a rare complication of the charcoal that was administered. You review the medical record and treatment sheets in detail after the call and discover that Dr. A's team accidentally administered a 10 times overdose of the charcoal, which you suspect caused the sodium imbalance and Brandy's death. You inform Dr. A of the outcome and your discovery and contact your liability company. They suggest you work internally with your team to prevent these sorts of errors in the future.

What should you do?

One of the author's (BK) was the owner of the practice in this case. I met with Dr. A to discuss my findings and Brandy's tragic demise. He expressed remorse and accountability. In discussing the stakeholders involved, while I was concerned with the consequences that disclosure might have for the practice's reputation, and Dr. A was concerned about a potential liability claim, we concluded that Brandy's owners had the most compelling interest in learning that the chocolate ingestion did not cause her death. Otherwise, they may have felt culpable. We agreed that I would meet with the clients and disclose the truth. It was the most difficult conversation with a client I had ever had. I did my best to convey my feelings of regret and responsibility for the error and vowed to modify our protocols to mitigate similar errors in the future. The clients thanked me for coming forward and chose not to pursue a liability claim. While some clients will not respond well, it has been our experience in similar circumstances that disclosure, honesty, and transparency regarding medical errors result in more satisfactory outcomes for both the veterinarian and the client than efforts to conceal and thwart admission of the truth.

Applying Ethics to Errors: The Ethics of Lying in Veterinary Practice

This book has emphasized the role of the veterinarian as animal advocate, where the veterinarian utilizes all available resources to promote the course of action that is most likely to provide the best outcome for the patient regardless of costs or concerns about the psychological wellbeing of the client [16, 17]. Veterinarians in practice also have a fiduciary duty to serve the animal owner because the client is paying them [14]. A pivotal means of fulfilling this responsibility is to acquire informed consent (see Chapter 3).

When considering whether to reveal a medical error to a client, some veterinarians may resort to dishonesty, lying, or non-disclosure: "To lie is to make an assertion that one knows to be false with the purpose of inducing another to believe that it is true. Honesty is more than not telling a lie or telling the truth when a client specifically requests information. Failing to inform a client about something they could not know, whether a client specifically asks or not, can also be dishonest" [14].

Veterinary medicine is viewed by the public as an honest and ethical profession [18]. Clients have placed great importance on the honesty and trustworthiness of the veterinarian [19]. Lying is in violation of the American Veterinary Medical Association (AVMA) Principles of Veterinary Medical Ethics, which state that a veterinarian shall be "honest in all professional interactions" [20].

Philosophy and Deception

The belief that deception is harmful and immoral has been promulgated by theologians such as St. Augustine, who claimed that "every lie is a sin," and philosophers such as Immanuel Kant, who argued that "The greatest violation . . . is lying" [21]. Deontologists maintain that one should never lie and therefore favor unconditional application of informed consent [22, 23]. Utilitarian theory emphasizes morality based on positive net outcomes; the ethical acceptability of lying depends on its consequences, and the obligation to tell the truth can be outweighed by the duty not to hurt others [14, 23]. The utilitarian would morally justify professional conduct such as being ambiguous or evasive, omitting facts, and lying so long as it promotes the patient's or client's wellbeing [23].

Paternalism and Dishonesty

Paternalism is the predominant communication style in veterinary practice, in which the practitioner makes decisions on behalf of the client [24–27]. Within this paradigm, a veterinarian may be inclined to pursue dishonest behavior because they do not want to cause unnecessary stress to the client [28].

Failing to Disclose as Dishonesty

Failing to disclose a medical error that results in increased client cost and/or the animal's decline or death is often driven by a desire to preserve one's self-interest [29]. This type of lying is difficult to justify in that it is intended to benefit the liar to the detriment of clients and/or animals.

Consequences of Lying

If a client were to somehow discover that their veterinarian did not disclose the truth about an error, consequences could include loss of trust in the profession and feelings of anger and betrayal. Lying also carries costs for the liar, such as feelings of guilt and entitlement, loss of credibility, pursuit of retribution by the client, and actions by regulatory authorities [28, 30].

Summary

Dishonesty, lying, and non-disclosure are routes that some veterinarians may follow when faced with a medical error. Lies based on self-interest are in violation of professional codes of conduct, can result in loss of trust in the veterinary profession, and may be harmful to the clinician, the profession, and the client. The decision to be professionally dishonest might be reconsidered if the veterinary practitioner felt compelled to defend such a decision to peers, clients, or the veterinary medical board. Divulging medical errors to clients requires courage, empathy, and excellent communication skills.

Communicating about Errors

Veterinary clients whose animals have been affected by an error want and deserve to know the cause. When veterinary clients learn of an error, they may experience two different types of disappointment: (i) with the error; (ii) with the *handling* of the error. In the authors' experience, clients tend to be less forgiving of mistakes in the handling of the situation. Once an event has occurred, we cannot change the facts, but we can influence how the event is managed.

Should a doctor apologize to their patient/client after an error? This is an important question with ethical implications that has been debated for years in the human and veterinary professions. There has been an evolution regarding this topic toward the use of an apology [31]. Although physicians have some legal protections for offering apologies to their patients, veterinarians have no such protections. Liability settlements, however, are likely far lower for veterinarians than for physicians.

One of the authors (JC), who co-owned several large emergency/specialty practices in California for many years and has interfaced with insurance representatives representing the AVMA and the California Veterinary Medical Association programs, has found that they consistently support disclosing errors and apologizing to veterinary clients who have suffered harm. Whether recommended or not by an insurance company, our recommendation is to disclose errors and offer apologies.

There are two forms of apology: (i) an apology of sympathy, which does not acknowledge accountability for the event; and (ii) an apology of responsibility. For example, "I'm so sorry this happened" is an apology of sympathy, whereas "I'm so sorry we made this error" is an apology of responsibility. Caregivers always have the option of offering an apology without acknowledging culpability. This may be very appropriate as an empathetic gesture before knowing the true cause(s) of an AE, or in situations where an AE has occurred but there was no fault by the medical personnel. Either way, it would be wise to note in the medical record exactly what type of apology was disclosed to the client.

If, however, a known error occurred, an apology of responsibility is warranted and important. A full apology should convey accountability and culpability, an explanation of the circumstances that led to the mistake, and a promise of corrective actions [32]. An apology should not include justifications that may be interpreted as denials of fault, and there should be no requests for forgiveness within the apology, which would shift the focus from the needs of the client to those of the clinician [32]. Further guidance on communicating about errors can be found in Clark and Kipperman [33].

Healing and Moving On

Considering the pervasiveness of medical errors in veterinary practice, it is likely that nearly every member of a veterinary healthcare team will at some point be directly affected by an error. In the authors' experience, very few practices take a proactive stance regarding medical errors and their aftermath. Policies, procedures, and systems can and should be put in place, ideally *before* they are needed. All members of the team share the common goal of patient safety. Therefore, when patient safety is compromised due to an error, all members of the team share collective responsibility and can learn from these events. If you have made mistakes in practice, you are not alone!

Perhaps most importantly, remember to approach every adverse event or medical error situation with sensitivity and empathy for all parties affected. With open dialogue, open minds, a desire to learn from others, and adherence to ethical principles and approaches, the veterinary profession's handling of medical errors will continue to evolve in a positive direction.

References

1 Shmerling, R.H. (2020). First, do no harm. Harvard Health Blog. https://www.health.harvard.edu/blog/first-do-no-harm-201510138421 (accessed August 22, 2022).

2 Wu, A.W., Folkman, S., McPhee, S.J. et al. (1991). Do house officers learn from their mistakes? *Journal of the American Medical Association* 265 (16): 2089–2094.

3 Wallis, J., Fletcher, D., Bentley, A. et al. (2019). Medical errors cause harm in veterinary hospitals. *Frontiers in Veterinary Science* 6: 12.

4 Kogan, L.R., Rishniw, M., Hellyer, P.W. et al. (2018). Veterinarians' experiences with near misses and adverse events. *Journal of the American Veterinary Medical Association* 252 (5): 586–595.

5 Alexander-Leeder, C.A., Guess, S.C., Waiting, D.K. et al. (2022). Medical errors: Experiences, attitudes and perspectives of incoming and outgoing final-year veterinary students in the USA. *Veterinary Record* 191(3): e1735. https://doi.org/10.1002/vetr.1735.

6 Schortz, L., Mossop, L., Bergstrom, A. et al. (2022). Type and impact of clinical incidents identified by a voluntary reporting system covering 130 small animal practices in mainland Europe. *Veterinary Record* 191(2): e1629. https://doi.org/10.1002/vetr.1629.

7 Petrou, E., Noble, P.J.M., Singleton, D. et al. (2022). Using electronic health records (EHRs) to identify medication errors occurring in veterinary practices (UK). In: *BSAVA Congress Proceedings 2022*. Quedgeley: British Small Animal Veterinary Association https://doi.org/10.2223 3/9781913859114.36.4.

8 Volk, J.O., Schimmack, U., Strand, E.B. et al. (2020). Executive summary of the Merck Animal Health Veterinarian Wellbeing Study II. *Journal of the American Veterinary Medical Association* 256 (11): 1237–1244.

9 Shapiro, D.E., Duquette, C., Abbott, L.M. et al. (2019). Beyond burnout: a physician wellness hierarchy designed to prioritize interventions at the systems level. *American Journal of Medicine* 132 (5): 556–563.

10 Scharf, V.F., McPhetridge, J.B., and Dickson, R. (2022). Sleep patterns, fatigue, and working hours among veterinary house officers: a cross-sectional survey study. *Journal of the American Veterinary Medical Association* 260 (11): 1377–1385.

11 Jurney, C. and Kipperman, B. (2022). Moral stress. In: *Ethics in Veterinary Practice*, ch. 22 (ed. B. Kipperman and B.E. Rollin). Hoboken, NJ: Wiley-Blackwell.

12 Oxtoby, C., Ferguson, E., White, K. et al. (2015). We need to talk about error: causes and types of error in veterinary practice. *Veterinary Record* 177 (17): 438.

13 Mamary, M.A. and Daniel, M. (2016). Medical error—the third leading cause of death in the US. *British Medical Journal* 353: i2139.

14 Tannenbaum, J. (1995). *Veterinary Ethics: Animal Welfare, Client Relations, Competition and Collegiality*, 2e. St. Louis, MO: Mosby YearBook.

15 Craven, R.F. and Hirnle, C.J. (2008). *Fundamentals of Nursing: Human Health and Function*, 6e. Philadelphia, PA: Lippincott Williams & Wilkins.

16 Main, D. (2006). Offering the best to patients: ethical issues associated with the provision of veterinary services. *Veterinary Record* 158(2): 62–66.

17 Kipperman, B. (2022). Veterinary advocacies and ethical dilemmas. In: *Ethics in Veterinary Practice*, ch. 7 (ed. B. Kipperman and B.E. Rollin). Hoboken, NJ: Wiley-Blackwell.

18 Kedrowicz, A.A. and Royal, K.D. (2020). A comparison of public perceptions of physicians and veterinarians in the United States. *Veterinary Sciences* 7 (2): 50.

19 Gordon, S., Gardner, D.H., Weston, J.F. et al. (2019). Quantitative and thematic analysis of complaints by clients against clinical veterinary practitioners in New Zealand. *New Zealand Veterinary Journal* 67 (3): 117–125.

20 American Veterinary Medical Association (n.d). Principles of veterinary medical ethics. https://www.avma.org/KB/Policies/Pages/Principles-of-Veterinary-Medical-Ethics-of-the-AVMA.aspx (accessed August 24, 2022).

21 Gaspar, J.P., Levine, E.E., and Schweitzer, ME. (2015). Why we should lie. *Organizational Dynamics* 44(4): 306–309.

22 Kant, I. (1959 [1785]). *Foundation of the Metaphysics of Morals*, trans. L.W. Beck. Indianapolis, IN: Bobbs-Merrill.

23 Richard, C., Lajeunesse, Y., and Lussier M.T. (2010). Therapeutic privilege: between the ethics of lying and the practice of truth. *Journal of Medical Ethics* 36(6): 353–357.

24 Bard, A.M., Main, D.C., Haase, A.M. et al. (2017). The future of veterinary communication: partnership or persuasion? A qualitative investigation of veterinary communication in the pursuit of client behavior change. *PLoS One* 12 (3): e0171380.

25 Svensson, C., Emanuelson, U., Bard, A.M. et al. (2019). Communication styles of Swedish veterinarians involved in dairy herd health management: a motivational interviewing perspective. *Journal of Dairy Science* 102 (11): 10173–10185.

26 Janke, N., Coe, J.B., Sutherland, K.A. et al. (2021). Evaluating shared decision-making between companion animal veterinarians and their clients using the observer OPTION 5 instrument. *Veterinary Record* 189(8): e778.

27 Enlund, K.B., Jennolf, E., and Pettersson, A. (2021). Small animal veterinarians' communication with dog owners from a motivational interviewing perspective. *Frontiers in Veterinary Science* 8: 772589.

28 Palmieri J.J., and Stern, T.A. (2009). Lies in the doctor-patient relationship. *Primary Care Companion to the Journal of Clinical Psychiatry* 11(4): 163–168.

29 Levine, E.E. and Schweitzer, M.E. (2014). Are liars ethical? On the tension between benevolence and honesty. *Journal of Experimental Social Psychology* 53: 107–117.

30 Bok, S. (1999). *Lying: Moral Choice in Public and Private Life*. New York: Vintage Books.

31 Bendix, J. (2019). Should doctors apologize for mistakes? *Medical Economics* 96(21): 17.

32 Petronio, S., Torke, A., Bosslet, G. et al. (2013) Disclosing medical mistakes: a communication management plan for physicians. *Permanente Journal* 17(2): 73–79.

33 Clark, J. and Kipperman, B. (2022). Medical errors. In: *Ethics in Veterinary Practice*, ch. 9 (ed. B. Kipperman and B.E. Rollin). Hoboken, NJ: Wiley-Blackwell.

Section 2

Principles of Diagnosis

11

The Influence of Patient Weight on Decision-Making

Barry Kipperman

Abstract

This chapter addresses the importance of acquiring and documenting patient body weights and recognizing changes in patient weights. Evaluating changes in weight as a percentage of previous body weight rather than as an absolute number is recommended. Early identification of weight gain or weight loss accompanied by appropriate action optimizes patient outcomes and minimizes poor quality of life and mortality. A flow chart is provided to guide clinicians as to when and how to intervene when weight loss is noted. An action plan is advised for weight gain or weight loss of 5% or more in asymptomatic patients.

Keywords: *body weight, weight, documenting weight, recognizing weight, overweight, obesity, weight loss, weight gain, proportional weight, medical records*

Why Obtaining and Documenting Patient Body Weights Is Imperative

Because significant changes in body weight in our patients usually occur over a period of weeks to months, it is very difficult for owners who see their animal every day to recognize weight gain or weight loss. As an analogy, I don't notice that my hair is receding; only when I look at pictures from years ago do I appreciate that I'm losing hair! I'm sure many readers have had the experience of seeing a patient and immediately observing a change in their body condition while the owner did not notice this difference. As a result, changes in patient weights are usually detected incidentally or ancillary to the reason for the veterinary visit.

Why is obtaining and documenting the body weight of every patient at every visit important? Because obesity is a modern-day epidemic. Dogs and cats are considered overweight when their weight is more than 10–20% above their ideal weight [1]. The American Veterinary Medical Association has endorsed defining obesity as present when a dog or cat is >30% above their ideal weight [2].

Over a 10-year period, Banfield® pet hospitals reported a 158% and 169% increase in the prevalence of overweight dogs and cats, respectively [3]. In the Association for Pet Obesity Prevention 2022 clinical survey, 59% of 880 dogs and 61% of 272 cats were classified as clinically overweight or obese by their veterinary healthcare professional [4]. A study in the United Kingdom classified 65% of adult dogs and 37% of juvenile dogs as overweight or obese [5]. Obese dogs and cats are more likely to be diagnosed with numerous co-morbidities, including diabetes mellitus and orthopedic conditions [6, 7]. Consequently, the median lifespan is shorter in overweight dogs [8] and cats [9].

Conversely, because our patients can't complain of nausea and reduced appetite, documentation and recognition of weight loss form a crucial step in the diagnosis of almost all serious disorders. In some diseases such as diabetes mellitus, or chronic enteropathy or hyperthyroidism in cats, energy level and appetite may be normal or greater than normal, hindering the owner's recognition of a problem. Because the poorer the patient body condition is at the time of diagnosis the poorer the prognosis, early detection of disease through documentation and recognition of weight loss is pivotal.

Documentation of Patient Weights in Veterinary Practice

A retrospective study of the primary care veterinary records of 148 dogs in the United Kingdom over an approximately 12-month interval found that only 70% of the medical record entries documented patient body weight [10]. The median frequency was of one weight measurement per four consultations. In an evaluation of the medical records of over 19 million cats, after the first year of life there was a precipitous decline in the proportion of body weight measurements for cats 1–2 years of age and a more gradual decline thereafter [11]. Only 29% of medical records submitted to the Dog Aging Project reported a numerical body condition score (BCS) [12]. In an assessment of over 129 000 feline visits, though 95% of visits recorded a weight, only 23% recorded a BCS [13].

While it can be challenging to obtain weights in certain cases such as fractious patients, large non-ambulatory dogs, and trauma patients, there is clearly room for improvement in the documentation of veterinary patient weights in medical records. To apply the Principle of Patient Advocacy, the goal for any practice should be to obtain and document weights for each patient at each visit.

Ensuring That Documented Weights Are Accurate

Another vital step is to ensure that documented patient weights are accurate. I encourage taking the time to educate your paraprofessional team obtaining patient weights as to why this is such an important task. This can be a challenge in some patients because puppies are often excited and seldom stay still, fearful patients may be shivering or trying to escape, and some giant-breed dogs may not fit on the scale.

Ideally, patients should be weighed on scales that are appropriate for their size. Exotic companions should be weighed on a scale that measures in smaller increments than for dogs and cats, such as a food scale that measures in grams. Dogs and cats weighing 2–20 lb (1–9 kg) should be weighed on a small scale that measures in pounds and ounces, and patients larger than 20 lb (9 kg) should be weighed on larger, step-on scales. To mitigate fear, patients should be weighed with their owners present. Veterinarians should never accept as being accurate the method of weight acquisition in which a human steps on the scale with the animal, then subtracts their own weight from the combined weight.

There will be instances when the documented weight is significantly different than what is expected based on prior weight recordings. In these cases, the clinician should not hesitate to request a second or third attempt to better ensure consistency and an accurate value (as we do with blood pressure measurements). Many times, the repeat weights will differ significantly from the originally reported weight.

Recognition of Patient Body Weights

The acquisition and documentation of patient body weights are only of value if the veterinary clinician recognizes the reported weight and compares this to previous weights. In my experience, it is very common for medical records to document significant changes in patient body weights over time with no acknowledgment of this trend by the clinician (the importance of noting serial trends in patient data is discussed in Chapter 15). Many software programs used in practice readily provide a visual chart of trends in recorded weights. Taking the time to review serial patient body weights is pivotal to fulfilling the Principle of Patient Advocacy.

Absolute versus Relative Patient Weights

It is common for practitioners to assess changes in patient body weights through a human-centric perspective. Countless times I've been told by a colleague about an animal patient, "It's only 1 or 2 lb, I'm not very concerned." Indeed, for most 100–200 lb (45–90 kg) humans, weight gain or loss of 1–2 lb (½–1 kg) is inconsequential. But if a previously 10 lb cat is now 9 lb, the patient has incurred a 10% weight loss. That's analogous to my losing 15 lb (7 kg)! To properly interpret changes in body weights of our animal patients, we must consider this as a percentage of their previous body weight.

When Changes in Body Weight Require Intervention

Weight Gain

Disclosure of increasing or declining patient weights is in keeping with our duty to obtain informed consent (see Chapter 3). In my experience, weight gain is often associated with a reduction in activity and exercise with age while the patient is ingesting the same number of calories as in years past. Owners of geriatric animals should be educated about this common and predictable scenario to mitigate weight gain.

Weight gain of 5% or more should initiate an action plan [14]. Because overweight and obesity in companion animals impairs quality of life, shortens lifespan, and once established are difficult to reverse, and a recent study found that pet owners who self-identified their pet as overweight or obese appeared to have low levels of willingness to change their behavior [15], preemptive monitoring to prevent obesity from developing is strongly encouraged. A combination of informing owners that their animal is or may become overweight, discussing the health and welfare implications of obesity, and providing information on how to achieve weight loss is the most effective mechanism for motivating animal owners to improve the health and welfare of their overweight or obese animal companions. An incremental approach including follow-up calls and serial weights may improve compliance with weight management plans.

Unfortunately, a recent report found that veterinarians in recorded visits used weight trends reactively (i.e. to illustrate a problem), rather than proactively (i.e. to prevent a problem) [16]. Veterinarians in that study infrequently explained the impact of weight status on the pet's health and wellbeing when discussing a weight trend with a client. In other investigations on disclosure of overweight or obese status, only 50% of 917 veterinary client–patient interactions contained an exchange involving the mention of a dog's or cat's weight [17], and only 7% of feline medical records used terms associated with overweight [13]. Another survey of veterinary professionals found that avoidance of discussing obesity with certain clients was common, and 25% indicated that client attitude or history influenced their willingness to discuss weight for an overweight pet, where negative attitudes or past experiences may lead to avoiding the topic [18]. Time constraints also influenced failure to discuss weight. These studies suggest a reluctance to discuss overweight and obesity with clients.

Weight Loss

A false assumption is prevalent among many pet owners (and some clinicians) that weight loss is normal and expected with aging. Weight loss is almost always associated with a disease. Any patient with less than or equal to 5% weight loss who has symptoms related to illness, or any patient with more than 5% weight loss regardless of whether symptoms are present, should undergo a diagnostic evaluation, which should include a minimum database (MDB) (see Chapter 17) and abdominal ultrasound if the MDB is inconclusive. In these subsets of patients, such diagnostic testing identifies a cause for the weight loss in about 80% of cases in my experience. Referral is advised if diagnostic testing is inconclusive. A flow chart for when and how to intervene relative to patient weight loss is summarized in Figure 11.1.

This recommendation is based on the premise that it is better to err on identifying disease sooner even if some of these evaluations are inconclusive. The earlier you intervene, the lower your diagnostic rate will be, while the prognosis for patients with identified disease will be better. The more advanced weight loss is before testing is performed, the diagnostic rate rises while patient

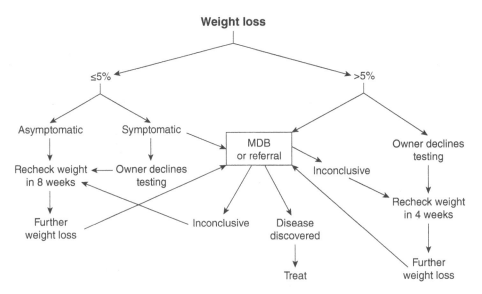

Figure 11.1 Clinical strategies based on patient weight loss. MDB, minimum database.

prognosis declines. While some clinicians may be concerned that prompt intervention as advised here may result in client complaints about the costs of negative investigations, the Principle of Patient Advocacy accepts this as an ancillary outcome of early diagnoses.

While some of the guidance in Figure 11.1 may seem apparent, let's discuss some of the more subtle concerns. When the veterinarian expresses concern about weight loss, it is common for animal owners to respond by either diminishing its importance or finding an excuse ("I think she's following me around the house more often"). Some owners will attribute weight loss to recent intentional efforts. Do not let these rationalizations dissuade you from encouraging intervention or appropriate monitoring.

Achieving client compliance with the recommendations in Figure 11.1 may be challenging. While it's easy to give up and concur with the owner's contention that all is well so as not to be perceived as pessimistic or confrontational, a common outcome of this situation is either no scheduled recheck or a recheck that doesn't provide a safety net for the patient. For example, scheduling the next visit in four months may discover a degree of weight loss that accompanies a poor prognosis if the mild weight loss recognized today continues. A strategy that was successful in my practice was to strike an agreement with the client: "Mrs. Y, can we agree that you'll bring Fluffy back in for a free recheck of her weight in four weeks? If her weight is stable, then we no longer need to be worried, but if she loses more weight, then we'll pursue testing at that time. Is that OK?" Compliance with these rechecks was high, as was approval of diagnostic testing, as the client had been prepared for this. This time frame is more conducive to ensuring a good prognosis if weight loss continues.

I commonly saw patients who had lost 25–40% of their body weight at the time of referral. While some of these cases were due to owner neglect in bringing their animal to their veterinarian in an advanced state of illness (see Chapter 5 for how to mitigate this concern), most of these cases were being treated and monitored by a colleague while the patient lost weight. The prognosis for these patients was very poor, as they cannot endure necessary diagnostic or therapeutic procedures (including anesthesia or surgery) without a major setback or death, and they often cannot survive long enough for appropriate therapies to take effect. Nutritional support via enteral feeding is often required to salvage patients with this degree of weight loss (Case Study 11.1).

Reliable acquisition, documentation, and recognition of patient body weights, followed by appropriate actions regarding changes in patient weights, are pivotal to fulfilling the Principle of Patient Advocacy.

Case Study 11.1   A Cat with Severe Weight Loss

Merlin, a 14-year-old female cat, is seen for routine annual evaluation. Present weight is recorded as 8 lb. The documented weight in the medical record one year before this was 10 lb. Vaccinations are provided. No mention of weight loss is noted. Four months later, Merlin is presented for weakness and anorexia. Weight is now 5.5 lb and Merlin is referred. She is cachectic and weakly ambulatory. Diagnostic testing suggests chronic enteropathy as the cause. While endoscopy is the preferred next step to stage the disease, which guides proper treatment, this was bypassed due to concern of anesthetic mortality or decline in condition because of her debilitated state. An esophagostomy tube was placed under sedation to facilitate nutritional support. Merlin received heat and intravenous fluid support and took all night to recover and regain ability to ambulate. Merlin was discharged on tube feedings and steroid suspension. She steadily gained weight and survived for 14 months.

References

1 German, A.J. (2006). The growing problem of obesity in dogs and cats. *Journal of Nutrition* 136 (7 Suppl): 1940S–1946S.

2 Burns, K. (2018). Taking on obesity as a disease. American Veterinary Medical Association. https://www.avma.org/javma-news/2018-10-01/taking-obesity-disease (accessed March 4, 2023).

3 Banfield (2017). State of pet health. Top issues: Obesity. https://www.banfield.com/state-of-pet-health/obesity (accessed March 4, 2023)

4 Association for Pet Obesity Prevention (2022). State of U.S. pet obesity: moving from awareness to treatment. https://static1.squarespace.com/static/6425ec5d33eaaa634113b2d4/t/6454f61c0cad1648 60799c8f/1683289630779/2022+State+of+US+Pet+Obesity+Report.pdf (accessed May 17, 2023).

5 German, A.J., Woods, G.R., Holden, S.L. et al. (2018). Small animal health: dangerous trends in pet obesity. *Veterinary Record* 182 (1): 25.

6 Lund, E.M., Armstrong, P.J., Kirk, C.A. et al. (2005). Prevalence and risk factors for obesity in adult cats from private US veterinary practices. *International Journal of Applied Research in Veterinary Medicine* 3 (2): 88–96.

7 Lund, E.M., Armstrong, P.J., Kirk, C.A. et al. (2006). Prevalence and risk factors for obesity in adult dogs from private US veterinary practices. *International Journal of Applied Research in Veterinary Medicine* 4 (2): 177–186.

8 Salt, C., Morris, P.J., Wilson, D. et al. (2019). Association between life span and body condition in neutered client-owned dogs. *Journal of Veterinary Internal Medicine* 33 (1): 89–99.

9 Teng, K.T., McGreevy, P.D., Toribio, J.-A.L. et al. (2018). Strong associations of 9-point body condition scoring with survival and lifespan in cats. *Journal of Feline Medicine and Surgery* 20 (12): 1110–1118.

10 German, A.J. and Morgan, L.E. (2008). How often do veterinarians assess the bodyweight and body condition of dogs? *Veterinary Record* 163 (17): 503–505.

11 Campigotto, A.J., Poljak, Z., Stone, E.A. et al. (2019). Investigation of relationships between body weight and age among domestic cats stratified by breed and sex. *Journal of the American Veterinary Medical Association* 255 (2): 205–212.

12 Dog Aging Project. https://dogagingproject.org (accessed August 13, 2023).

13 Taylor, S., Roberts, G., Evans, M. et al. (2022). Recording of body weight and body condition score of cats in electronic health records from UK veterinary practices. *Journal of Feline Medicine and Surgery* 24 (10): e380–e393.

14 Kipperman, B.S. and German, A.J. (2018). The responsibility of veterinarians to address companion animal obesity. *Animals* 8 (9): 143. https://doi.org/10.3390/ani8090143.

15 Sutherland, K.A., Coe, J.B., and O'Sullivan, T.L. (2023). Assessing owners' readiness to change their behaviour to address their companion animal's obesity. *Veterinary Record* 192 (3): e1979.

16 Janke, N., Coe, J.B., Bernardo, T.M. et al. (2022). Use of health parameter trends to communicate pet health information in companion animal practice: a mixed methods analysis. *Veterinary Record* 190 (7): e1378.

17 Sutherland, K.A., Coe, J.B., Janke, N. et al. (2022). Veterinary professionals' weight-related communication when discussing an overweight or obese pet with a client. *Journal of the American Veterinary Medical Association* 260 (9): 1076–1085.

18 Sutherland, K.A., Coe, J.B., and O'Sullivan, T.L. (2022). Exploring veterinary professionals' perceptions of pet weight-related communication in companion animal veterinary practice. *Veterinary Record* 192 (4): e1973.

12

The Influence of Age and Aging on Decision-Making
Barry Kipperman

Abstract

This chapter provides data comparing the lifespan of humans with that of dogs and cats. One implication of the rapid aging process for companion animals is that decisions about whether to intervene when they are ill may be influenced by a patient's expected lifespan. Ageism is a potential outcome of such considerations. The principle of A Day Is Really a Week – a day of illness for pets is comparable to a week for sick humans – is proposed. Veterinarians should ensure their clients understand this principle to encourage immediate visits to the hospital when pets are ill. The rapid progression of disease in pets requires veterinary clinicians to assume an aggressive diagnostic posture.

Keywords: *lifespan, age, aging, ageism, quality of life, advocacy, allocating resources*

It is common knowledge that the lifespan of dogs and cats is far lower than that of humans. In 2021, human life expectancy in the United States was 76 years [1] (this has been reduced by the Covid pandemic). By comparison, the median longevity of dogs from different studies ranges from 10 to 15 years of age (the variability in reported lifespans may be due to differing populations studied) [2–5]. Veterinarians also know that large-breed dogs develop illnesses and die at younger ages compared to small-breed dogs [6]. The median lifespan of cats in one study was 14 years [7]. The fact that most pets die from euthanasia (which may be elected for reasons unrelated to declining quality of life) may lead to underestimation of natural life expectancy [8].

Aging has been defined as the process in which "individuals experience progressive loss of function, greater risk of certain types of disease, and a greater likelihood of death as their chronological age increases" [9]. The Dog Aging Project is conducting research to attempt to assess influences on aging to enhance the period of life spent free of disease or the healthspan, via a longitudinal study of over 41 000 dogs [10].

Clinical Implications of Patient Age

There are numerous implications of patient age for the veterinary clinician. The first relates to managing risk. When making decisions about whether to initiate an intervention for an ill patient, four factors are often considered:

- Likelihood of restoration of a good quality of life
- Pain and side effects
- Estimated quantity of life
- Costs

Sentient animals experience a quality of life that can be assessed as poor, neutral, or good. Since animals cannot comprehend the idea of a future life, an animal's interest relates to present welfare concerns, in other words how the animal "feels." Therefore, if the patient's interest is being prioritized, veterinarians might discount client costs as a factor. This still results in difficult decisions. For example, do the nausea and lethargy related to chemotherapy treatments justify remission of lymphoma?

Most sick humans desire both a good quality and duration of life, as noted by Kuhse and Singer: "When we want to evaluate a treatment's efficacy, we are interested not only in whether a treatment can 'save a life,' but also for *how long* it can save a life, and what the *quality* of that life will be like" [11]. As veterinarians serve both animals and humans, short-term improvements in quality of life may not be enough to satisfy our clients. This concern is heightened by the reality that some clients perceive their decision to pursue treatment as an investment, and a poorer than expected quantity of life may leave animal owners with feelings of buyer's remorse and dissatisfaction.

Consequently, in my experience pet owners are far more likely to approve chemotherapy for lymphoma in dogs (median survival time of 12 months) than for cats (median survival time of 4–5 months). In some cases, despite good intentions, we are unable to provide both quality and quantity of life. I've had the misfortune of having senior patients die or decline within hours or days of receiving chemotherapy, surgery, or pericardiocentesis. My own feelings of doubt over the shared decisions made for these patients were worsened by some clients' sentiments of regret and anger that we pursued an intervention for an aged patient.

One of the consequences of client expectations that the clinician provides both an improved quality of life and an enduring lifespan to justify the cost is that practitioners may not advise diagnostic tests or treatment (and may therefore recommend euthanasia) if the sick patient is believed to be near the end of their natural lifespan. Therefore, a 14-year-old German shepherd dog with a gastric dilatation-volvulus may not have corrective surgery, while a 10-year-old schnauzer with a gall bladder mucocele may be more likely to receive a cholecystectomy, despite good prognoses for both patients. A clinician may be more inclined to persuade a client to pursue diagnosis and treatment for a curable disease in a 2-year-old dog compared to a 15-year-old dog. A veterinarian might consider euthanasia of a young dog to be more morally problematic then ending the life of a dog near the end of its natural lifespan, as the young dog is believed to have not yet lived a full life, while the older dog is perceived to have "had a good life." Pragmatically, a pet owner can acquire a new animal for a fraction of the cost of a life-saving procedure. I knew a colleague who used to ask his clients in these settings, "Do you want this dog, or any dog?"

One of the liabilities of these estimations by veterinarians is that the wide variation in the reported median lifespans of pets makes such decisions uncertain. At what age should we decide that a particular dog or cat is "too old" to intervene? Should we be making these decisions at all? Ideally, such decisions should of course be shared with our clients. We all know of animals who far exceeded these median lifespans, such as cats living to 18–20 years of age. Such considerations can result in discrimination based on age or ageism (see Chapter 4) (Case Study 12.1).

Case Study 12.1 Whether to Perform Testing for a Senior Cat

You see Felix, an 18-year-old cat presented to an emergency service for progressive lethargy and declining appetite. Physical exam reveals thin body condition. Vital signs are stable. You offer diagnostic tests to assess the cause and severity of the problem, starting with blood and urine testing. The owner declines your counsel and brings Felix to her regular veterinarian, who contends that Felix is too old to be helped and that euthanasia is the only humane alternative. The owner accuses you of trying to take advantage of her by offering the testing, since "even I and my vet knew there wasn't any hope." What the regular veterinarian told the pet owner is uncertain, but whatever it was seemed to reinforce the notion that offering non-invasive testing for Felix was immoral or wrong. What should you do? How should this influence your recommendations for senior patients?

Another problem with basing decisions on age is that body condition and co-morbidities should also factor into these decisions. For example, if you are seeing two 12-year-old golden retrievers with the same illness, but one is in good body condition with no other co-existing diseases and the other is obese with co-morbidities, wouldn't you be more likely to intervene on behalf of the former patient? What about when you don't know the age of your patient?

Quality-adjusted life-years (QALY) have been used in human medicine as a measure of distributing care that reflects both lives saved and patients' valuations of quality of life. QALY combines expected survival with expected quality of life in a single metric [12]. Is it morally defensible to have a medical policy that favors younger patients over older ones [11]? Numerous problems arise when considering adapting this concept to veterinary medicine. Veterinary patient preferences cannot be accurately assessed by others, nor is there a valid, commonly utilized metric to assess quality of life for all disease conditions. Such a paradigm violates client autonomy if veterinary clinicians do not offer all available options to their clients. The ethical principle of justice suggests treating "like cases alike," which would not be the case using QALY. Finally, if veterinarians were to systematically deny diagnostics or care to senior patients, not all these animals would have their suffering ended via euthanasia. Do we have the knowledge and resources to provide suitable palliative and hospice care for all these patients?

In a setting of limited financial or physical resources, policies favoring younger patients seem morally appropriate. For example, consider the situation where two dogs from the same family ingest ethylene glycol (which is nephrotoxic), one dog is 2 years old and the other is 10 years old, and there is only a single dialysis machine available; or two dialysis machines are available, but the owner can only afford treatment for one of the dogs. In my experience, seldom do these conditions apply in veterinary medicine. In some circumstances, availability of blood products may be limited, requiring the clinician to decide how to allocate a limited resource. Finally, when relevant, one can argue that investing costs into caring for an older patient may divert limited resources from provision of food or veterinary care to other family pets. Of course, clients rather than the clinician should decide whether this is a valid concern.

Age is not a disease, but it is one of many factors clinicians must consider when making decisions about senior patients. In these circumstances, it would be important for the owner to know that you can likely provide more certainty regarding short-term improvement in quality of life as compared to quantity of life, as none of us can predict the future. You should also provide clients with evidence-based epidemiologic data of survival times associated with select diagnoses and treatments when available.

Clinical Implications of Patient Aging

The fact that pets' lifespans are about one-seventh that of humans has profound implications for veterinarians' clinical approach to patients. The first concern relates to educating our clients, so they understand the need to view their pet's illness from a pet-centric perspective. Countless times in my career, clients justified monitoring sick patients instead of pursuing testing or intervention because "it's only been a few days or a week." From a human-centric perspective, a few days or even a week are indeed considered to be an acute phase of illness. In fact, humans with lower back pain of up to six weeks in duration are considered to have acute disease.

It should be apparent why such a human-centered time frame does not serve our patients well. If we waited for weeks of clinical signs of illness before acting, our patient mortality rates would be near 100%! When I explained the "a day for a pet is really a week for humans" rule to my clients, their response suggested that they had never considered this in making decisions about when to see the veterinarian. If we are not routinely educating our clients that A Day Is Really a Week, we cannot expect them to promptly bring their sick animal companion to the veterinarian.

The other ramification of rapid aging in pets relates to veterinarian recommendations. Veterinary clinicians too often utilize a conservative diagnostic approach (Case Study 12.2) to patients that belies the A Day Is Really a Week principle. This can prolong patient illness and result in poorer prognoses and higher costs when (or if) a diagnosis is made. A one-week duration of illness for our patients is analogous to a one or two-month course of human illness. Consequently, practitioners should view each patient visit as a precious opportunity accompanied by a sense of urgency. We should not assume that a second or third visit will occur. The presumption that clients will reliably return if symptomatic treatment fails does not consider client availability, the stress (for both clients and patients) of travel to the hospital, nor the costs of another visit. "Get it right the first time" should be our motto.

It is quite understandable why our clients may prefer symptomatic treatment to diagnostic testing due to costs. The Principle of Optimizing Patient Outcomes compels the clinician to explain to clients why a more aggressive approach is warranted for sick pets compared to ill humans. The fact that some of our patients have mild disease that is self-limiting and recover without testing does not detract from this argument. Based on the Principle of Patient Advocacy, it is better to inform a client that diagnostic testing of their sick animal companion found no evidence of serious illness (error of commission) than to presume that they will recover spontaneously (error of omission), potentially resulting in underdiagnosis or missed diagnosis (see Chapter 16). The aphorism "hope is not a strategy" also applies to veterinary practice. The rapid aging process in veterinary patients demands an aggressive diagnostic approach by clinicians to mitigate suffering and improve prognoses.

Case Study 12.2 A Conservative Approach to a Sick Dog

You see Milly, a four-year-old female standard poodle, on Monday for lethargy and reduced appetite of one or two days' duration. You advise symptomatic treatment with subcutaneous fluids and an appetite stimulant. You advise Milly's owner that if she is not feeling better in another day or two to return for tests. A callback the next day reveals no change in condition. Milly returns on Friday afternoon collapsed and moribund and is immediately referred to a local internist. She makes a full recovery after two days of intensive care for hypoadrenocorticism.

References

1 Arias, E., Tejada-Vera, B., Kochanek, K.D. et al. (2022). Provisional life expectancy estimates for 2021. Vital Statistics Rapid Release, no. 23. Hyattsville, MD: National Center for Health Statistics. https://doi.org/10.15620/cdc:118999.

2 O'Neill, D.G., Church, D.B., McGreevy, P.D. et al. (2013). Longevity and mortality of owned dogs in England. *Veterinary Journal* 198 (3): 638–643.

3 Lewis, T.W., Wiles, B.M., Llewellyn-Zaidi, A.M. et al. (2018). Longevity and mortality in Kennel Club registered dog breeds in the UK in 2014. *Canine Genetics and Epidemiology* 5 (1): 1–17.

4 Urfer, S.R., Kaeberlein, M., and Promislow, D.E.L. (2020). Lifespan of companion dogs seen in three independent primary care veterinary clinics in the United States. *Canine Medicine and Genetics* 7: 7. https://doi.org/10.1186/s40575-020-00086-8.

5 Teng, K.T.Y., Brodbelt, D.C., Pegram, C. et al. (2022). Life tables of annual life expectancy and mortality for companion dogs in the United Kingdom. *Scientific Reports* 12 (1): 1–11.

6 Harvey, N.D. (2021). How old is my dog? Identification of rational age groupings in pet dogs based upon normative age-linked processes. *Frontiers in Veterinary Science* 8: 643085.

7 O'Neill, D.G., Church, D.B., McGreevy, P.D. et al. (2015). Longevity and mortality of cats attending primary care veterinary practices in England. *Journal of Feline Medicine and Surgery* 17 (2): 125–133.

8 Pegram, C., Gray, C., Packer, R. et al. (2021). Proportion and risk factors for death by euthanasia in dogs in the UK. *Scientific Reports* 11 (1): 1–12.

9 McKenzie, B.A., Chen, F., and LaCroix-Fralish, M.L. (2022). The phenotype of aging in the dog: how aging impacts the health and well-being of dogs and their caregivers. *Journal of the American Veterinary Medical Association* 260 (9): 963–970.

10 Dog Aging Project. https://dogagingproject.org (accessed September 6, 2022).

11 Kuhse, H. and Singer, P. (1992). Allocating health care resources and the problem of the value of life. In: *Death and the Value of Life* (ed. D. Cockburn). Lampeter: Trivium Publications.

12 La Puma, J. and Lawlor, E.F. (1990). Quality-adjusted life-years: ethical implications for physicians and policymakers. *Journal of the American Medical Association* 263 (21): 2917–2921.

13

The Day of the Week Matters

Barry Kipperman

Abstract

This chapter discusses the potential association between the limited availability of advanced veterinary procedures on weekends and poor patient outcomes. Multiple case studies are provided for consideration. While veterinary clinicians cannot control when patients become ill and when clients seek care, they must be aware of the day of the week, the limitations associated with weekend care, and its impacts on patient outcomes when making clinical decisions and obtaining informed consent from clients. A more aggressive diagnostic approach is warranted as the weekend nears due to limited access to specialists.

Keywords: *day of the week, specialists, referral practices, practice hours, availability, weekends, weekend effect*

Although the veterinary profession can offer increasingly sophisticated care to patients, in practice such care is not equitably distributed. Advanced and critical care is usually provided by veterinary specialists, who constitute only about 10% of all veterinarians in the United States [1]. Most specialists work in private referral practices or in teaching hospitals that provide care 24 hours a day. Owners must be able to transport their animal companions to these practices to receive these services. As many of these practices are concentrated in urban and suburban locations, those in rural settings or without a means of transportation may have difficulty accessing such services. As noted in Chapter 8, the quality of veterinary care for patients is also often limited by an owner's capacity and willingness to purchase these resources.

While the impacts of economic limitations on veterinary care and access to care are being discussed in veterinary schools and academic publications [2–5], another limitation to care is seldom discussed or considered. Most private veterinary practices are closed from Friday at 6 p.m. (or from Saturday at noon) until Monday morning. This means that on weekends sick patients are either not seen at all or must be seen by a local emergency hospital. But many specialists such as radiologists, oncologists, surgeons, and internists have limited to no availability on weekends. While ultrasound studies and certain surgeries may be available during this period, the full range of services are not accessible. Decisions affecting patients (and consequently patient outcomes) are quite often influenced by this 60-hour interval of relative inaccessibility of care leading to patient vulnerability.

This chapter will discuss my observations of common practices prompted by this reality, their consequences on patient outcomes, and how we can improve patient outcomes by recognizing that The Day of the Week Matters. Let's consider a few examples (Case Studies 13.1–13.3).

Case Study 13.1 A Sick Dog Seen on Thursday Morning

Winston, a five-year-old male pug, is seen on Thursday morning for acute onset of lethargy. No history of trauma, recent anesthesia, or vomiting is noted. Physical exam reveals low-grade fever. Winston's owner is convinced he is ill and requests an explanation. You advise a minimum database (MDB) of testing (see Chapter 17), which reveals leukocytosis and consolidation of Winston's left cranial lung lobe on radiographs. The radiology report suggests aspiration pneumonia as the most likely cause. As Winston is still eating, you prescribe an antibiotic for pneumonia and advise that Winston should return if he is not significantly improved in 2–3 days' time. Winston returns Saturday morning for dyspnea and anorexia and radiographs now reveal pleural effusion, confirmed via thoracocentesis to be hemorrhage. Options provided to the owner include:

- Euthanasia based on Winston's lack of response to treatment, the uncertain cause, and his declining condition.
- Sending the pleural fluid out to the lab for analysis. Results would not be expected for at least another 48–60 hours as clinical pathology services are limited on weekends. Hemorrhagic fluid often yields inconclusive results.
- Referring Winston to an emergency hospital for supportive care and chest taps as needed until he can see an internal medicine specialist on Monday (which would be the fifth day of his illness).

Differential diagnoses for acute lung lobe consolidation include pneumonia, edema, atelectasis, hemorrhage, contusion, abscess, and torsion. Some of these conditions would be expected to respond to medications and/or time, while others require lobectomy to resolve. A thoracic CT scan would likely identify the etiology. As CT scans (and the qualified personnel to perform them) and thoracic surgery are generally not available on weekends, the plan for Winston's care disregarded the Principle of Optimizing Patient Outcomes by providing a suboptimal safety net if the antibiotic trial failed.

Had Winston presented on a Monday, then a 2–3-day therapeutic trial for pneumonia would have allowed him access to all available resources if he didn't improve. Because he presented on Thursday and The Day of the Week Matters, the clinician in this case should have recognized the limitations to Winston's care posed by the temporal proximity to the weekend and enacted a more aggressive posture. Disclosing to the client the limitations to care (in this case, CT and thoracic surgery) caused by the impending weekend is a compelling component of acquiring informed consent. Although brachycephalic dogs commonly develop aspiration pneumonia, the absence of risk factors in this case should have prompted enough skepticism regarding the radiologist's diagnosis to offer referral for a consultation and/or CT scan on Thursday, the day of presentation.

Young pugs are predisposed to lung lobe torsion [6]. CT scans are diagnostic, and lung lobectomy is curative. Had Winston's torsion been identified on Thursday afternoon, then a corrective lobectomy could have been scheduled for Friday. Rapid referral in this case may have prevented a euthanasia decision, a more prolonged period of illness, and reduced medical costs.

Case Study 13.2   A Sick Dog Seen on Saturday Morning

Charley, an 11-year-old male mastiff, presents on a Saturday morning for acute onset of lethargy and anorexia. Examination is unremarkable. You advise blood work, which reveals leukocytosis and elevated alkaline phosphatase (ALP), and dispense an antibiotic over the weekend for a possible infection. Charley is seen again on Monday for progressive decline. No food intake was noted all weekend. Radiographs reveal a large volume of ascites. Centesis retrieved turbid fluid and Charley is referred for further evaluation. A diagnosis of septic peritonitis is made at the referral hospital and Charley dies during laparotomy to discern the cause.

The most common causes of this presentation include infectious, metabolic, or anatomic (gastrointestinal obstruction, neoplasia) conditions. Once metabolic causes were ruled out by the lab work, it was irrational to assume that prescribing an antibiotic to a senior anorexic patient would provide a good chance of success. It is common for clinicians to perform therapeutic trials (see Chapter 22) with antibiotics, antiemetics, and/or appetite stimulants as the weekend approaches on the premise that, "This will get him [the patient] through the weekend." The recognition of your practice's limited weekend hours should encourage referrals to hospitals providing more comprehensive services during this period, rather than a tendency to conduct therapeutic trials to bridge this gap.

This trial violated the principle that The Day of the Week Matters. At the time of referral on Monday, the owner informed the emergency clinician that she delayed bringing Charley in over the weekend because she wanted to give the medication time to take effect. Clients may be so hopeful that therapy will succeed that they are often reluctant to admit failure of the trial: the patient may decline during this period, often to the point where it becomes too late to help. In some respects, no therapy is better than unsuccessful therapy, as any therapy often leads to delayed recognition of the patient's lack of response. Once the lab work was inconclusive, either imaging or referral for further testing should have been strongly advised.

Case Study 13.3   A Sick Dog Seen on Tuesday

Tippy, a 10-year-old female Dalmatian, is seen by her regular veterinarian on Tuesday for declining appetite of five days' duration. Exam reveals suspicion of an enlarged spleen. Lab testing reveals hypoalbuminemia and moderate anemia (packed cell volume [PCV] = 27%). Imaging is not advised. An antibiotic is dispensed, and the owners are advised to call if she is not significantly improved in 2–3 days' time. A progress report on Thursday reveals no improvement. An ultrasound study is scheduled for Friday afternoon, which reveals a splenic mass and hemoabdomen. Tippy's PCV is now 17%. She is referred for emergency surgery, which reveals metastases. Euthanasia is elected. On receiving an update regarding Tippy's outcome, the referring veterinarian states, "Thanks for the update. I guess the outcome would have been poor even if I had diagnosed this earlier."

Clinicians may be inclined to take a conservative approach when patients are seen early in the week. The practitioner may assume that there is time remaining in the week for rechecks if the patient does not improve. As occurred with Tippy, this often results in prolonged patient suffering and in frequent referrals to specialists on Friday. While this avoids running into the weekend that officially begins at the end of Friday, numerous patient limitations arise with Friday referrals: specialists are usually quite busy and their availability to see patients may be limited. If your patient can be seen as with Tippy, the availability of ancillary specialties (such as radiology and clinical pathology) may also cause delays in diagnosis and treatment (Case Study 13.4). In this case, the ultrasound study should have been performed on Thursday at the time of the progress report, even if referral was necessary, rather than delaying this until Friday afternoon.

Case Study 13.4   A Dog with Lymph Node Enlargement Seen on Tuesday

Posey, a six-year-old female Labrador retriever, is seen on Tuesday for lethargy and declining appetite for 2–3 days. Examination confirms generalized lymphadenopathy. The medical record notes, "Discussed possible lymphoma. Advise antibiotic trial x one week. If lymphoma, nodes will continue to enlarge." Posey returns on Friday for labored breathing. Exam reveals stertor due to markedly enlarged cervical and retropharyngeal lymph nodes compressing her trachea, and Posey is referred to an oncologist. A likely diagnosis of lymphoma is discussed, and the owner wishes to proceed with diagnostic testing followed by chemotherapy. Aspirates from multiple lymph nodes are obtained, but cytology results will not be available until Monday afternoon. Should the oncologist send Posey home until lymphoma is confirmed knowing that labored breathing could worsen? Should they begin chemotherapy treatment immediately assuming a diagnosis of high-grade lymphoma, knowing that the treatment may interfere with acquiring a diagnosis if the results from the aspirates are inconclusive? Ideally, a progress report on Posey should have been scheduled for Thursday; referral at that time would have mitigated the limitations associated with Friday referrals.

In human medicine, the association between weekend healthcare delivery and poor outcomes is known as the "weekend effect." After controlling for patient risk and surgery type, human patients undergoing non-emergency major surgery on the weekends had a significantly increased risk of death and major complications compared with patients undergoing surgery on weekdays [7]. In another human study, postoperative mortality rose as the day of the week of elective surgery approached the weekend, and was higher after admission for emergency surgery on the weekend compared with weekdays [8]. It seems reasonable to presume that comparable outcomes apply in veterinary practice.

In veterinary medicine, while there are many highly qualified and board-certified emergency clinicians working weekends, at many hospitals weekend hours are preferentially staffed by less experienced clinicians and interns, which may also influence patient outcomes. A recent study revealed that the euthanasia rates of dogs with non-traumatic hemoabdomen were significantly higher when they were seen by interns [9]. The authors concluded that euthanasia rates in these patients may be influenced by the experience of the clinician.

While veterinary clinicians cannot control when patients become ill and when clients seek care, they must be aware of the day of the week and the limitations associated with weekend care and its impacts on patient outcomes when making clinical decisions and acquiring informed consent from clients. These detrimental impacts on patient care also likely have pernicious influences on the mental health of the veterinary team caring for patients over the weekend. A more aggressive diagnostic approach or referral is warranted as the weekend nears due to limited access to specialists.

References

1 American Veterinary Medical Association (AVMA) (2020). Veterinary specialists 2020. https://www.avma.org/resources-tools/reports-statistics/veterinary-specialists-2020 (accessed September 11, 2022).

2 Kipperman, B.S., Kass, P.H., and Rishniw, M. (2017). Factors that influence small animal veterinarians' opinions and actions regarding cost of care and effects of economic limitations on patient care and outcome and professional career satisfaction and burnout. *Journal of the American Veterinary Medical Association* 250 (7): 785–794.

3 LaVallee, E., Mueller, M.K., and McCobb, E. (2017). A systematic review of the literature addressing veterinary care for underserved communities. *Journal of Applied Animal Welfare Science* 20 (4): 381–394.

4 Stull, J.W., Shelby, J.A., Bonnett, B.N. et al. (2018). Barriers and next steps to providing a spectrum of effective health care to companion animals. *Journal of the American Veterinary Medical Association* 253 (11): 1386–1389.

5 Kipperman, B., Block, G., and Forsgren, B. (2022). Economic issues. In: *Ethics in Veterinary Practice*, ch. 8 (ed. B. Kipperman and B.E. Rollin). Hoboken, NJ: Wiley-Blackwell.

6 Holmes, A.C., Tivers, M., Humm, K. et al. (2018). Lung lobe torsion in adult and juvenile pugs. *Veterinary Record Case Reports* 6 (3): e000655.

7 Glance, L.G., Osler, T., Li, Y. et al. (2016). Outcomes are worse in US patients undergoing surgery on weekends compared with weekdays. *Medical Care* 54 (6): 608–615.

8 Smith, S.A., Yamamoto, J.M., Roberts, D.J. et al. (2018). Weekend surgical care and postoperative mortality: a systematic review and meta-analysis of cohort studies. *Medical Care* 56 (2): 121.

9 Molitoris, A., Pfaff, A., Cudney, S. et al. (2022). Early career clinicians euthanize more dogs with nontraumatic hemoabdomen but not gastric dilatation and volvulus than more experienced clinicians. *Journal of the American Veterinary Medical Association* 260 (12): 1514–1517.

14

The Time of Day Matters

Barry Kipperman

Abstract

This chapter considers the relationship between the time of day that veterinary procedures are begun and patient outcomes. Multiple case studies are provided for reflection. Indications for applying the Principle of Optimizing Patient Outcomes should be considered by the clinician when evaluating how the time of day may influence patient outcomes. This requires the fortitude to reschedule patient procedures to ensure that the timing reduces risks and enhances benefits. Most veterinary procedures should ideally be performed during the day, and specific, evidence-based criteria should be utilized to justify the potential increased risks to patients and costs to clients from performing procedures after hours.

Keywords: *time of day, procedures, optimizing patient outcomes, postponing, rescheduling, after hours, communication*

At most veterinary practices, scheduled appointments are seen in the morning, patients are admitted to the hospital as warranted, and diagnostic and therapeutic procedures and surgeries are performed in the afternoon. In Chapter 9, one of the "nine rights" for optimizing patient outcomes relates to the time of day that procedures are performed. Ideally, the time of day of procedures should align with other patient rights, including right doctor state of mind, right staff, and right equipment, which may also be influenced by the time of day. For example, I am not a "morning person." My capacity for decision-making improved as the workday progressed. The standard schedule of conducting procedures in the afternoons suited me well, while an emergency ultrasound-guided pericardiocentesis at 7 a.m. did not. Other clinicians may schedule workdays where no appointments are seen and procedures are started in the morning, requiring a different circadian rhythm to be at their best.

In the morning, I often inherited the care of patients from the overnight emergency service. I had to complete these evaluations either before my appointments started at 9 a.m. or between appointments. After evaluating critical patients first, my goal in deciding the sequence of patients to examine was to expeditiously diagnose patients who would benefit from procedures earlier that day rather than later. So, for example, a dyspneic cat with pleural effusion needing thoracocentesis, a weak, large-breed dog with cardiac tamponade needing pericardiocentesis, or a vomiting patient who may need corrective surgery to resolve an obstruction I could confirm via ultrasound would be prioritized. A cat with chronic weight loss or a dog with chronic nasal discharge whose procedures were deemed to be less urgent and could be postponed without compromising prognosis would be seen later. I did my best to avoid a scenario where a delayed diagnosis of a patient who needed a procedure promptly would result in postponement of that procedure to later in the day or to the following day.

As another example, procedures on high-risk patients (liver shunt surgery, thoracotomy, senior patients) should ideally be performed in the morning to give them most of the day to recover from anesthesia and be closely monitored, which may avoid the need for transfer of care between shifts or for overnight care. But an early procedure time may not coincide with the doctor's preferred state of mind or with the preferred experience of the technicians needed to maximize patient survival from the procedures. What if a mobile surgeon cannot arrive to start one of these procedures until 4 p.m.? In these cases, the clinician is often at the mercy of the mobile vet regarding scheduling. This may result in suboptimal patient outcomes.

Let's say you have a dental procedure scheduled for 1 p.m. after lunch on a frail, geriatric cat considered to be a high-risk patient. You schedule all subsequent procedures accordingly. You then find out that the technician you prefer to manage the anesthesia who provides the best chance for a positive outcome will be on her break then. Should you proceed with a less experienced technician/anesthetist? Reschedule this procedure so that this case is started later with the preferred technician? Postpone this elective procedure to another day? Eliminate or postpone the technician's lunch break?

Case Studies 14.1–14.3 highlight considerations associated with the principle that The Time of Day Matters. (See Case Studies 9.8–9.10 for other examples related to the time of day.)

Case Study 14.1   A Cat with Pyometra Diagnosed Late in the Afternoon

Buffy, a two-year-old female intact cat, is referred to you for lethargy. Lab work at the referring veterinary practice reveals leukocytosis and exam confirms fever. You perform an abdominal ultrasound study immediately after this appointment that identifies a pyometra. It is now 4 p.m. You call the referring veterinarian (RDVM) to discuss this diagnosis and the treatment options. You suggest having your board-certified surgeon perform ovariohysterectomy at 5 p.m. and keeping Buffy overnight for supportive care and pain management. The RDVM requests that you have the client and Buffy return to his practice, where he will perform the surgery before closing time and send her right back to your hospital for overnight care. You believe that this plan will be more stressful for Buffy and the client due to the need for two more trips, but this may save the client costs by having a general practitioner perform the surgery instead of a specialist. This plan also pleases an important source of your income.

Should you accept this plan and advise that the client return to their regular practice? Should you dispute this suggestion and argue for keeping Buffy at your practice? Should you inform the client of the two available options including costs and let them choose which one they prefer? Might such full disclosure upset your colleague?

If we consider the indications for applying the Principle of Optimizing Patient Outcomes in Table 9.1 to this case, the drawbacks of proceeding with the suggested plan include that the client may complain if they learn that the surgery could have been performed at the referral hospital and this was not disclosed, which may result in a negative perception of the profession; or that client distress may be caused by the need to continue transporting Buffy. It seems unlikely that team members would develop moral stress or that the patient would endure prolonged pain, suffering, or an increased risk of mortality because of the decision suggested by the RDVM. If the RDVM rushes the surgery to be able to complete it before closing time, this could have negative implications for Buffy's outcome (but the specialist surgeon may be subject to the same concern at the end of their workday even when their hospital doesn't close). Ideally, the specialist and RDVM would agree to be as transparent as possible entailing full disclosure and leave the decision in the hands of the client.

Case Study 14.2   A CT Scan Performed at Night

You refer Dolly, a stable, eupneic 12-year-old beagle with a solitary pulmonary mass, coughing, and normal lab results, to a surgeon at another practice for a CT scan for preoperative screening for local metastases. A morning appointment is scheduled. You receive a phone call from the surgeon at 8:00 p.m. informing you that Dolly died under anesthesia. On further inquiry, the surgeon states that the anesthesia and CT scan were started at 7:30 p.m. When you ask why the procedure was started so late in the evening and whether this was a typical time for performing CTs at their practice, the surgeon states, "Do you know how many cases I've seen today? I performed four major surgeries and stayed late to get this CT and lobectomy done. I'm sorry about the outcome, but you should be thankful I got it done."

As you also work in referral practice, you are aware that CT scans are considered an advanced imaging procedure that requires a high level of proficiency from the anesthetist or technician supervising the patient, as thoracic scans require that patients hold their breath during the scan. You also know that this procedure is usually completed during daytime hours, and that most technicians responsible for performing CT scans end their workdays at 5–6 p.m. You wonder if a technician with less or no experience with thoracic CTs was entrusted with your patient given the delayed start time. You also question whether the surgeon was in the proper state of mind to supervise the procedure given the nature of the discussion. You are troubled by doubts as to whether these factors may have contributed to Dolly's negative outcome. Should you press this concern further and request that a systematic investigation be conducted to determine the cause of Dolly's death (see Chapter 10) and jeopardize your relationship with a colleague? Should you disclose your concerns to Dolly's owner or to the veterinary medical board?

If we consider the indications for applying the Principle of Optimizing Patient Outcomes, the drawbacks of the instituted plan included prolonged patient pain or suffering; patient fatality; client distress; client complaint or malpractice suit; moral stress for the team; and poor reputation for the profession. Given the circumstances in this case, it is difficult to justify performing this non-emergency CT study and lung lobectomy after hours when the attending doctor had had a difficult day with many procedures.

At many referral practices, cases considered to be emergencies (gastric dilatation-volvulus [GDV], non-traumatic hemoabdomen, pyometra) may undergo surgery after hours. In many of these cases, a surgeon who worked all day is disturbed from sleep, comes into the hospital to perform a high-risk procedure, and then may have to work the following day. It seems logical that such conditions may result in poorer patient outcomes compared to the same operations performed during the day. In one study of human patient outcomes related to daytime versus after-hours surgery, after-hours surgery was associated with significantly increased postoperative mortality and morbidity, which might be related to the critical nature of these patients, availability of resources, and/or fatigue factor of the personnel [1]. A recent study adjusting for case acuity in human patients concluded that night surgery (5 p.m.–7 a.m.) was associated with an increased risk of postoperative mortality and morbidity [2].

Time-honored assumptions regarding which conditions require emergency care in veterinary medicine are being challenged, to some extent because of the financial burdens associated with emergency procedures (there are usually additional fees) and the potential for economic euthanasia. A recent study found no difference in mortality rates in dogs with GDV who had surgery a mean of 22 hours after presentation and gastric decompression compared with those who had surgery at the time of decompression [3], and multiple reports found good outcomes in cases of pyometra when patients were operated on the day after presentation [4, 5]. Veterinary procedures should ideally be performed during the day and specific, evidence-based criteria should be utilized to justify the potential increased risks to patients and costs to clients from performing procedures after hours (Case Study 14.3).

Case Study 14.3   Whether to Perform a Liver Biopsy on a Cat Late in the Afternoon

You see Gordon, a two-year-old cat, for one week of lethargy and anorexia. Physical exam reveals jaundice and lab work shows moderately elevated liver enzymes and bilirubin. You advise liver biopsies to best determine the cause of the problem, and discuss the costs, pros, and cons of referral for laparoscopic biopsies versus ultrasound-guided biopsies, which can be done at your practice. The client approves the ultrasound-guided biopsies. The mobile radiologist provides a window for arrival between 1 and 4 p.m. and arrives at 4 p.m. The ultrasound study suggests that hepatic biopsies are indicated. You call the owner to discuss the results of the ultrasound and the sedation and biopsy procedure is approved. It is now 5 p.m.

You realize hemorrhage is a potential side effect of the procedure. A study found 57% of cats had significant bleeding associated with percutaneous ultrasound-guided liver biopsies [6]. You wonder if it is wise to proceed with the biopsies as the hospital closes at 6 p.m., which limits your capacity to monitor Gordon after the procedure. You could proceed with the biopsies and hope that internal bleeding does not occur and send Gordon home for further observation. You could call the owner to request she transfer Gordon's care to an emergency hospital for monitoring, but these costs were not factored in to your original estimate, and this may prompt doubt in the owner's mind about the starting time of the procedure. You could postpone the biopsies, but the radiologist may charge another fee for a second visit, and this may disappoint Gordon's owner. What should you do?

If we consider the indications for applying the Principle of Optimizing Patient Outcomes, the risks of internal bleeding after the biopsy procedure are significant. This could result in patient fatality or suffering; increased client costs; client distress or complaints (especially if they must bring Gordon to an emergency hospital for weakness or collapse); moral stress for the team; and disgrace for the profession. Given these factors, it is difficult to justify starting Gordon's non-emergency percutaneous ultrasound-guided liver biopsy procedure at 5 p.m. The degree of owner dissatisfaction would likely be much higher if a major complication arose that endangered Gordon's life compared to rescheduling the biopsy procedure.

The advantages of delaying or rescheduling select procedures to optimize patient outcomes are peace of mind, reduced stress levels for you and your staff, and possibly reduced overtime costs for staff who may be asked to work late. Drawbacks are primarily related to client communication. Having been in this position many times in my career, I can attest that clients are apt to express their disappointment. While honesty is an inherent aspect of ethical behavior, it is not necessary to tell your client "I scheduled too many procedures" or "The radiologist showed up late." While honesty is usually laudable, in these circumstances this level of candor is likely to discredit you, your practice, and the profession, and will probably exacerbate client dismay with the decision to postpone or reschedule.

In these situations, it is quite reasonable to explain to clients the negative implications of starting a procedure in proximity to the closing time of the hospital. Hospital hours are commonly displayed on websites and the front doors of many practices. Even in settings where the hospital does not close, you can explain that unanticipated circumstances arose that were beyond your control, and you believe that delaying the procedure is in their animal's best interest. While clients often complain that they are being inconvenienced and that their companion missed a meal while fasting, remind them that "Unlike a blood test, we only want to do this procedure once and I want to ensure that (animal name) has the best chance of a successful outcome." Most clients will understand if the cause of the postponement is related to patient emergencies that disrupted your schedule, and many have told me, "Of course, if my animal had an emergency, I'd want her care to be prioritized."

Because the workdays of veterinary clinicians are often prolonged due to unexpected visits and/or emergencies, rescheduling the start time of procedures to adhere to the Principle of Optimizing Patient Outcomes is sometimes required to fulfill your role as patient advocate. A reconsideration of which conditions mandate care after hours to achieve positive outcomes is being prompted by novel studies that should inform such decisions.

References

1 Yang, N., Elmatite, W.M., Elgallad, A. et al. (2019). Patient outcomes related to the daytime versus after-hours surgery: a meta-analysis. *Journal of Clinical Anesthesia* 54: 13–18.

2 Althoff, F.C., Wachtendorf, L.J., Rostin, P. et al. (2021). Effects of night surgery on postoperative mortality and morbidity: a multicentre cohort study. *BMJ Quality and Safety* 30 (8): 678–688.

3 White, R.S., Sartor, A.J., and Bergman, P.J. (2021). Evaluation of a staged technique of immediate decompressive and delayed surgical treatment for gastric dilatation-volvulus in dogs. *Journal of the American Veterinary Medical Association* 258 (1): 72–79.

4 McCallin, A.J., Hough, V.A., and Kreisler, R.E. (2021). Pyometra management practices in the high quality, high volume spay-neuter environment. *Topics in Companion Animal Medicine* 42: 100499.

5 McCobb, E., Dowling-Guyer, S., Pailler, S. et al. (2022). Surgery in a veterinary outpatient community medicine setting has a good outcome for dogs with pyometra. *Journal of the American Veterinary Medical Association* 260 (S2): S36–S41.

6 Pavlick, M., Webster, C.R., and Penninck, D.G. (2019). Bleeding risk and complications associated with percutaneous ultrasound-guided liver biopsy in cats. *Journal of Feline Medicine and Surgery* 21 (6): 529–536.

15

Serial Monitoring of Laboratory Results

Barry Kipperman

Abstract

There are compelling medical reasons why veterinary clinicians should be routinely performing laboratory testing in at-risk asymptomatic patients, and serially monitoring laboratory data in asymptomatic and symptomatic patients with chronic diseases. Yet evidence suggests poor compliance with these evidence-based practices. Possible reasons for insufficient patient testing and monitoring include inadequate understanding of the health benefits to patients, lack of time, poor communication skills to elicit client compliance, and costs. This chapter discusses the importance of interpreting acquired data serially (evaluating multiple sets of data) to improve capacity to diagnose patients in the earliest phases of disease and improve health outcomes.

Keywords: *trends, laboratory testing, compliance, monitoring, asymptomatic, symptomatic, chronic disease, serial trends, spreadsheets*

Veterinary practitioners routinely acquire data including patient weights (see Chapter 11) and laboratory test results that provide valuable information about patient health. This chapter discusses the indications for performing laboratory testing in at-risk asymptomatic patients and in patients with chronic disease, and why it is important to interpret patient data serially (evaluating multiple sets of data) to improve capacity to diagnose patients in the earliest phases of disease and optimize patient outcomes.

Rationale for Performing Testing in Asymptomatic Patients

Patients are often presented to veterinarians in advanced stages of illness, such as senior cats with chronic renal failure and severe azotemia. Clients in these settings often ask us: "Is there something that could have been done to identify this earlier?" In order not to magnify any sense of guilt, we may reply that animals are adept at hiding their symptoms in early stages of illness. It is precisely for this reason that laboratory testing in at-risk asymptomatic patients is warranted. The American Association of Feline Practitioners feline senior care guidelines advise performing baseline diagnostics at least annually starting at 7–10 years of age, with frequency increasing with age [1].

The American Animal Hospital Association (AAHA) Senior Care Guidelines [2] advise laboratory testing (see Chapter 17) for senior patients (defined as dogs in the last 25% of their predicted lifespan and cats greater than 10 years old) every 6–12 months.

Even the routine utilization of laboratory testing has limitations to identifying metabolic diseases early. Consider chronic kidney disease (CKD), where inadequate urine concentrating ability reflects 66% loss of functioning nephrons, and azotemia reflects 75% loss of function [3]. The symmetric dimethylarginine (SDMA) blood test provides better sensitivity, increasing when only 40% of function has been lost [4]. In my experience, when clinicians perform testing in both asymptomatic and ill patients, urine acquisition is uncommon. This is unfortunate, as loss of concentrating ability may be an early sign of CKD, and proteinuria is often associated with hypertension and CKD and is associated with progression of CKD [5].

As clients may not understand the value in performing testing on an animal companion who they perceive to be normal, it is imperative that we be able to articulate why this is necessary to enhance compliance. The basis for justifying testing in at-risk asymptomatic patients is twofold: it establishes a baseline of normal data that facilitates detection of subtle changes that may indicate disease in the future; and when we can diagnose disease before symptoms arise, our ability to slow progression of disease, provide effective treatment, and prolong lifespan is enhanced. With my clients I use the example of blood pressure in humans, which is commonly measured at physician visits because hypertension can lead to strokes and other undesirable sequelae without overt symptoms.

Waiting until our patients are ill to perform testing often results in high rates of diagnoses and poor patient prognoses due to advanced stages of illness. Routinely performing testing in at-risk asymptomatic patients will result in lower diagnostic rates and improved capacity to intervene earlier when disease is identified. Client compliance and satisfaction with testing of asymptomatic patients are dependent on the initiative and communication skills of the practitioner.

Compliance with Testing Asymptomatic Patients

In a study of medical records of over 353 000 cats attending 244 primary care clinics in the United Kingdom, only 11% of diagnoses of CKD were made following a routine geriatric health check [6]. Cats were most commonly diagnosed with CKD following presentation due to clinical signs compatible with CKD. The authors concluded, "The limited proportion of cats diagnosed following a health check suggests that these are not carried out routinely, indicating there may be many older cats that have undiagnosed subclinical CKD."

In a study evaluating medical record confirmation of blood pressure assessments in cats, only 4% of cats nine years of age and older had their blood pressure measured [7]. Presentation with clinical signs compatible with hypertension was the most common reason for a cat to have its blood pressure assessed. The authors noted, "Blood pressure measurement is not commonly used to screen cats known to be at risk of developing hypertension (e.g. the aging cat, those with CKD, and those with hyperthyroidism)." A recent survey found that 81% of Canadian veterinarians did not routinely recommend blood pressure evaluation during senior feline wellness examinations [8]. The American College of Veterinary Internal Medicine consensus statement on systemic hypertension suggests annual screening of blood pressure in dogs and cats nine years of age and older [5] and the AAHA Senior Care Guidelines [2] recommend annual blood pressure screening of all senior cats and dogs.

Rationale for Recognizing Serial Trends in Laboratory Results

When interpreting laboratory test results during a busy day, rather than evaluate each result individually, to save time clinicians may instead look for any results flagged by the laboratory to be either above or below reference intervals. The problem with this approach is that for some patients, results designated as abnormal may be normal for that patient, while other patients can have important changes in results that still lie within the reference range and may therefore go unidentified by the clinician.

Examples of patients whose results may be flagged as abnormal but may be normal include elevated packed cell volume (PCV) in greyhounds, low mean corpuscular volume (MCV) in Akitas, high MCV in poodles, and low platelet counts in cavalier King Charles spaniels. Evaluation of serial trends in these patients over time may reveal persistently abnormal values of these analytes, suggesting these are unlikely causes for concern as dangers to patient health.

Examples of patients where results deemed to be normal by the lab may instead be abnormal for the patient include a PCV at the low end of the reference interval in a dehydrated patient (where we would expect hemoconcentration) or in a greyhound; a potassium value at the low end of the reference range in a patient with diabetic ketoacidosis, metabolic acidosis, and severe hyperglycemia (which should elevate extracellular potassium); or a high–normal T4 value in a cat ill with CKD (which should cause a low T4). Evaluation of serial trends in these patients may also allow earlier recognition of a problem.

As with changes in body weight, test results in some patients may seem innocuous when evaluated alone, but trends may suggest a more concerning pattern. One of the best ways to improve diagnostic sensitivity is by interpreting test results in a serial fashion, evaluating the latest results in comparison with prior results (Case Studies 15.1–15.2). Many electronic lab reports provide serial results to facilitate more complete evaluations.

Case Study 15.1 A Dog with a Declining Packed Cell Volume

Gertie is a 12-year-old female golden retriever. Annual lab work has been performed for the past three years and was interpreted to be normal. She presents in August for vague signs of illness. Lab work revealed a PCV of 38%, and all other results were normal. She was discharged on a non-steroidal anti-inflammatory drug (NSAID) for possible arthritis. One month later, Gertie presents for lethargy and anorexia and is referred. Lab testing reveals anemia (PCV of 32%). Abdominal ultrasound reveals a splenic mass with metastases. Serial evaluation of Gertie's lab testing from one and two years ago reveals a PCV of 51% and 55%, respectively. Had Gertie's veterinarian recognized that a "normal" PCV for her was 51–55%, then the decline to 38% in August would have been more likely to be interpreted as problematic, despite this being identified as normal by the lab's reference range. The earlier recognition of anemia might have allowed diagnosis of the mass before metastases occurred.

Case Study 15.2   A Dog with a Declining Albumin

Rocky is a 10-year-old cocker spaniel. Routine geriatric lab work reveals moderately elevated liver enzymes and an albumin of 3.2 g/dl. Bile acids testing is normal. As Rocky is asymptomatic, no further action is taken. One year later, liver enzymes are still elevated, and the albumin is now 2.5 g/dl, which is within the low end of the lab's reference interval. Rocky is still asymptomatic, and no action is taken. Three months later, Rocky presents for anorexia and abdominal distension. Ascites is confirmed and Rocky is referred. Abdominal ultrasound reveals diffusely coarse liver architecture. The albumin is now 1.4 g/dl, bile acids are elevated, and liver biopsies confirm end-stage hepatic cirrhosis. Treatment is initiated with a poor prognosis.

Had Rocky's veterinarian serially evaluated test results, the decline in albumin from 3.2 to 2.5 g/dl would have been recognized as a potential harbinger of hepatic failure, as albumin is an indicator of synthetic liver function. A bile acids test could have been advised to address this concern, or another chemistry panel could have been advised in one month to reevaluate the liver enzymes and albumin. Earlier recognition of hepatic failure might have allowed treatment to be initiated sooner, resulting in a better prognosis for Rocky.

Discussion of Serial Trends with Clients

Once a clinician appreciates the value of serial monitoring of patient trends in laboratory data, it should be easier to convince your clients to pursue testing in at-risk asymptomatic patients. Once a concerning trend in patient data is recognized, it is logical that a clinician would discuss this with the client. Yet in a recent study of over 900 recorded veterinary visits, fewer than 10% of visits included a discussion of any health parameter trend [9]. Lack of time was a reported barrier. The majority of health parameter trends discussed were focused on body weight (74%), followed by blood work (20%). These results suggest either that veterinarians are not commonly performing routine lab work, are not evaluating and acknowledging trends in laboratory data over time, or do not discuss recognized trends with their clients.

Rationale for Serial Monitoring of Patients with Chronic Disease

The more lab work that veterinary clinicians perform in at-risk patients, the more often diagnoses of chronic diseases will be made. While in some cases this recognition will not require any action be taken, in many cases serial monitoring of these patients is indicated, either to assess the effects of an intervention or to decide when to intervene to slow disease progression and prevent clinical signs of illness. Examples would include the use of medication to control hypertension, to prevent progressive proteinuria, or to lower thyroid hormone concentration in feline hyperthyroidism. Serial monitoring of patients with chronic disease often entails evaluating the organ of origin of the disease (the kidney in CKD, the thyroid in hyperthyroidism), but also any detrimental effects on other organs (renal disease from diuretics treating congestive heart failure [CHF], cytopenias from treating hyperthyroidism).

Examples of common diseases requiring serial monitoring and monitoring parameters are outlined in Table 15.1. Clinicians should ideally create a suitable spreadsheet displaying serial results of relevant data in the medical record. Examples of spreadsheets for monitoring patients with common diseases are found in Tables 15.2–15.4.

Table 15.1 Common diseases requiring serial monitoring in veterinary medicine and monitoring parameters.

Disease	Monitoring parameters
Weight gain/loss	Weight, clinical signs
Diabetes mellitus	Weight, serial glucose, clinical signs
Hyperthyroidism	Weight, T4, BUN, creat, CBC, clinical signs
Chronic kidney disease	Weight, BUN, creat, PO_4, BP, proteinuria, PCV, K, HCO_3, clinical signs
Proteinuria	Weight, BP, UPC, BUN, creat, PCV
Hypertension	BP, BUN, creat, UPC, clinical signs
Anemia	Weight, PCV, MCV, MCHC, BP, clinical signs
Congestive heart failure	Weight, BUN, creat, clinical signs
Protein-losing enteropathy	Weight, alb, vit B_{12}, ascites/edema, clinical signs
Hypoadrenocorticism	Weight, Na, K $\pm$ glucose, alb, Ca, clinical signs

Alb, albumin; BP, blood pressure; BUN, blood urea nitrogen; Ca, calcium; CBC, complete blood count; creat, creatinine; HCO_3, bicarbonate; K, potassium; MCHC, mean corpuscular hemoglobin concentration; MCV, mean corpuscular volume; Na, sodium; PCV, packed cell volume; PO_4, phosphate; T4, thyroid hormone; UPC, urine protein–creatinine ratio; vit B_{12}, cobalamine.

Table 15.2 Spreadsheet for a cat with chronic kidney disease, hypertension, and proteinuria.

Date	Telmisartan dose (mg/d)	Weight	BP	PCV	BUN	Creat	PO_4	HCO_3	K	UPC
February 2022	None	10.0	200	25	50	2.6	6.6	12	3.5	1.2
February 2022	10	10.2	160	–	–	–	–	–	–	–
March 2022	10	10.2	140	24	40	2.4	6.2	14	3.6	0.8

BP, blood pressure; BUN, blood urea nitrogen; creat, creatinine; HCO_3, bicarbonate; K, potassium; PCV, packed cell volume; PO_4, phosphate; UPC, urine protein–creatinine ratio.

Table 15.3 Spreadsheet for a dog with congestive heart failure.

Date	Furosemide dose (mg/d)	Enalapril dose (mg/d)	BUN	Creatinine
September 2022	None	None	22	0.8
September 2022	12.5	2.5	28	1.0
October 2022	25	2.5	62	2.8
October 2022	18.75	2.5	48	2.2

BUN, blood urea nitrogen.

Table 15.4 Spreadsheet for a dog with epilepsy.

Date	Phenobarbital dose	Phenobarbital level (ug/ml)	Seizures (wk)	ALT	ALP	Albumin	Bilirubin	Bile acids
October 2022	–	–	2–4	100	50	3.0	0.1	–
October 2022	0.5 g BID	22	1–2	–	–	–	–	–
November 2022	0.5 g BID	25	0	120	70	2.9	0.1	10

ALP, alkaline phosphatase; ALT, alanine aminotransferase; BID, twice a day.

Compliance with Serial Monitoring of Patients with Chronic Disease

Despite medically compelling reasons to perform serial monitoring of patients with chronic disease, evidence suggests there is ample room for improvement. In a report evaluating monitoring of hyperthyroid cats, 29% of veterinarians did not measure renal parameters routinely after initiating treatment, despite evidence that treatment can worsen renal function, and only 47% stated that they routinely measure a complete blood count (CBC) in the early stages of management, despite evidence that anti-thyroid therapy can cause life-threatening cytopenias [10].

In another study of veterinary records confirming a diagnosis of feline hypertension, the median number of blood pressure measurements after diagnosis was one, and the urine protein/creatinine ratio (UPC) was measured in a minority of cats, despite the association between both UPC at diagnosis and the time-averaged UPC after treatment and survival after hypertension diagnosis [7]. The authors concluded, "Blood pressure monitoring of cats after diagnosis was limited, which may mean that control of blood pressure was inadequate in some cats and did not result in a decrease in blood pressure that would decrease the cat's risk of TOD [target organ damage]." As cats with hypertension diagnosed before associated clinical signs occur have improved survival, as do cats that have regular blood pressure monitoring after diagnosis and institution of treatment, these care patterns do not align with evidence-based practices [7].

One more investigation of records confirming CKD in cats found that repeated biochemistry was carried out in only 33% of cats, blood pressure measured in 26%, and UPC measured in 14% of cases [6]. These studies documenting limited laboratory monitoring after diagnoses reflect my experience reviewing the medical records of referring veterinarians.

Conclusion

There are compelling medical reasons why veterinary clinicians should be performing laboratory testing in at-risk asymptomatic patients, and for serial monitoring of laboratory results in asymptomatic and symptomatic patients with chronic diseases. Yet evidence suggests poor compliance with these evidence-based practices, resulting in underdiagnosis. Possible reasons for insufficient patient testing and monitoring include inadequate understanding of the health benefits to patients, lack of time, poor communication skills to elicit client compliance, and costs. While economic limitations may result in the need to compromise preferred patient monitoring, these can often be surmounted by the conviction of the practitioner that such measures are needed and the capacity to convey this to clients. Improving veterinarian compliance with these practices would not only improve patient health outcomes, but would also have economic benefits for the practitioner.

References

1 Ray, M., Carney, H.C., Boynton, B. et al. (2021). AAFP Feline Senior Care Guidelines. *Journal of Feline Medicine and Surgery* 23 (7): 613–638.
2 Dhaliwal, R., Boynton, E., Carrera-Justiz, S. et al. (2023). AAHA Senior Care Guidelines for Dogs and Cats. https://www.aaha.org/globalassets/02-guidelines/2023-aaha-senior-care-guidelines-for-dogs-and-cats/resources/2023-aaha-senior-care-guidelines-for-dogs-and-cats.pdf (accessed January 20, 2023).

3 Brown, S.A., Crowell, W.A., Brown, C.A. et al. (1997). Pathophysiology and management of progressive renal disease. *Veterinary Journal* 154 (2): 93–109.

4 Idexx (n.d). Why include SDMA? https://www.idexx.com/en/veterinary/reference-laboratories/sdma/why-sdma-matters (accessed September 19, 2022).

5 Acierno, M.J., Brown, S., Coleman, A.E. et al. (2018). ACVIM consensus statement: Guidelines for the identification, evaluation, and management of systemic hypertension in dogs and cats. *Journal of Veterinary Internal Medicine* 32 (6): 1803–1822. https://doi.org/10.1111/jvim.15331.

6 Conroy, M., Brodbelt, D.C., O'Neill, D. et al. (2019). Chronic kidney disease in cats attending primary care practice in the UK: a VetCompass™ study. *Veterinary Record* 184 (17): 526.

7 Conroy, M., Chang, Y.M., Brodbelt, D. et al. (2018). Survival after diagnosis of hypertension in cats attending primary care practice in the United Kingdom. *Journal of Veterinary Internal Medicine* 32 (6): 1846–1855.

8 Prost, K. (2023). Under pressure: a survey of Canadian veterinarians in the diagnosis and treatment of feline hypertension. *Canadian Veterinary Journal* 64 (1): 45–53.

9 Janke, N., Coe, J.B., Bernardo, T.M. et al. (2022). Use of health parameter trends to communicate pet health information in companion animal practice: a mixed methods analysis. *Veterinary Record* 190 (7): e1378. https://doi.org/10.1002/vetr.1378.

10 Higgs, P., Murray, J.K., and Hibbert, A. (2014). Medical management and monitoring of the hyperthyroid cat: a survey of UK general practitioners. *Journal of Feline Medicine and Surgery* 16 (10): 788–795.

16

Overdiagnosis and Useful Diagnosis
Barry Kipperman

Abstract

This chapter considers *overdiagnosis*, which causes more harm than good for patients. Causes and consequences of overdiagnosis are discussed. Case studies are provided to illustrate clinical overdiagnoses. Diagnoses that result in more benefits than harms to patients or clients are *useful diagnoses*. Criteria for useful diagnoses include (i) testing will influence the diagnostic plan; (ii) testing will influence the prognosis; (iii) testing will influence the treatment; or (iv) testing will influence the animal owner's decision. Examples are provided for each of these goals. The Veterinary Ethics Tool is presented as a framework to facilitate clinical decision-making and reach useful diagnoses.

Keywords: *overdiagnosis, useful diagnosis, harms, overtreatment, diagnostic plan, prognosis, therapy, Veterinary Ethics Tool, criteria*

Definitions

In Chapter 15, evidence was cited suggesting that veterinary clinicians do not perform testing of asymptomatic at-risk patients or patients with chronic disease often enough to comply with clinical practice guidelines. An important consequence of undertesting is *underdiagnosis or missed diagnosis*, in which patients with harmful or potentially harmful disease states do not have the disease(s) detected. This is distinct from *misdiagnosis*, the incorrect attribution of a disease. *Delayed diagnosis* occurs when a diagnosis is delayed even though sufficient information was available [1]. Underdiagnosis and delayed diagnosis can result in numerous patient harms, including suffering and premature death.

Some practitioners may instead conduct too many tests on patients, which can be equally problematic. *Overdiagnosis* refers to conditions where the correct identification of disease or its subsequent treatment causes patients more harm than good [2]. Overdiagnosis has been defined as "The detection and diagnosis of a condition that would not go on to cause symptoms or death in the patient's lifetime" [3].

Causes of Overdiagnosis

One possible cause of overdiagnosis is the "cool or novelty factor." This refers to a natural propensity to want to use newly acquired skills, equipment, or treatments, or a desire to make uncommon diagnoses. I can attest that after completing laparoscopy training and purchasing the requisite

Decision-Making in Veterinary Practice, First Edition. Barry Kipperman.

equipment, I may have been biased in my advice to clients to pursue biopsies via this method. After acquiring a continuous glucose monitoring system for the practice, I may have advised more glucose monitoring in my diabetic patients. In a geriatric cat with severe hypokalemia and an adrenal gland mass, I advised aldosterone testing even if the rare diagnosis of an aldosterone-secreting tumor could have been strongly inferred without this. Having the documentation of the elevated aldosterone level also enhanced my capacity to use the case for teaching purposes.

Another reason for overdiagnosis may be tied to our identity and self-esteem. Simply put, diagnosis is "what we do." In school, we are trained to translate patient symptoms into clinical diagnoses. For many clinicians, making diagnoses provides us with a sense of purpose and becomes our raison d'être. In the early period of my career, I viewed my patients as metaphorical puzzles and perceived my role as problem solver. Many of my clients implored me to "find the problem." It has been asserted that the identity of the veterinarian is tied to perfectionism and omniscience [4]. We may receive greater satisfaction from doing something compared to doing nothing (i.e. commission bias). In fact, we may perceive that our clients prefer action over inaction.

Consequently, when we identify a mass or a tumor in a patient, a natural inclination is to sample it via an incisional biopsy or aspirates. Some inexperienced clinicians may not recognize that the implications of making certain diagnoses may cause harm. For example, you may diagnose a large hepatic tumor in an older, asymptomatic small dog and consult your staff surgeon, who encourages you to advise hepatectomy. Severe hemorrhage occurs during the procedure and your patient dies. Your intentions were good, but you learned that this procedure in this subset of patients carries risk of mortality.

Some clinicians may order tests so as to be perceived by clients as thorough or competent or to defend themselves against concerns of malpractice. Specialists may feel compelled to perform testing if a patient was referred for that reason (i.e. for an endoscopy), to meet the expectations of the referring veterinarian. In the future, artificial intelligence algorithms may enhance diagnostic sensitivity and contribute to overdiagnosis [5].

Finally, economic incentives may influence clinician decisions to pursue testing and diagnoses. This tendency is promoted by marketing efforts from commercial laboratories that encourage testing. Diagnostic testing is a profit center for many practices [6] and an employer may expect you to perform a new assay purchased by the practice to justify its acquisition. In addition, the compensation of many clinicians is tied to their revenue production [7].

Consequences of Overdiagnosis

Overdiagnosis is one of the most harmful and costly problems in human healthcare [8]. The consequences of overdiagnosis include overtreatment, financial harms, and psychological harms [9]. Overtreatment is "the application of therapeutic interventions that provide no net benefit or do more harm than good for patients" [3] and refers to treatment that is unnecessary. Overtreatment may cause or prolong patient suffering and result in premature death. Overdiagnosis and overtreatment cause unnecessary costs for clients, which is burdensome and may cause misallocation of resources that are better spent on necessary care or on other animal companions, or conserved.

Clients may perceive being exploited by the clinician through overdiagnosis and overtreatment, which can irrevocably result in loss of trust. Overdiagnosis may cause clients emotional harm due to the stigma associated with a loved one "having a disease." For example, the disclosure of a heart murmur in an asymptomatic 14-year-old dog may cause clients to worry more than is warranted by the diagnosis of heart disease. Overtreatment causes emotional burdens for animal caretakers [10] and emotional exhaustion may lead to unwarranted euthanasia decisions.

Examples of Overdiagnosis in Human Medicine

The most controversial practices involving medical conditions of humans that may elicit overdiagnoses include routine prostate-specific antigen (PSA) screening for prostate cancer in men [11] and mammogram screening for breast cancer in women [12]. PSA screening in asymptomatic men does not affect the number of deaths from prostate cancer [9] and subjects many patients to unneeded biopsies. As a result, measures to curtail routine PSA testing in certain populations have been proposed [13]. In a review of overdiagnosis, imaging tests for cancer screening were the most common type [14].

Examples of Overdiagnosis in Veterinary Medicine

McKenzie [2] questions whether the routine pre-anesthetic screening of healthy, asymptomatic patients results in more benefits than harms. Innovation in genetics now allows for screening of the presence of 30 different cancers via a blood test detecting cell-free DNA known as "liquid biopsies" [15]. Results are reported as cancer signal detected or not detected [16]. This test does not identify the location or type of cancer (in most cases). While there may be significant benefits to detecting cancer before clinical signs arise, it is conceivable that the widespread utilization of this technology in veterinary patients may also result in overdiagnosis and overtreatment.

Case Studies 16.1–16.10 provide examples of overdiagnosis and serve as a reminder that "just because we can doesn't mean we should."

Case Study 16.1 Routine Ultrasound Screening of Geriatric Large-Breed Dogs

Given the frequency with which you diagnose splenic and liver cancers in advanced stages in older large-breed dogs, you decide to offer routine ultrasound screening in these asymptomatic patients in conjunction with their annual lab work. Your rationale is that ultrasound is non-invasive and may discover these tumors at an earlier stage, which may optimize patient outcomes. But this information also leads to difficult decisions: Should all patients with incidentally discovered hepatic or splenic masses have surgery to remove them?

One of the unanticipated consequences of this new practice is that you are diagnosing adrenal gland tumors in 5% of these patients. This has resulted in additional testing, including hormonal assays, electrocardiograms (EKGs), blood pressure measurements, and CT scans in some of these cases. Incidentally discovered adrenal masses or "incidentalomas" [17] create challenging decisions for the clinician. It can be difficult to classify whether these tumors are functional or non-functional and whether they are benign or malignant. While adrenalectomy is the treatment of choice, mortality rates are 0–22% and frequent intraoperative and postoperative complications occur [18].

Currently there are no standard, evidence-based recommendations to guide the treatment of incidental adrenal gland masses. How should you decide whether to advise testing and treatment or no intervention in patients with incidentalomas? What if you advise not to pursue testing and the patient dies from this? What if the patient dies from the surgery? Would you be held responsible? Numerous factors may have an impact on this decision, including tumor size, metastases, clinical signs, owner goals and willingness to accept risk, and costs. Finally, the increased recognition of incidental abdominal masses may cause animal owners psychological harm.

Case Study 16.2   To Treat or Not to Treat Cushing's Disease

When I was a resident, I developed an interest in hyperadrenocorticism (Cushing's disease) in dogs. As a result, in my first year in practice I made it a point that I would do my best to detect as many cases of dogs with this disease as I could, believing that this adhered to the Principle of Patient Advocacy. In virtually every dog I saw with diffuse hepatomegaly, elevated alkaline phosphatase (ALP) or cholesterol, and dilute urine, I advised additional testing including an adrenocorticotropic hormone (ACTH) stimulation test or dexamethasone suppression testing, and abdominal ultrasound. In addition to finding adrenal incidentalomas, I diagnosed dozens of patients with the common, pituitary-dependent form and I advised treating all these patients.

You can probably infer the result of these actions: I made lots of dogs sick from treatment with mitotane (trilostane was not available) and many clients noted, "He really didn't have a problem until you made him sick." It didn't take me long to appreciate that almost all these patients had no symptoms that affected their quality of life, few (if any) died from Cushing's disease, and "benign neglect" was the wiser approach in almost all these patients. At the start of my career, making these diagnoses was a source of pride. After these experiences, I found satisfaction in *not* pursuing a presumptive diagnosis of Cushing's disease in asymptomatic patients and in those whose symptoms did not affect their quality of life.

Case Study 16.3   Whether to Diagnose and Treat Subclinical Bacteriuria

When performing urinalyses on asymptomatic patients, some of them will have evidence of a urinary tract infection (UTI; i.e. bacteriuria, active sediment). It seems counterintuitive and perhaps neglectful to bypass urine culture and treatment in patients with subclinical bacteriuria, especially if the patient is immunocompromised such as those on systemic corticosteroids or chemotherapy, or in patients with diabetes mellitus, renal failure, or hyperadrenocorticism. What if this were to develop into a pyelonephritis and cause systemic illness?

The risk of development of infectious complications in patients with subclinical bacteriuria is small [19, 20], and this reflects my experience. The International Society for Companion Animal Infectious Diseases guidelines for the diagnosis and management of bacterial UTIs in dogs and cats [20] advise that culture of urine from animals that do not have lower urinary tract signs is not indicated because treatment is discouraged. Antibiotic stewardship to mitigate bacterial resistance is a point of contemporary emphasis.

Case Study 16.4   A Hepatic Mass in an Older Dog

When I was a resident, I saw Loki, an asymptomatic 12-year-old husky who presented for an abdominal ultrasound to elucidate the cause of elevated liver enzymes on an annual blood panel. The study revealed a large hepatic mass, suspected to be a hepatoma (benign) based on its appearance. Because of the size of the tumor, I advised resection/hepatectomy with biopsy. The client adamantly declined my counsel. I pressed further, suggesting that Loki's lifespan was likely to be shortened by ongoing growth of the tumor with inevitable illness. My persuasion did not change the decision to watch and wait. I was concerned about Loki's potential demise, feeling quite certain I had provided the right advice.

Once a year for the next three years, Loki's owner made it a point to find me as I changed jobs (this took some effort before the internet) and mailed me a photo of a happy Loki, proclaiming "Still doing fine ... no surgery!" Clients teach us many lessons if we are willing to learn from them, and I received a lesson in humility and the realization that providing guidance for geriatric patients with asymptomatic tumors is fraught with uncertainty. Sometimes, "nothing" is better than "something." I also learned that clients love to remind the vet when we are wrong!

Case Study 16.5   Coagulation Screening Before a Liver Biopsy

Because advanced hepatic disease can cause coagulopathies, it is routine for veterinarians to perform screening of coagulation function via prothrombin time (PT) and partial thromboplastin time (PTT) testing before a liver biopsy procedure to assess patient risk of bleeding, as the most common complication after ultrasound-guided percutaneous liver biopsies is hemorrhage. In an investigation of results of laparoscopic liver biopsies, 89% of dogs had coagulation profiles performed: no dog with coagulopathy had excessive hemorrhage associated with the biopsy procedure [21]. In another study, no association between conventional tests for coagulation and complications or decline in packed cell volume (PCV) was noted post ultrasound-guided liver biopsy in cats [22]. Present evidence does not support screening PT and PTT testing as indicators of risk of bleeding in patients having liver biopsies.

Case Study 16.6   Diagnosis and Treatment of Hypothyroidism

Hypothyroidism is one of the most common endocrinopathies in dogs. While a basal total thyroid hormone (T4) assay is a sensitive screening test, many diseases and medications will cause a low value, creating the potential for overdiagnosis if this test is relied on as the sole or primary determinant. In one study, the prevalence of a low T4 in healthy, middle-aged dogs tested for routine procedures was 13% [23].

The most common setting associated with overdiagnosis, and resultant overtreatment of hypothyroidism, is in older dogs with dilute urine, elevated ALP and cholesterol, and low T4. These dogs likely have hyperadrenocorticism with cortisol-associated reductions in basal T4 values. Many of these dogs are asymptomatic, but some may have symptoms that overlap with hypothyroidism, including lethargy and endocrine alopecia. As hypothyroidism is not fatal or painful, there is no indication to prescribe thyroid hormone in the absence of compelling clinical signs.

If there is uncertainty whether your patient with a low T4 has clinical signs of hypothyroidism and would benefit from treatment, a 1–2-month therapeutic trial with thyroid hormone does no harm, provided that a convincing response to treatment is relied on as the goal of a successful trial. Many of my clients could not ascribe any benefits to their dog from long-term thyroid hormone treatment prescribed by a referring veterinarian, disclosing instead that "My vet said he needed it."

Case Study 16.7   A Dog with a Urinary Bladder Mass and Local Lymphadenopathy

You see Gretel, a 12-year-old female mixed-breed dog, for signs of lower urinary tract disease that are not responding to antibiotic treatment for a presumptive UTI. Abdominal ultrasound reveals a luminal urinary bladder mass in the region of the trigone and iliac lymph node enlargement suggestive of local metastases. The mobile radiologist asks if you want to aspirate the mass and/or enlarged lymph nodes. In my experience, such requests are usually granted, I suspect for four reasons: (i) you may feel compelled to have the radiologist perform the procedure because you are reliant on their equipment and expertise to do this; (ii) you may assume the procedure is indicated if the radiologist is offering it; (iii) there is a natural tendency to "see lesions and sample lesions"; and (iv) the client wants to know what is wrong with Gretel.

In this case, a strong presumption can be made that Gretel's symptoms are due to a transitional cell carcinoma (TCC) that has metastasized to local lymph nodes. The chance of cure or disease resolution is very poor, even with attempted surgical extirpation of the mass and lymph nodes. Surgical resection of trigonal masses is typically incomplete, with recurrence in a few months [24]. Percutaneous aspirates of the mass or lymph nodes have the potential to seed further metastases while providing knowledge that could have been surmised without this risk. Procedures that cause more harm than good are overdiagnoses and should not be performed. Although histologic confirmation of the mass can possibly be achieved via cystoscopy, traumatic catheterization, or laparoscopic-assisted cystotomy, the availability of a sensitive and specific urine test (*BRAF* mutation) is the preferred, non-invasive means of diagnosing TCC [25].

In most cases like this (with or without lymphadenopathy), presumptive medical management of TCC (without a cytologic or histologic diagnosis) with a non-steroidal anti-inflammatory drug (NSAID) is reasonable and may provide short-term relief of clinical signs; in some cases, partial remissions can be achieved with chemotherapy for 3–9 months.

Case Study 16.8   A Dog with a Solitary Pulmonary Mass

You see Waldo, a 13-year-old dog, for coughing. Thoracic radiographs reveal a solitary caudal lobe pulmonary mass. The remainder of routine testing is unremarkable. Should you advise aspirating the mass to attempt to make a cytologic diagnosis? Should you advise a thoracic CT scan to stage the extent of the mass and screen for local nodal metastases? Should you advise lobectomy to excise the mass?

Based on Waldo's signalment and the radiographic finding, a primary lung tumor (adenocarcinoma) is by far the most likely cause of the cough. Definitive treatment requires lobectomy. Palliative care including anti-tussives and anti-inflammatories would be helpful, but the mass and cough would be expected to progress over time. The fundamental question for Waldo's owner is whether they are willing to consider lobectomy. Harms include anesthetic risks, pain associated with the surgery, and significant costs. Benefits include the potential for cure of the neoplasm and temporary or permanent resolution of the cough without the side effects of medications.

Aspirates of the mass should only be considered if lobectomy is a consideration: even so, given the small chance that the lesion is non-neoplastic, the harms including pneumothorax, and costs, outweigh the benefits. This would be an example of overdiagnosis. If lobectomy is to be pursued, a CT scan to stage the tumor is reasonable, only provided that the costs also allow for completion of the lobectomy. If the client cannot afford the CT and surgery, then the surgery must be prioritized as the definitive treatment. As with any potential illness, the sooner definitive intervention occurs, the better the prognosis. If the client wishes not to pursue lobectomy, then palliative medical management is indicated without further testing.

Case Study 16.9   Whether to Pursue a Liver Biopsy in a Dog with Hepatic Failure

You see Penny, a 10-year-old female Doberman pinscher, for abdominal distension, lethargy, and declining appetite. Lab tests reveal elevated liver enzymes, hypoalbuminemia, and isosthenuria. Bile acids results are above the reference range. Abdominal ultrasound reveals small liver size with irregular architecture and a moderate volume of anechoic ascites. Abdominocentesis yields a pure transudate. You refer Penny to an internist for hepatic biopsies.

Laparoscopic biopsies are obtained with no complications and Penny is discharged the same day on an analgesic and a diuretic. Penny never fully recovers from the anesthesia and dies at home four days later. Penny's owner is quite upset and feels that the biopsy procedure hastened Penny's demise and caused her death. You feel badly about this case and wonder whether the biopsy procedure was warranted.

Chronic hepatic disease is common in Dobermans. It was clear from the testing performed that Penny had hepatic failure, as indicated by the elevated bile acids, ascites, and low albumin. The ultrasound findings also suggested an advanced stage of disease. Unfortunately, evidence of survival times and prognostic indicators in dogs with chronic hepatopathy is limited. One report found ascites to be a negative prognostic indicator [26]. Systemic signs of illness also usually worsen prognosis relative to a patient with no symptoms. The very serious nature of this disease and the uncertainty as to whether Penny's condition could be improved at all, and if so for how long, should have been communicated to Penny's owner by the internist before the biopsy procedure.

The rationale of the biopsy procedure is that it presumes that Penny will survive, that any setbacks are temporary, and it takes the "long view," i.e. the histologic diagnosis guides which specific treatments (such as anti-fibrotics and chelators) can optimize Penny's outcome. While it is easy to conclude that the biopsy procedure was not worthwhile for Penny, what about patients who do survive and exceed expectations with treatment? Penny's negative outcome shortly after the laparoscopy reflects my own experience in symptomatic dogs with hepatic failure. I consider hepatic biopsy procedures in these cases as overdiagnoses, as steroid with or without diuretics is the foundation of therapy in almost all cases of chronic hepatopathy in dogs. Other medications that would be indicated based on a histologic diagnosis are ancillary to patient survival and clinical improvement.

The take-home message is that the clinician must utilize their experience with disease conditions and guide their client based on these outcomes. Given my experiences with negative outcomes in this subset of patients, I often advised bypassing hepatic biopsies in ill dogs with hepatic failure in lieu of therapeutic trials for chronic hepatitis.

Case Study 16.10   Whether to Perform Diagnostic Endoscopy in a Dog with Diffuse Enteropathy

You see Missy, a 10-year-old female Yorkshire terrier, for abdominal distension, weight loss, and diarrhea. Appetite and attitude are normal. Lab testing reveals pan-hypoproteinemia, hypocalcemia, and low cholesterol. Urine protein is negative. There is no response to a 10-day antibiotic trial, and you refer Missy to the same internist as in Case Study 16.9. Intestinal mycoses are not endemic in your practice region. Abdominal ultrasound reveals changes consistent with diffuse enteropathy and anechoic ascites, confirmed as a transudate. The internist advises a diagnostic endoscopy procedure and calls you after offering this to Missy's owner.

Considering your experience with a poor outcome after Penny's liver biopsies in Case Study 16.9, you ask the internist to justify the rationale for this recommendation. The anesthetic and procedural risks and mortality rates from an endoscopy procedure are very small compared with more invasive measures such as laparoscopy and laparotomy. You are told that the histologic diagnosis *may* influence treatment and prognosis, but do not perceive a great deal of conviction for this recommendation. You consult with Missy's owner, who declines the endoscopy and wishes to begin treatment based on the most likely diagnosis.

There are numerous histologic diagnoses that may be acquired via intestinal biopsies in patients with protein-losing enteropathy (PLE). The premier question to be considered is: Will the diagnosis meaningfully change patient treatment or prognosis? Unlike in cats where diffuse intestinal lymphoma is common and requires oral chemotherapy to optimize outcomes, this condition is very rare in dogs. Hypoproteinemia has been found to be a negative prognostic indicator in dogs with chronic enteropathy [27, 28]. Consequently, a strong case can be made that diagnostic endoscopy with biopsies of dogs with PLE is overdiagnosis, as treatment involves a combination of dietary management and anti-inflammatory and anti-thrombotic treatments in almost all cases regardless of the histologic diagnosis.

Criteria for Useful Diagnosis

Chapter 15 and this chapter have discussed definitions, examples, and harms related to *underdiagnosis*, *delayed diagnosis*, and *overdiagnosis*. Diagnoses that result in more benefits than harms to patients or clients should be referred to as *useful diagnoses*. One or more of the following criteria should be considered as requirements to justify a useful diagnosis:

- *Testing will influence the diagnostic plan*: Examples include:
  - Ultrasound of cats with chronic vomiting to determine diagnostic endoscopy vs. lymph node aspirates vs. surgery.
  - Blood pressure measurement in hypertensive patients with CKD.
  - UPC to quantify proteinuria in patients with protein-losing nephropathy.
  - ACTH stimulation test in symptomatic patients with biochemical evidence of hyperadrenocorticism.
  - Insulin–glucose ratio in senior dogs with persistent hypoglycemia and clinical signs.
- *Testing will influence the prognosis*. Examples include:
  - Imaging to screen for metastases prior to surgery or chemotherapy in patients with neoplasia.
  - Documenting concurrent cardiac and renal failure in senior patients.
  - Bone biopsy in dogs with bone swelling to distinguish osteomyelitis from osteosarcoma.
  - Thoracic ultrasound in cats with pleural effusion to distinguish heart failure from neoplasia.
  - Serial complete blood count to screen for neutropenia in dogs with parvoviral enteritis [29].
  - Documenting atrial fibrillation in a Doberman pinscher with dilated cardiomyopathy and congestive heart failure [30].
- *Testing will influence the treatment*. Examples include:
  - Serial blood pressure measurements determine fluid resuscitation doses in patients with hypovolemic shock.
  - Total protein measurements determine the need for colloids in patients with hemorrhagic shock.
  - Thoracic imaging in dyspneic patients determines if effusion is present requiring therapeutic thoracocentesis.
  - UPC and blood pressure testing in a patient with CKD to determine the need for treatment of protein-losing nephropathy or hypertension.
  - Therapeutic drug monitoring to determine drug dosing.
  - Urine culture in symptomatic patients with recurrent UTIs to determine antibiotic choice.

- Serial PCVs to determine need for blood transfusion in a patient with hemorrhage.
- Vitamin B_{12} assay in cats with suspected chronic enteropathy to determine the need for supplementation.
- *Testing (non-invasive) will influence the animal owner's decision.* Examples include:
  - MRI of the brain in a senior dog with seizures to screen for a brain tumor.
  - Nasal CT in a senior dog with nasal discharge to screen for a nasal tumor.
  - BUN/creatinine testing in an ill senior cat with uremic breath to confirm CKD.
  - Abdominal ultrasound to confirm a splenic mass in a dog with non-traumatic hemoabdomen.
  - Thoracic radiographs to confirm cardiomegaly to support a diagnosis of aortic thromboembolism in a cat with paraplegia.
  - Cardiac ultrasound to confirm pericardial effusion in a dog with ascites and weakness.
  - MDB (Chapter 17) in senior patients, which may influence the decision to proceed with elective anesthetic procedures (i.e. dental or mass excisions).

If you are considering testing that does not meet any of these criteria, you should reassess this decision. The Veterinary Ethics Tool offers a framework to facilitate decision-making in clinical veterinary medicine (Table 16.1) [31]. While the tool uses the term "treatments" related to professional responsibilities, it applies just as well to whether to perform tests on patients.

Table 16.1 The Veterinary Ethics Tool (VET) offers a framework to facilitate decision-making in clinical veterinary medicine.

	Relationship	Questions to facilitate ethical deliberation	No	I don't know	Possibly	Definitely
Animal-centered factors (justificatory reasons)	**Clinician–patient** (clinical responsibility)	*A.* Do you perceive the proposed treatment to be in the best interests of the patient?	×	–	✓	✓
		A1. Will the proposed treatment improve the patient's health?	×	–	✓	✓
		A2. Will the proposed treatment improve the patient's quality of life: *(a)* immediately	×	–	✓	✓
		(b) long term	×	–	✓	✓
		B. Is the proposed treatment option the one with the least potential to cause harm and suffering while still achieving the intended clinical goal?	–	–	✓	✓
		C. Have measures been taken to minimize the potential for harm and suffering?	–	–	✓	✓
		D. Do the expected benefits outweigh the potential harm and suffering inflicted on the animal or are they at least in balance?	×	–	✓	✓

(Continued)

Table 16.1 (Continued)

	Relationship	Questions to facilitate ethical deliberation	No	I don't know	Possibly	Definitely
Secondary factors (explanatory reasons)	**Clinician–profession** (professional responsibility)	E. Does the primary clinician/team have experience in carrying out the proposed treatment and/or is it a well-documented recognized treatment?	–	–	✓	✓
		F. Is this case an example of good ethical decision-making for students/trainees/colleagues?	–	–	✓	✓
		G. Would you feel comfortable justifying the proposed treatment to professional colleagues?	–	–	✓	✓
	Client–patient	H. Would proceeding with the proposed treatment have a positive impact on the owner–animal relationship?	–	–	✓	✓
		I. Would proceeding with the proposed treatment have a positive impact on the client's quality of life and/or financial benefits (e.g. the proposed treatment will allow breeding from a valuable animal)?	–	–	✓	✓
	Clinician–client	J. Is the proposed treatment financially viable for the client?	×	–	✓	✓
		K. Is the client capable of providing a suitable home environment and/or administrating medication during the recovery period?	×	–	✓	✓
Priority check	**Professional responsibility**	L. Are the secondary factors E–K (explanatory reasons) more influential in your clinical decision than the animal-centered factors A–D (justificatory reasons)?	✓	–	×	×

×	Consider alternative treatment options.
–	Reconsider procedure and the clinician's responsibility.
✓	Valid reasons for clinical procedure.

Source: [31]/John Wiley & Sons.

References

1 Car, L.T., Papachristou, N., Bull, A. et al. (2016). Clinician-identified problems and solutions for delayed diagnosis in primary care: a PRIORITIZE study. *BMC Family Practice* 17 (1): 1–9.

2 McKenzie, B.A. (2016). Overdiagnosis. *Journal of the American Veterinary Medical Association* 249 (8): 884–889.

3 Carter, J.L., Coletti, R.J., and Harris, R.P. (2015). Quantifying and monitoring overdiagnosis in cancer screening: a systematic review of methods. *British Medical Journal* 350: g7773.

4 Hobson-West, P. and Jutel, A. (2020). Animals, veterinarians and the sociology of diagnosis. *Sociology of Health & Illness* 42 (2): 393–406.

5 Coghlan, S. and Quinn, T. (2023). Ethics of using artificial intelligence (AI) in veterinary medicine. *AI & Society* http://dx.doi.org/10.1007/s00146-023-01686-1.

6 Covetrus (2019). Can wellness plans generate revenue for veterinary practices? https://software. covetrus.com/apac/veterinary-insights/article/client-solutions/can-wellness-plans-generate-revenue-for-veterinary-practices (accessed September 24, 2022).

7 Opperman, M. (2019). Pro on ProSal. *Today's Veterinary Business*, February/March. https:// todaysveterinarybusiness.com/pro-on-prosal (accessed September 24, 2022).

8 Brodersen, J., Schwartz, L.M., Heneghan, C. et al. (2018). Overdiagnosis: what it is and what it isn't. *BMJ Evidence-Based Medicine* 23 (1): 1–3.

9 Kale, M.S. and Korenstein, D. (2018). Overdiagnosis in primary care: framing the problem and finding solutions. *British Medical Journal.* 362: k2820. https://doi.org/10.1136/bmj.k2820.

10 Spitznagel, M.B., Jacobson, D.M., Cox, M.D. et al. (2017). Caregiver burden in owners of a sick companion animal: a cross-sectional observational study. *Veterinary Record* 181 (12): 321.

11 Barry, M.J. (2009). Screening for prostate cancer—the controversy that refuses to die. *New England Journal of Medicine* 360 (13): 1351.

12 Shepardson, L.B. and Dean, L. (2020). Current controversies in breast cancer screening. *Seminars in Oncology* 47 (4): 177–181.

13 Barry, M.J. and Albertsen, P.C. (2016). Is prostate-specific antigen screening "proven ineffective care"? *Annals of Internal Medicine* 164 (10): 687–688.

14 Jenniskens, K., De Groot, J.A., Reitsma, J.B. et al. (2017). Overdiagnosis across medical disciplines: a scoping review. *British Medical Journal Open* 7 (12): e018448.

15 PetDx. https://petdx.com (accessed February 9, 2023).

16 O'Kell, A.L., Lytle, K.M., Cohen, T.A. et al. (2023). Clinical experience with next-generation sequencing–based liquid biopsy testing for cancer detection in dogs: a review of 1,500 consecutive clinical cases. *Journal of the American Veterinary Medical Association* 261 (6): 827–836. https://doi. org/10.2460/javma.22.11.0526.

17 Myers, N.C. III (1997). Adrenal incidentalomas: diagnostic workup of the incidentally discovered adrenal mass. *Veterinary Clinics of North America: Small Animal Practice* 27 (2): 381–399.

18 Cavalcanti, J.V., Skinner, O.T., Mayhew, P.D. et al. (2020). Outcome in dogs undergoing adrenalectomy for small adrenal gland tumours without vascular invasion. *Veterinary and Comparative Oncology* 18 (4): 599–606.

19 Wan, S.Y., Hartmann, F.A., Jooss, M.K. et al. (2014). Prevalence and clinical outcome of subclinical bacteriuria in female dogs. *Journal of the American Veterinary Medical Association* 245 (1): 106–112.

20 Weese, J.S., Blondeau, J., Boothe, D. et al. (2021). International Society for Companion Animal Infectious Diseases (ISCAID) guidelines for the diagnosis and management of bacterial urinary tract infections in dogs and cats. *Journal of Japanese Association of Veterinary Nephrology and Urology* 13 (1): 46–63.

21 McDevitt, H.L., Mayhew, P.D., Giuffrida, M.A. et al. (2016). Short-term clinical outcome of laparoscopic liver biopsy in dogs: 106 cases (2003–2013). *Journal of the American Veterinary Medical Association* 248 (1): 83–90.

22 Pavlick, M., Webster, C.R., and Penninck, D.G. (2019). Bleeding risk and complications associated with percutaneous ultrasound-guided liver biopsy in cats. *Journal of Feline Medicine and Surgery* 21 (6): 529–536.

23 Dell'Osa, D. and Jaensch, S. (2016). Prevalence of clinicopathological changes in healthy middle-aged dogs and cats presenting to veterinary practices for routine procedures. *Australian Veterinary Journal* 94 (9): 317–323.

24 Fulkerson, C.M. and Knapp, D.W. (2015). Management of transitional cell carcinoma of the urinary bladder in dogs: a review. *Veterinary Journal* 205 (2): 217–225.

25 Antech (n.d). CADET BRAF and CADET BRAF-PLUS. Accurate canine bladder and prostate cancer test. https://www.antechdiagnostics.com/cadet-braf-plus (accessed October 1, 2022).

26 Raffan, E., McCallum, A., Scase, T.J. et al. (2009). Ascites is a negative prognostic indicator in chronic hepatitis in dogs. *Journal of Veterinary Internal Medicine* 23 (1): 63–66.

27 Benvenuti, E., Pierini, A., Bottero, E. et al. (2021). Immunosuppressant-responsive enteropathy and non-responsive enteropathy in dogs: prognostic factors, short-and long-term follow up. *Animals* 11 (9): 2637.

28 Pietra, M., Galiazzo, G., Bresciani, F. et al. (2021). Evaluation of prognostic factors, including duodenal p-glycoprotein expression, in canine chronic enteropathy. *Animals* 11 (8): 2315.

29 Eregowda, C.G., De, U.K., Singh, M. et al. (2020). Assessment of certain biomarkers for predicting survival in response to treatment in dogs naturally infected with canine parvovirus. *Microbial Pathogenesis* 149: 104485.

30 Friederich, J., Seuß, A.C., and Wess, G. (2020). The role of atrial fibrillation as a prognostic factor in doberman pinschers with dilated cardiomyopathy and congestive heart failure. *Veterinary Journal* 264: 105535.

31 Grimm, H., Bergadano, A., Musk, G.C. et al. (2018). Drawing the line in clinical treatment of companion animals: recommendations from an ethics working party. *Veterinary Record* 182 (23): 664.

17

The Minimum Database

Barry Kipperman

Abstract

This chapter introduces the minimum database (MDB) of testing for sick patients and considers its components, rationale, benefits, and drawbacks. An implicit assumption for the recommendation of an MDB is that veterinarians have a greater duty to prevent animal suffering than to preserve client resources. Potential causes and consequences of not completing the MDB when seeing sick patients are considered. Clinicians should advise an MDB for all sick patients when the diagnosis cannot be confirmed from a history and physical examination. Case examples are provided to support the MDB as a diagnostic standard of care for sick patients.

Keywords: *minimum database, testing, costs, diagnosis, underdiagnosis, delayed diagnosis, complaints, incremental approach, spectrum of care*

During my internship, I was taught that a minimum database (MDB) of diagnostic testing should be recommended for any patient deemed to be seriously or critically ill. Most of these patients are brought to the hospital because of anorexia, lethargy, vomiting, weight loss, weakness, or collapse. The components of an MDB are listed in Table 17.1.

Table 17.1 Components of a minimum database for testing sick patients.

Complete blood count
Chemistry panel (including electrolytes)
Urinalysis
Thoracic radiographs
Abdominal radiographs and/or ultrasound
Thyroid hormone (T4) in senior cats
Feline leukemia virus in cats

Although the wisdom of or basis for these recommendations was not clear to me at the time, I tried to follow my mentor's teachings and faced peer pressure if I did not. I recall a fellow intern who admitted to the hospital a male dog that had sustained vehicular trauma, but did not recommend or perform abdominal radiographs. The animal died the next morning, and an autopsy revealed uroperitoneum secondary to a ruptured urinary bladder. If I wasn't convinced of the value of obtaining an MDB before seeing this case, I was soon after.

As the principal of a referral emergency and specialty hospital, I interviewed recent veterinary graduates regularly over a period of about 20 years for internships and emergency positions on our staff. During many of these interviews, I offered the following scenario and asked the veterinarian what they would advise: "A dog is brought to you for acute onset of lethargy and declining appetite. The owner is very concerned and relays to you how subdued the dog is compared with its normal behavior. Physical examination reveals only mild pyrexia. The owner tells you the dog is a family member and finances are not a concern."

In almost every instance, the young veterinarian recommended performing a complete blood count (CBC) and serum biochemical testing. When I replied that testing reveals only mild neutrophilia, only about half the candidates then suggested performing radiographs, while the remainder suggested providing supportive care and assessing patient response. When I asked these veterinarians why radiographs and a urinalysis were not advised initially, they typically answered that there was no indication for these tests based on the history or physical examination findings.

I believe that obtaining an MDB as a starting point for diagnostic testing of sick patients has fallen out of favor. Before we examine the causes and consequences of its decline, let us consider its purpose.

Merits of the Minimum Database

Although there is no evidence supporting the benefits of obtaining an MDB of diagnostic testing in sick veterinary patients, several rationales for doing so are advanced here.

First, the MDB represents a battery of tests most likely to result either in a diagnosis or a presumptive diagnosis based on exclusion. In my experience, the MDB met these goals in approximately 75% of sick patients. Diagnostic efficiency is improved in contrast with an incremental approach (i.e. performing tests individually over several days). Keep in mind that this is a *minimum* database; that is, this is the minimal amount of information about a sick patient that is required to make a diagnosis and fulfill our duties to obtain informed consent and optimize patient outcomes. Implicit assumptions for the routine use of the MDB are that (i) the goal for clinicians and most clients of testing sick patients is an expeditious, *useful diagnosis* (see Chapter 16); and (ii) a useful diagnosis can lead to specific treatment or euthanasia to mitigate patient suffering.

Second, patients often have multiple diseases, and the MDB helps in identifying all the conditions present. This improves capacity to render an accurate prognosis (see Chapter 20). As an example, I examined a geriatric cat that had been evaluated by its primary veterinarian for weight loss. Laboratory testing revealed high thyroid hormone concentration, but the cat did not improve over the next four weeks despite treatment with methimazole. At the time of referral, ascites secondary to abdominal neoplasia was confirmed via ultrasonography.

Third, the MDB provides a framework to ensure that standards of care for diagnostic testing of sick patients are consistent between veterinarians. Particularly for multi-doctor practices, reducing doctor-to-doctor variability in diagnostic approach seems a reasonable goal, and such an approach would, I believe, serve training programs as well.

Fourth, the risks to patients of obtaining an MDB are negligible.

Drawbacks of the Minimum Database

The most important potential concern with obtaining an MDB of diagnostic testing in every sick patient is client cost. The costs of diagnostic testing associated with the MDB are likely to be higher than the costs associated with an incremental diagnostic strategy. An ethical approach to address this concern is to preface the recommendation of an MDB by stating, "To maximize the chance of discovering the problem or problems today, I advise a comprehensive battery of tests including ..." This provides owners with limited resources or those who prefer that incremental testing be performed (such as those considering euthanasia) the opportunity to "opt out" of the MDB. This proposal does not sanction exploiting clients (i.e. performing an MDB unnecessarily when the diagnosis is apparent in the exam room, such as in a cat with an abscess or in a dog with generalized lymphadenopathy whose owner does not wish to pursue chemotherapy).

Obtaining an MDB may create client displeasure if the test results are negative or inconclusive. Clinicians know that reporting that results of diagnostic testing were normal will occasionally result in owners wondering why you advised all those tests; replying that the negative results tell you that the patient is healthy or that more testing may be necessary to discover the cause of the problem does not always change the owner's demeanor.

Finally, obtaining an MDB can yield unexpected results, such as incidental uroliths or masses, and a decision must then be made as to whether to pursue these findings, particularly when they may not be relevant to the presenting complaint (see Chapter 16).

The Case for the Minimum Database

Some veterinarians feel uncomfortable advising a battery of tests for patients. Consider, however, what must occur for a client to make an appointment to bring an animal to the hospital. Most importantly, the owner must first recognize that the animal is ill or is behaving in an unusual manner. Because our patients cannot directly communicate or complain about pain, headaches, nausea, or weakness, and because animals often conceal signs of disease, owners may not recognize that there is a problem until later in the course of an illness.

Many owners, on recognizing that something is wrong with a beloved animal companion, will retreat into denial, causing them to delay making an appointment. Moreover, because of concerns about the cost of veterinary care or after consulting "Dr. Google," some owners may decide to wait to see whether the problem resolves on its own. Finally, once owners have made the decision to bring their pet to a veterinarian, they must then call and schedule an appointment that suits their schedule, which could take additional time.

Given all of this, the duration of illness for any sick animal may be much longer than is reported or acknowledged. Therefore, assuming a conservative diagnostic posture is illogical.

Causes of Circumventing the Minimum Database

Many factors have contributed to the demise of the MDB [1]. Of particular concern is that with the onset of economic downturns, veterinarians who suggest obtaining an MDB of diagnostic testing may find that higher percentages of owners decline than when disposable incomes are higher. It is likely that many veterinarians feel awkward offering tests that clients decline, and it would be a natural response, when clients regularly decline our advice, to stop offering the MDB to all owners of sick pets.

When I completed my internship and residency, one could be reasonably certain that any veterinarian who had completed postgraduate training would have been taught to recommend that an MDB be obtained for any ill patient. This may no longer be true, as when I have asked newly trained veterinarians why a step-by-step diagnostic approach was advised in select cases, I was told that their training programs advocated this approach to spend as few client resources as possible.

It seems to me that many veterinarians, either because of training or a belief that preserving resources is more important to clients than finding the cause of their animal's illness, see protecting client finances as one of their premier responsibilities.

The veterinary clinician should not be the limiting factor in whether sick patients receive thorough testing: our duty to relieve animal suffering (in the Veterinarian's Oath) is more compelling than protecting client resources (not in the Oath). The recent focus on spectrum of care [2], defined as "Providing a continuum of acceptable care that considers available evidence-based medicine while remaining responsive to client expectations and financial limitations," may also contribute to an incremental approach to testing sick patients over several days.

Unfortunately, there are virtually no clinical practice guidelines from leading veterinary associations regarding a standard of care for testing sick patients [3, 4]. Guidelines from the American Animal Hospital Association (AAHA) cite a CBC, urinalysis, and chemistry as tests to be included in the MDB for sick senior animals; imaging studies are considered elective [5].

Finally, in my experience clients are apt to complain when a veterinarian has performed tests that yield inconclusive results. We are viewed by clients as far more responsible for errors of commission (i.e. recommending tests that yield negative results) than errors of omission (i.e. not recommending testing when it was necessary). As a result, veterinarians may over time develop a conservative diagnostic approach. A survey of small animal internal medicine specialists found that the most common reason for a client complaint was related to cost of care, and 72% reported changing the way they practice medicine to avoid a client complaint [6].

Consequences of Circumventing the Minimum Database

There are limitations to what conditions can be diagnosed based on the results of a CBC and serum biochemical panel alone, resulting in *underdiagnosis* and *delayed diagnosis* for many animals with serious conditions (Case Studies 17.1–17.4). I have seen far more patient morbidity because of failure to obtain an MDB than I have from completing this battery of tests.

Case Study 17.1   A Dog with Vague Symptoms and Pleural Effusion

You work in a multi-doctor general practice. Winston, a five-year-old male pug, is seen by your associate on Tuesday morning for acute onset of lethargy. Physical exam reveals low-grade fever. Blood testing is advised and completed, which reveals leukocytosis. Winston is discharged on an antibiotic for a presumptive infection. You see Winston on Friday for progressive decline, and he is dyspneic. You advise thoracic radiographs, which reveal pleural effusion.

Thoracocentesis is advised and performed, yielding bloody fluid. Post-centesis thoracic radiographs reveal consolidation of Winston's left cranial lung lobe. The radiology report suggests a focal lung abscess, hematoma, granuloma, or torsion as the most likely causes given the poor response to antibiotic. You advise coagulation testing and lobectomy. Winston's owner asks you if the fluid in his chest or the lung problem was present at the time of his previous visit. You respond that you cannot answer this question because chest x-rays were not taken at that time, as Winston had no signs of labored breathing then.

Case Study 17.2   A Dog with Vomiting

You work in a multi-doctor general practice. Jazz, a two-year-old shih tzu, is seen by your associate on Monday for vomiting. Abdominal radiographs are advised, which are unremarkable. Jazz is discharged on a dietary plan of nothing per os (NPO) for 12 hours, followed by bland diet in frequent increments. You see Jazz on Thursday for progressive vomiting, lethargy, and anorexia. Physical exam reveals ptyalism. You advise repeat abdominal radiographs and thoracic radiographs due to concern of possible aspiration pneumonia secondary to persistent vomiting. Chest x-rays confirm an esophageal foreign body. The owner confirms Jazz had eaten a steak bone before his initial presentation. You advise immediate referral for endoscopic retrieval of the bone with a guarded prognosis. Jazz's owner inquires as to why this was not discovered on Monday's x-rays, and whether his prognosis would have been better had this problem been identified then.

Case Study 17.3   A Dog with Gastric Dilatation-Volvulus

You work in a multi-doctor general practice. Eddie, a 10-year-old German shepherd dog, is seen by your associate for non-productive retching and abdominal distension. Abdominal radiographs confirm gastric dilatation-volvulus (GDV). Eddie's owner is informed that this is a life-threatening condition, but that the prognosis is excellent with corrective surgery. Surgery is approved and preoperative blood testing is unremarkable. Eddie's stomach is de-rotated and adhered to his body wall, and recovery is uneventful. You see Eddie four weeks after surgery for coughing. You advise thoracic radiographs, which reveal multifocal pulmonary nodules consistent with metastatic neoplasia or fungal disease. Eddie's owner asks if these lesions were present when surgery for the GDV was approved. You reply that you cannot answer this question because chest x-rays were not taken at that time, as Eddie had no signs of coughing then.

Case Study 17.4   A Cat with Chronic Kidney Disease (CKD)

You work in a multi-doctor general practice. Jennifer, a 14-year-old female cat, is seen on Tuesday by your associate for lethargy and declining appetite. Examination reveals small kidneys. Blood testing is advised and performed, which reveals azotemia consistent with CKD. Intravenous fluid diuresis is advised, which is declined, and subcutaneous fluids are prescribed. You see Jennifer on Friday for progressive decline and loss of vision. Examination confirms fever, bilateral mydriasis, and retinal detachments. Systolic blood pressure is 240 mmHg. Urinalysis confirms a urinary tract infection (UTI). You inform Jennifer's owner that her fever may be due to a kidney infection and her blindness due to high blood pressure. Her owner asks you if these were present on Tuesday and whether her blindness could have been prevented. You respond that you cannot answer this, as these tests were not performed then because Jennifer did not have a fever or blindness at that time.

An incremental diagnostic approach over multiple days often results in clients having to make multiple visits to the veterinarian or to an emergency center to resolve their animal's illness, possibly leading to emotional or financial stress. Such an approach also results in the performance of therapeutic trials with symptomatic treatments (see Chapter 22) in animals with non-specific signs of illness when a diagnosis cannot be determined, to see whether treatment or time alone will yield improvement. Although this may be sufficient for dogs and cats with some illnesses, these trials can delay acknowledgment of inadequate patient response as well as the institution of appropriate treatments, affect patient prognosis because of delayed treatment, provide false hope to owners of animals with terminal or non-responsive conditions, prolong patient suffering, or interfere with subsequent diagnostic testing. I have seen countless cases of hemangiosarcoma that temporarily appeared to "respond" to antimicrobials and gastrointestinal tract obstructions that temporarily appeared to "respond" to antacids.

Conclusion

As a result of multiple factors, it seems that the initial strategy of testing for many sick veterinary patients is limited to a CBC and serum biochemical profile. But doing so limits our knowledge regarding our patients and means that many patients with conditions such as pneumonia, pulmonary metastasis, cardiac disease, esophageal foreign bodies, pericardial effusion, gastrointestinal tract obstruction, abdominal neoplasia, UTI, urolithiasis, and protein-losing nephropathy will be underdiagnosed or diagnosed late in the course of their illness, resulting in increased patient morbidity and mortality.

Although the proliferation of in-house laboratory equipment and digital radiography means it is easier than ever before to obtain diagnostic test results, clinicians too often are not taking advantage of these resources. In the absence of an MDB, obtaining informed consent is not possible, because we do not have sufficient information to provide animal owners with an accurate diagnosis or prognosis. It is in our interests and our patients' interests to revisit the MDB as a standard of care in ill patients and to modify our instruction of veterinary students and interns accordingly. Despite all the dramatic changes in small animal medicine over the past 35 years, the MDB in sick patients remains as vital and valuable as ever.

References

1 Kipperman, B.S. (2014). The demise of the minimum database. *Journal of the American Veterinary Medical Association* 244 (12): 1368–1370.

2 Brown, C.R., Garrett, L.D., Gilles, W.K. et al. (2021). Spectrum of care: more than treatment options. *Journal of the American Veterinary Medical Association* 259 (7): 712–717.

3 Block, G. (2018). A new look at standard of care. *Journal of the American Veterinary Medical Association* 252 (11): 1343–1344.

4 Pugliese, M., Voslarova, E., Biondi, V. et al. (2019). Clinical practice guidelines: an opinion of the legal implication to veterinary medicine. *Animals* 9 (8): 577. https://doi.org/10.3390/ani9080577.

5 Dhaliwal, R., Boynton, E., Carrera-Justiz, S. et al. (2023). AAHA Senior Care Guidelines for Dogs and Cats. https://www.aaha.org/globalassets/02-guidelines/2023-aaha-senior-care-guidelines-for-dogs-and-cats/resources/2023-aaha-senior-care-guidelines-for-dogs-and-cats.pdf (accessed January 20, 2023).

6 Bryce, A.R., Rossi, T.A., Tansey, C. et al. (2019). Effect of client complaints on small animal veterinary internists. *Journal of Small Animal Practice* 60 (3): 167–172.

18

In What Order Should Tests Be Performed?

Barry Kipperman

Abstract

The order in which diagnostic tests are performed has implications for client costs and satisfaction, staff safety, patient safety and survival, and ethical behavior. This chapter provides guidance for the sequence of testing patients in critical condition, including hypotension/shock and dyspnea/respiratory distress. Tests in these patients can often cause their demise and even death, and therefore an incremental diagnostic posture is typically necessary to optimize patient outcomes. Various strategies are also proposed for the sequence of completing testing in stable patients. Judicious sedation can facilitate testing in fractious and dyspneic patients. Case examples are provided to illustrate an ethical approach to diagnostic testing.

Keywords: *testing order, testing sequence, incremental testing, critical patients, respiratory distress, dyspnea, stress, sedation*

The benefits of performing laboratory testing in at-risk asymptomatic patients and in patients with chronic diseases were discussed in Chapter 15 and Chapter 17 considered a minimum database (MDB) of testing for sick patients. Once a clinician has concluded that a patient should receive testing, an ancillary decision relates to the order in which testing should be completed. This has implications for client costs and satisfaction, staff safety, patient safety and survival, and ethical behavior. There is no empirical data guiding veterinary clinicians when choosing the sequence of testing. Typically, the tests to be performed are directed by the clinician and the order is often left to the discretion of the technician(s) working with the patient. Let's examine this decision based on patient characteristics.

Patients in Critical Condition

The risks of testing patients in critical condition are considerably higher than those in stable condition. Tests in these patients must often be performed incrementally and decisions about the order of testing are especially consequential, requiring clear communication between the clinician and their team. Let's consider two categories of this subset of veterinary patients.

Hypotension/Shock

The most common causes of hypotension or shock are trauma and non-traumatic hemorrhage. While all hypotensive patients are clearly sick and therefore warrant an MDB of testing, their critical condition renders them very susceptible to death from stress related to testing. I have witnessed iatrogenic, stress-induced death in these patients when inexperienced clinicians attempted to perform radiographs or ultrasonography prior to restoration of blood pressure via fluid resuscitation. Initial diagnostic efforts in patients in shock must be minimized until they are stable to limit worsening their condition. Moreover, clients may perceive it unethical for the clinician to perform an MDB and then inform them that the patient expired immediately thereafter.

The only essential diagnostic test to initiate life-saving measures in these patients is blood pressure monitoring, which seldom, if ever, causes patient decline. While acquiring pretreatment blood testing is ideal prior to intravenous (IV) fluid administration, this can be challenging in hypotensive patients, and should be immediately aborted if the patient resists to the point that survival is in question (this is more common in cats and small dogs due to the need for jugular venipuncture). If blood samples can be obtained, performing a PCV/total protein test is beneficial to guide treatment and prognosis. All other tests on blood samples should be delayed until the patient is responding to treatment and informed consent can be obtained. Routine acquisition of a urine sample is often stressful to patients and is not indicated until after systolic blood pressure is over 90 mmHg.

While it may be appealing to perform imaging studies during fluid resuscitation, these patients should never be moved to other areas of the hospital while hypotensive, as this is stressful and may result in death. If an imaging unit can be brought to the patient and imaging is performed without placing the patient in a supine position, then it can be considered. Once hypotension has resolved and the patient's condition is deemed to be stable (including reductions in heart rate and improved alertness), this is the time to meet with the owner, discuss a diagnostic plan, then initiate remaining testing. Continued monitoring of blood pressure and vital signs is necessary during testing to identify signs of relapse that would warrant aborting testing and reinitiating IV fluid treatment.

Respiratory Distress

The most common causes of respiratory distress are congestive heart failure (CHF), asthma, and pleural effusion. As with hypotensive patients, patients in respiratory distress are at high risk of death and decisions to subject them to tests and in what order have profound implications. Use of pulse oximetry to evaluate for hypoxia is a benign test and should be performed immediately. Rectal probes should be avoided as rectal insertion is stressful. Thoracic imaging is pivotal in determining potential causes and a prognosis. With film-based radiography, some patients (especially cats) may arrest and die from the stress of being handled and transported to the x-ray room multiple times to acquire satisfactory images. With the advent of digital radiography, this outcome is much less likely.

As a veterinary student, I was instructed by the attending resident to provide oxygen supplementation to a dyspneic cat until he returned. I complied with this order, but as I placed the mask over the cat's nose, the patient resisted and repeatedly moved away from me. I tried restraining the patient to continue the treatment, but the cat arrested and expired before I could page the resident to return. I still feel guilty that I did not know better than to stop the treatment that led to the cat's demise. Veterinary staff should always be cautioned and trained that if they believe a patient's dyspnea is much worse due to interventions, abort and have the clinician evaluate the patient immediately.

Use of thoracic ultrasonography as a primary method of imaging patients in respiratory distress has expanded in the past few years [1, 2], and may be able to provide diagnoses without transporting the patient and without the need to place the patient in lateral recumbency or in a supine position for radiographs. This is a more rapid and safe means of screening patients for pleural and pericardial effusions compared to radiography.

In large dogs with pleural effusion, diagnostic and therapeutic thoracocentesis can often be accomplished without sedation. In small dogs and cats with pleural effusion, sedation is often necessary (the IV route is preferred) before thoracocentesis to prevent stress-related deaths. While it may seem paradoxical to sedate a patient in respiratory distress, the benefits of completing a life-saving procedure almost always outweigh the risks of judicious sedation. If sedation is needed, this is a great opportunity to complete all desired tests and this should be communicated to the client.

On-site N-terminal pro B-type natriuretic peptide (NT-pro BNP) testing can be helpful in the rapid diagnosis of CHF in cats [1], but acquiring blood in these patients is stressful and requires a high degree of supervision and judicious monitoring to avoid iatrogenic mortality. Attempts to acquire enough blood for a complete blood count and chemistry panel in dyspneic patients should await significant improvement in dyspnea or sedation, even if the patient will receive medications (such as diuretics) that may confound the interpretation of test results.

Asymptomatic at-Risk Patients

The rationales for laboratory testing of asymptomatic at-risk patients include establishing a baseline of normal data that facilitates detection of subtle changes that may indicate disease in the future, and diagnosing disease before symptoms arise, which can improve our capacity to slow progression of disease, provide effective treatment, and prolong lifespan. Let me divulge a story to provide advice regarding the sequence in which these tests should be performed.

During my residency, I was holding a feline patient who I suspected had diabetes mellitus while blood was being drawn from their jugular vein. After the procedure, my student noted that the cat had voided urine all over the bottom portion of my tie. I took off the tie and requested that the student wring as much urine as possible out onto a urine dipstick, prioritizing glucose and ketone measurements (students always get the dirty work). The next step was to throw away the necktie! The take home message is: Always try to obtain urine samples via cystocentesis *before* blood samples and diagnostic imaging.

Sick Patients in Stable Condition

Chapter 17 outlined the case for performing an MDB of testing for all sick patients. Once this has been advised and approved by the client, blood, urine, and imaging tests are of course not performed simultaneously. Let's consider four different strategies regarding the sequence of the MDB.

Least to Most Costly

To keep client costs as low as possible, some clinicians may elect to begin with the least expensive tests and save the costliest tests for last. Adherence to this strategy would mean performing laboratory testing prior to imaging studies, which tend to cost more (especially ultrasound examinations). This plan requires receiving laboratory test results before imaging studies are completed.

Staff Convenience and Safety

In my experience, many practices are more reluctant to perform imaging studies on large- and giant-breed dogs compared to smaller patients. This is likely caused by the difficulties for veterinary staff in lifting and moving these dogs onto the x-ray or ultrasound table and placing them in a supine position. It is not uncommon for staff to be kicked, bitten, or urinated on while they and patients struggle with this process. In the days before ultrasound studies were routinely used, I can recall many technicians giving me a dirty look when I requested an upper gastrointestinal (GI) barium series on a large dog. If staff convenience and safety should dictate the sequence of the MDB, then imaging studies in large-breed dogs would be performed last (or the patient can be sedated if deemed safe). If the patient is fractious, sedation facilitates completing testing for both the patient and the staff. All tests must be completed rapidly in this circumstance before the patient recovers.

Third-Party Influences

In some cases, the sequence of the MDB may be influenced by factors beyond your control. For example, if lab samples are sent out to a commercial laboratory and the lab picks up at your practice at noon, then the clinician seeing a patient at 11 a.m. may expedite blood and urine samples before imaging to ensure the results are returned the same day. If you admit a patient for an MDB at 3 p.m. and the mobile radiologist can only arrive at 3:15 or the next day, you may advise an ultrasound study before laboratory testing.

Diagnostic Sensitivity or Positive Predictive Value

While utilizing any of these strategies for sequencing testing of sick patients may be reasonable, to adhere to the Principle of Patient Advocacy, ideally the order of testing should be based on either diagnostic sensitivity (the proportion of patients with the disease that correctly test positive) or positive predictive value (the probability a patient with a positive test has the disease) [3].

While veterinary clinicians are not expected to be clairvoyant, when a reasonable prediction of the patient's diagnosis can be surmised, it is best to perform the test that will yield that diagnosis first (Case Studies 18.1–18.4). This strategy allows the clinician to truncate the MDB as needed. For example, in Case Study 18.1, it would be unethical to perform imaging studies after identifying severe azotemia if the client cannot afford or does not wish to pursue hospitalization for diuresis or placement of a subcutaneous ureteral bypass system for ureteral obstruction considering the poor prognosis. In Case Study 18.4, it would be ethically problematic to complete the full MDB after seeing the thoracic radiographs given the grave prognosis associated with an abdominal mass and pulmonary metastases, unless the client wishes to proceed with surgery and chemotherapy.

Case Study 18.1 A Senior Cat with Uremic Breath

You see Mr. SpongeBob, a 14-year-old cat, for weight loss, lethargy, and anorexia. Physical examination reveals uremic breath and ulcers on the margins of his tongue. You suspect a severe case of chronic renal failure (CRF). As the most direct path to this diagnosis, you advise a urine specific gravity and renal panel to start, which confirms isosthenuria and severe azotemia. Before advising and completing the MDB, you discuss the ramifications of severe CRF with the client.

Case Study 18.2   A Two-Year-Old Labrador with Vomiting

You see Forest, a two-year-old male Labrador, for vomiting and anorexia of three days' duration. The owner reports that the dog is very inquisitive and "likes to put everything in his mouth." Exam is unremarkable. You suspect GI obstruction as the most likely cause. As the most direct path to this diagnosis, you advise abdominal radiographs as the first test to be performed, which reveal changes consistent with intestinal obstruction. Before advising and completing the MDB, you discuss the diagnosis and need for surgery with the client.

Case Study 18.3   A Puppy with Diarrhea

You see Henry, a four-month-old, unvaccinated puppy, for lethargy, anorexia, and diarrhea. Fever is confirmed on examination. You suspect parvoviral enteritis. As the most direct path to this diagnosis, you advise a fecal test for parvovirus as the first test to be performed, which is positive. Before advising and completing the MDB, you discuss the diagnosis and prognosis with the client.

Case Study 18.4   A Senior Dog with an Abdominal Mass and Cough

You see Wendy, a 13-year-old mixed-breed dog, for lethargy, reduced appetite, and coughing. Examination confirms an abdominal mass and coughing. You suspect pulmonary metastases as the cause of the cough. As the most direct path to this diagnosis, you advise thoracic radiographs as the first test to be performed, which reveal multifocal pulmonary nodules. Before advising and completing the MDB, you discuss the diagnosis and poor prognosis with the client.

Because clinicians cannot always (or even usually) predict which test within the MDB will provide a diagnosis, the sequence of tests may not be relevant in these cases, and the entire MDB will need to be completed to adequately inform the client (provided a urine sample is obtained first).

References

1 Ward, J.L., Lisciandro, G.R., Ware, W.A. et al. (2018). Evaluation of point-of-care thoracic ultrasound and NT-proBNP for the diagnosis of congestive heart failure in cats with respiratory distress. *Journal of Veterinary Internal Medicine* 32 (5): 1530–1540.

2 Cole, L., Pivetta, M., and Humm, K. (2021). Diagnostic accuracy of a lung ultrasound protocol (Vet BLUE) for detection of pleural fluid, pneumothorax and lung pathology in dogs and cats. *Journal of Small Animal Practice* 62 (3): 178–186.

3 McKenzie, B.A. (2021). Rational use of diagnostic and screening tests. *Journal of Small Animal Practice* 62 (11): 1016–1021.

19

Diagnostic Errors

Barry Kipperman

"The greatest mistake is to imagine that we never err."

Thomas Carlyle

"Error is not a fault of our knowledge, but a mistake of our judgment giving assent to that which is not true."

John Locke

Abstract

Diagnostic errors may occur when interpreting test results, often caused by inherent prejudices related to our experiences. This chapter discusses types of decision-making in practice and common cognitive biases that lead to diagnostic errors. Case examples are provided to illustrate anchoring bias, availability bias, commission bias, confirmation bias, overconfidence bias, search satisfaction/premature closure bias, and diagnostic momentum bias. Strategies for mitigating biases and reducing diagnostic errors are outlined, including recognition, slowing down, skepticism, routine use of the minimum database, using diagnostic and treatment algorithms and lists of differential diagnoses, and seeking independent advice.

Keywords: *system 1 thinking, system 2 thinking, cognitive bias, anchoring bias, availability bias, commission bias, confirmation bias, overconfidence bias, search satisfaction/premature closure bias, diagnostic momentum bias*

As veterinary clinicians attempt to interpret patient clinical signs and results of laboratory testing and/or imaging into a *useful diagnosis*, inherent prejudices related to our experiences can lead us astray, resulting in *misdiagnoses* or *diagnostic errors*.

Incidence of Diagnostic Errors

Numerous reports of the incidence of diagnostic errors are available in human medicine. A retrospective review of over 2000 electronic health records of primary care patients found a diagnostic error to be likely in 4% of consultations [1]. In an investigation of primary care pediatric patients, an 11% diagnostic error rate was noted in patients with abnormal laboratory values [2], and the frequency of diagnostic error in inborn neonatal intensive care unit patients during the first seven days of admission was 6% [3]. It is reasonable to believe that diagnostic error

Decision-Making in Veterinary Practice, First Edition. Barry Kipperman.
© 2024 John Wiley & Sons, Inc. Published 2024 by John Wiley & Sons, Inc.

rates are comparable or even higher in veterinary practice given the limitations of time and resources clinicians are often faced with.

Decision-Making Processes

A common mechanism to understand decision-making is based on dual process theory, characterized by two discrete types [4]. System 1 thinking is a rapid, unconscious process during which conclusions are reached based on heuristics or mental shortcuts [5, 6]. System 1 thinking relies on intuition, allowing us to reach a diagnosis quickly based on past experiences without using a formal reasoning process. This method is utilized most often by experienced practitioners [7]. The merits of this system are that it is often effective for routine cases, and the clinician is typically satisfied with the outcome [5]. Liabilities of system 1 processing are that efficiency is gained at the sake of completeness, errors are more likely, and we are less apt to acknowledge these errors [5, 8].

System 2 thinking is more deliberate, time-consuming, and analytical [7], using differential diagnosis lists or algorithms [5]. This method is more amenable to solving unfamiliar cases, is used more often by inexperienced clinicians, and may be more accurate. System 2 thinking is more reliant on correct information, which may not be readily available.

System 1 thinking may be considered as more *reflexive* and system 2 thinking as more *reflective*. Veterinarians in one study usually used a system 1 approach to make decisions [9]. While system 2 thinking is taught to students as the ideal approach to addressing clinical cases, system 1 thinking is believed to be a necessary adaptation to the realities of practice where time and information limitations are common, and veterinarians perceive owner expectations for quick diagnoses. Canfield et al. have proposed that systems 1 and 2 thinking are not mutually exclusive and that using them sequentially may be optimal: "The key to improved diagnostic acumen is to learn to trust your intuition in System 1 thinking but recognize when it might need to be supported by more methodical System 2 thought processes" [7].

Cognitive Biases

Bias is "the psychological tendency to make a decision based on incomplete information and subjective factors rather than empirical evidence" [10]. All clinicians are likely susceptible to diagnostic errors deriving from biases. Ironically, it is typical to lack an awareness of one's own bias [8]. It has been asserted that most diagnostic errors result from cognitive biases that are ingrained in our decision-making processes rather than a lack of knowledge [5, 11]. Cognitive error caused by bias may be more prominent with system 1 thinking, which may be the predominant type of problem-solving in veterinary practice [12, 13]. Up to 75% of errors in human internal medicine practice are thought to be cognitive in origin [14], and in a review of 225 insurance claims of veterinary practices in the United Kingdom, cognitive limitations accounted for 51% of the errors [15].

Types of cognitive biases relevant to veterinary practice are described in Table 19.1 with associated case studies. Some of these biases may overlap or occur concurrently.

Case Studies 19.1 and 19.2 are examples of anchoring bias. In Case Study 19.1, it is likely that Priscilla's initial symptoms were due to pyometra and pyelonephritis (kidney infection). The focus on pyometra as the probable cause resulted in bypassing submission of a urinalysis, which precluded recognition of the concurrent UTI, and thorough imaging, which prevented discovery and

Table 19.1 Types of cognitive biases [5, 8, 11, 13, 16, 17].

Type of bias	Description	Case studies
Anchoring	Overemphasis on a single diagnosis or disease	19.1–19.2
Availability	Favoring conditions recently seen or easily remembered	19.3–19.4
Commission	Tendency toward action rather than inaction	19.5–19.6
Confirmation	Inclination to pursue evidence to confirm a preconceived hypothesis or diagnosis	19.7–19.8
Overconfidence	Exaggerated belief in your diagnostic skills	19.9–19.10
Search satisfaction/ premature closure	Limiting diagnostic inquiry to the first plausible explanation discovered	19.11
Diagnostic momentum	Propensity to accept a diagnosis without questioning its accuracy or reluctance to change a treatment plan initiated by a colleague	19.12–19.14

Case Study 19.1   A Dog with Fever and Polyuria/Polydipsia

You see Priscilla, a 12-year-old female intact Yorkshire terrier, for lethargy, anorexia, and polyuria/polydipsia (PU/PD). Fever is confirmed on examination. You are convinced she has an infected uterus (pyometra) and a cursory ultrasound confirms this suspicion. Blood testing reveals leukocytosis and elevated alkaline phosphatase (ALP). Urine is not obtained. She recovers well from ovariohysterectomy and short-term antibiotic treatment. Priscilla's symptoms recur at home shortly after treatment is discontinued. Urinalysis and urine culture confirm isosthenuria and a urinary tract infection (UTI) and radiographs reveal uroliths in her kidneys and urinary bladder.

Case Study 19.2   Another Dog with Polyuria/Polydipsia

You see Woody, a four-year-old Labrador retriever, for acute onset of lethargy and PU/PD. As you are an internal medicine specialist, you interpret Woody's temperature of 102.4 °F as a fever, and azotemia and isosthenuria discovered on lab work with no evidence of a UTI lead you to a tentative diagnosis of leptospirosis and acute renal failure. Woody is treated with intravenous (IV) fluids and antibiotic, but his condition is worse the next day. Your colleague with an emergency medicine background suggests screening for ethylene glycol (EG), which is positive for antifreeze toxicity.

---

removal of the uroliths. In Case Study 19.2, the internist's training created a bias toward infectious disease, which diminished consideration of toxic causes including EG.

Case Studies 19.3 and 19.4 are examples of availability bias, in which an inexperienced clinician's diagnoses were influenced by the recollection of unusual conditions. It's human nature to preferentially remember uncommon diagnoses we have missed relative to more common, mundane conditions: "Conditions we have failed to diagnose correctly in the past are readily available to memory, and this encourages us to look for these conditions more aggressively" [16].

But these cool cases are often metaphorical "zebras," which relate to the common aphorism in medicine that "if you hear hoofbeats, think horses [more common conditions] rather than zebras

---

Case Study 19.3   A Cat with Cervical Ventroflexion and Weakness

You are an intern at a teaching hospital. You see Pandora, a 12-year-old cat, for severe weakness. Examination reveals cervical ventroflexion and generalized weakness. The last time you saw a cat with these symptoms during your internal medicine rotation they were caused by hypokalemia from an aldosterone-secreting adrenal gland tumor, and the symptoms resolved after surgical excision. Pandora's lab work reveals moderate azotemia and hypokalemia (2.5 mmol/l). You schedule an abdominal ultrasound study for the next day to screen for an adrenal tumor and send Pandora home. The next day, Pandora's weakness is worse. The ultrasound study reveals small kidneys consistent with chronic renal failure (CRF) and normal adrenal glands. Pandora's potassium level is now 2.0 mmol/l due to hypokalemic nephropathy.

Case Study 19.4   A Dog with Dyspnea

You are an intern at a teaching hospital. You see Warren, a 14-year-old West Highland terrier, for acute-onset cough and dyspnea. The last Westie you saw on your internal medicine rotation with these symptoms was diagnosed with idiopathic pulmonary fibrosis (IPF) and was euthanized due to a poor prognosis. You remember this because you had tentatively diagnosed pneumonia before the internal medicine consultation was completed. You order thoracic radiographs, and you see lesions like those of the dog with IPF. You discuss your suspicion of IPF with Warren's owner, and euthanasia is elected. The following day the radiology report suggests cardiogenic pulmonary edema as the probable cause of Warren's symptoms.

[rare conditions]." What makes Case Studies 19.3 and 19.4 more tragic is that more treatable conditions (CRF and heart failure) were ignored. When faced with diagnostic uncertainty, a strategy to counter availability bias is to "treat for the treatable," meaning we should attempt to ensure that conditions with easier treatments and better prognoses are not ignored.

Case Studies 19.5 and 19.6 are examples of commission bias. In Case Study 19.5, the clinician ordered tests that are unnecessary given the benign nature of Peanut's symptoms, the recognition that hyperadrenocorticism is not painful, an imminent health threat, or fatal, and the acknowledgment that treatment is not warranted. Possible rationales for unwarranted testing include satisfying the clinician's curiosity and allaying uncertainty, projecting the impression that testing somehow justifies the visit, or to defend the practitioner from client accusations of malpractice [16]. In Case Study 19.6, action is taken that is not supported by evidence that such cases are very seldom due to UTIs in young cats and are therefore responsive to time rather than treatment.

Case Study 19.5   A Dog with Hair Loss and Abdominal Distension

You see Peanut, a 13-year-old dachshund, for hair loss, PU/PD, and a pot-bellied appearance. Appetite is voracious. Examination reveals truncal alopecia and abdominal distension. You strongly suspect these signs are all due to hyperadrenocorticism. To confirm your suspicion, you order an adrenocorticotropic hormone (ACTH) stimulation test and abdominal ultrasound, which confirm pituitary-dependent hyperadrenocorticism. As quality of life is not affected by these problems based on the history, you are not inclined to advise treatment, which you know carries risks.

Case Study 19.6   A Cat Urinating in the House

You see Buster, a two-year-old cat living in a multi-cat household. Buster has inappropriate urination, pollakiuria, and stranguria a week after a new cat was introduced to the household. You strongly suspect idiopathic cystitis secondary to stress as the most likely cause of the problem. The client tells you: "Many of my cats have had this in the past, and they all improved after antibiotic treatment." You dispense a one-week course of antibiotic.

While dispensing antibiotic may be viewed as a benign act that placates the client, such behaviors are not in keeping with antibiotic stewardship.

In Case Studies 19.7 and 19.8, the attending clinician attempted to make common diagnoses based on incomplete and insufficient evidence. Veterinarians often feel the weight of client expectations to "find the problem," frequently with limited diagnostics. This perceived pressure creates a recipe for confirmation bias, interpreting information to fit a preconceived diagnosis.

Case Studies 19.9 and 19.10 are examples of overconfidence bias. As clinicians gain experience, it is common to apply intuitive, system 1 thinking to cases. As we make diagnoses, treat patients,

---

Case Study 19.7   See That Pneumonia Lesion?

Your intern comes into your office and asks if you'll "take a look at some rads." You are told that the thoracic radiographs are of a 14-year-old Chihuahua with severe dyspnea and hypoxia. Before you respond, you ask the intern to interpret the images and her face almost touches the monitor screen as she points to an indiscernible speck of white in the lungs, which she interprets as consistent with pneumonia. You point out that a patient with such severe symptoms should have a lesion commensurate with those symptoms and that it should not require "squinting" to account for the problem. This patient had underlying diseases on lab work and a blood gas profile consistent with pulmonary thromboembolism.

Case Study 19.8   It Must Be Kidney Failure

You see Toby, a 13-year-old cat, for severe weight loss and declining appetite. You advise a minimum database (MDB) of testing, but radiographs are declined. Lab results reveal a blood urea nitrogen and creatinine slightly above the upper end of the reference range and isosthenuria. Phosphate levels are normal. You make a diagnosis of CRF and advise hospitalization for IV fluid diuresis. After three days of no clinical improvement, Toby is referred for an ultrasound, which confirms an intestinal tumor.

Case Study 19.9   It Must Be a Foreign Body

You see Benny, a one-year-old Bernese mountain dog, for acute onset of lethargy and vomiting. Lab results are unremarkable, and you interpret radiographs as being consistent with intestinal obstruction. You inform the client that Benny likely ingested a foreign object as the cause of the problem, despite the owner telling you that this is unlikely. Rather than wait for the radiologist's report, you advise immediate laparotomy and provide an excellent prognosis. During surgery, you discover no abnormalities.

Case Study 19.10   It Must Be Cognitive Changes

You see Palmer, a 15-year-old Lhasa apso, for pacing, inability to get comfortable, and declining appetite. Lab tests are unremarkable. Based on Palmer's age and symptoms, you make a diagnosis of cognitive dysfunction or a pituitary macrotumor with a poor prognosis. Palmer's owner seeks a second opinion. Abdominal radiographs reveal bilateral large nephroliths, which were attributed as the cause of his symptoms.

---

and see them improve, it's inevitable that overconfidence in our diagnostic skill may develop. This may lead us to believe that we can take shortcuts to diagnosing cases based on our experience. I can recall bypassing thoracic radiographs of dogs with ascites, assuring my client that ultrasound of the abdomen would find the cause, and quickly discovering dilated hepatic veins suggestive of a cardiogenic etiology. I tried to ease my embarrassment by joking that "I was shopping in the wrong department."

Case Study 19.11 is an example of search satisfaction or premature closure bias. This diagnostic error resulted in prolonged patient suffering and client dissatisfaction. The attribution of a minimal or mild abnormality in diagnostic results as the cause of significant patient symptoms is a frequent bias in practice. One means of limiting this error is to attempt to objectively assess whether the severity of the lesion or abnormality relied on to make the diagnosis is commensurate with the patient's symptoms. One of the important rationales for completing an MDB of testing is that geriatric patients often have multiple conditions. Consequently, an incomplete evaluation frequently leads the clinician to incorrect conclusions and prognoses. In my experience, as lab results are relied on and performed more often than imaging, metabolic and endocrine diseases are overdiagnosed, while anatomic and neoplastic conditions are underdiagnosed.

Case Studies 19.12–19.14 are examples of diagnostic momentum bias. In Case Study 19.12, multiple emergency clinicians had the opportunity to question the diagnosis made by the primary

---

Case Study 19.11   A Diagnosis of Hyperthyroidism

You see Bugsy, a 10-year-old cat, for weight loss of 20% of his body weight and declining appetite. Lab tests reveal a T4 value slightly above the reference range. You diagnose hyperthyroidism, prescribe medication, and advise a recheck in three weeks. Further weight loss and decline are noted, and Bugsy is referred. Abdominal ultrasound reveals an intestinal mass and ascites.

Case Study 19.12   A Labrador Diagnosed with Pancreatitis

Shane, a four-year-old male Labrador retriever, is seen on Monday by a local veterinarian for lethargy, vomiting, and declining appetite for five days. Dietary indiscretion is reported. Abdominal radiographs, lab tests, and hospitalization are advised and approved, and supportive care with IV fluids and an antiemetic is initiated for a tentative diagnosis of pancreatitis. Shane is transferred for four consecutive days and nights between the clinician's practice and a local emergency clinic with instructions for supportive care, with no improvement. On Friday afternoon, Shane is referred to your internal medicine practice for evaluation. The previous radiographs reveal an intestinal foreign body. Surgery is advised with a guarded prognosis. The owner approves all necessary care. An intestinal resection and anastomosis is required to remove a corn cob from Shane's small intestine.

Case Study 19.13   When to Discontinue Oxygen Supplementation

Tiger, a one-year-old male cat, is seen by your colleague in a 24-hour practice on Saturday morning for acute onset of dyspnea. A tentative diagnosis of asthma/bronchitis is made based on radiographs and NT-BNP testing. Oxygen supplementation is initiated in a small, specialized cage and continues until Monday morning due to a rapid respiratory rate, when his care is transferred to you. You suspect that Tiger's persistent tachypnea may be due to stress and move him to a normal cage. The rapid breathing resolves and Tiger is sent home.

Case Study 19.14   A Cat with an Intestinal Foreign Body

Toby, a six-month-old cat, is seen by your colleague on Saturday morning in a 24-hour practice for acute onset of vomiting. The owner relays a concern that he may have eaten a ribbon. Physical exam reveals a fever. Diagnostic evaluation including lab tests and radiographs is inconclusive, but a feline pancreatic lipase result is elevated, suggestive of pancreatitis. Toby receives supportive care and antiemetics all weekend for a diagnosis of pancreatitis despite multiple episodes of vomiting daily. His care is transferred to you on Monday morning, at which time Toby arrests and expires. A postmortem approved by the client confirms intestinal perforation and peritonitis from a ribbon.

---

veterinarian, but instead proceeded with the requested treatment plan. The primary clinician also chose to adhere to the inaccurate diagnosis. In Case Study 19.13, dyspnea in most cats with asthma resolves after 24 hours of supportive care. Tapering of the oxygen supplementation was warranted over the weekend, but this was perceived as risky by the other clinicians, especially when the patient's respiratory rate remained rapid and no instructions for tapering were left by the diagnosing clinician. Serial pulse oximetry or repeat radiographs could have supported a decision to taper and withdraw the oxygen. In Case Study 19.14, the original clinician put more weight on a single test result than on the compelling history provided by the owner. Again, numerous clinicians had the opportunity to question the original diagnosis considering the poor response to supportive care and change the plan, but did not do so.

This is a common bias in my experience, perhaps because it is easier and less confrontational to simply follow a colleague's plan. This behavior is far more likely if the other veterinarians are either economically dependent on the primary diagnostician (i.e. an employee or those in a referral practice) or perceive that it is not safe to "speak up." To satisfy the Principle of Optimizing Patient Outcomes, practitioners should be encouraged to question a colleague's diagnosis, especially if the patient is failing or not responding to care. When patients are transferred to your care, you are not obliged to continue a plan that seems inappropriate. Addressing diagnostic momentum bias requires courage, a culture of "leaving egos at the door," and an expectation of responsibility for each patient by each veterinarian involved in patient care. In our practice, new clinicians inheriting a case from a colleague were encouraged to review the medical records, call the client to introduce themselves, modify diagnostic or treatment plans as needed, and update estimates.

Strategies for Mitigating Biases and Reducing Diagnostic Errors

Several strategies for mitigating cognitive biases and reducing diagnostic errors have been proposed:

- *Education*: Teaching about bias has not proven to be helpful. A review paper concluded that educational efforts toward recognizing biases in human medicine were ineffective in reducing errors [18].
- *Recognition*: Acknowledge the presence of bias and embrace the possibility that it may influence your diagnostic reasoning [13].
- *Slowing down*: Use system 2 thinking and critical reflection when warranted, especially if the patient is not responding to treatment [8, 13].
- *Skepticism*: Challenge yourself to consider other possible diagnoses and to question the diagnoses of colleagues when suitable [13].
- *Routine use of the MDB*: Use the MDB (Chapter 17) as a diagnostic foundation or checklist to increase the chances of detecting co-morbidities.
- *Diagnostic and treatment algorithms*: Use evidence-based guidelines [5, 13] when available, such as the American College of Veterinary Internal Medicine consensus statements [19], and refer to lists of differential diagnoses applicable to patient symptoms. "You will not find what you are not looking for."
- *Seek independent advice*: Many methods of checks and balances are available, including informal consults with colleagues ("Can I run a case by you?"), speaking with pathologists and clinical pathologists, use of patient rounds to solicit feedback and counsel from team members, ensuring a radiologist interprets all imaging studies, medical records review by a supervisor [13], and referrals to those with greater expertise.

References

1 Cheraghi-Sohi, S., Holland, F., Reeves, D. et al. (2018). The incidence of diagnostic errors in UK primary care and implications for health care, research, and medical education: a retrospective record analysis of missed diagnostic opportunities. *British Journal of General Practice* 68 (suppl 1): bjgp18X696857. https://doi.org/10.3399/bjgp18X696857.

2 Rinke, M.L., Singh, H., Heo, M. et al. (2018). Diagnostic errors in primary care pediatrics: project RedDE. *Academic Pediatrics* 18 (2): 220–227.

3 Shafer, G.J., Singh, H., Thomas, E.J. et al. (2022). Frequency of diagnostic errors in the neonatal intensive care unit: a retrospective cohort study. *Journal of Perinatology* 42 (10): 1312–1318.

4 Kahneman, D. (2011). *Thinking, Fast and Slow*. New York: Farrar, Straus and Giroux.

5 McKenzie, B.A. (2014). Veterinary clinical decision-making: cognitive biases, external constraints, and strategies for improvement. *Journal of the American Veterinary Medical Association* 244 (3): 271–276.

6 Whitehead, M.L., Canfield, P.J., Johnson, R. et al. (2016). Case-based clinical reasoning in feline medicine: 3: use of heuristics and illness scripts. *Journal of Feline Medicine and Surgery* 18 (5): 418–426.

7 Canfield, P.J., Whitehead, M.L., Johnson, R. et al. (2016). Case-based clinical reasoning in feline medicine: 1: intuitive and analytical systems. *Journal of Feline Medicine and Surgery* 18 (1): 35–45.

8 O'Sullivan, E.D. and Schofield, S.J. (2018). Cognitive bias in clinical medicine. *Journal of the Royal College of Physicians of Edinburgh* 48 (3): 225–232.

9 Vandeweerd, J.M., Vandeweerd, S., Gustin, C. et al. (2012). Understanding veterinary practitioners' decision-making process: implications for veterinary medical education. *Journal of Veterinary Medical Education* 39 (2): 142–151.

10 Tversky, A. and Kahneman, D. (1974). Judgment under uncertainty: heuristics and biases. *Science* 185 (4157): 1124–1131.

11 Yuen, T., Derenge, D., and Kalman, N. (2018). Cognitive bias: its influence on clinical diagnosis. *Journal of Family Practice* 67 (6): 366–372.

12 May, S.A. (2013). Clinical reasoning and case-based decision making: the fundamental challenge to veterinary educators. *Journal of Veterinary Medical Education* 40 (3): 200–209.

13 Canfield, P.J., Whitehead, M.L., Johnson, R. et al. (2016). Case-based clinical reasoning in feline medicine: 2: managing cognitive error. *Journal of Feline Medicine and Surgery* 18 (3): 240–247.

14 Graber, M.L., Franklin, N., and Gordon, R. (2005). Diagnostic error in internal medicine. *Archives of Internal Medicine* 165 (13): 1493–1499.

15 Oxtoby, C., Ferguson, E., White, K. et al. (2015). We need to talk about error: causes and types of error in veterinary practice. *Veterinary Record* 177 (17): 438.

16 McKenzie, B.A. (2021). Rational use of diagnostic and screening tests. *Journal of Small Animal Practice* 62 (11): 1016–1021.

17 Madison, J.E., Volk, H.A., and Church, D.B. (2022). *Clinical Reasoning in Veterinary Practice: Problem Solved!* 2e. Hoboken, NJ: Wiley-Blackwell.

18 Norman, G.R., Monteiro, S.D., Sherbino, J. et al. (2017). The causes of errors in clinical reasoning: cognitive biases, knowledge deficits, and dual process thinking. *Academic Medicine* 92 (1): 23–30.

19 American College of Veterinary Internal Medicine (ACVIM) (n.d.) Consensus statements. https://onlinelibrary.wiley.com/page/journal/19391676/homepage/free_reviews_and_consensus_statements.htm (accessed May 29, 2023).

20

Providing a Prognosis

Barry Kipperman

"Medicine is a science of uncertainty and an art of probability."

William Osler

Abstract

Little attention has been given to the chronological step between acquisition of a diagnosis and initiation or declining of treatment, providing a prognosis. This chapter discusses what a prognosis is and the rationale for providing a prognosis to clients, including client expectations of veterinarians. Evidence for reluctance to provide a prognosis and for an optimistic bias among physicians presenting a prognosis is provided. Barriers to discussing a prognosis and the components of a prognosis are provided with case studies. Advice is offered for communicating prognosis using candor, compassion, and precise, understandable terms.

Keywords: *prognosis, barriers, components, communication, optimism, pessimism, emotions, adjectives, clients*

This book has addressed many of the responsibilities of the veterinary clinician in chronological order, including acquiring a patient history (Chapter 2), obtaining informed consent from clients (Chapter 3), and performing tests and interpreting test results to reach a *useful diagnosis* (Chapters 15–19). Acquiring informed consent is initially enacted after history-taking and physical examination. At this point in the consultation, the clinician has formulated a list of patient problems, differential diagnoses, and a diagnostic and/or therapeutic plan of action tailored to that patient. The information provided to clients at this stage is often preliminary.

While considerable instruction and resources are available for making a diagnosis and treating patients, there is scant literature in clinical veterinary medicine devoted to the step between acquisition of a diagnosis and initiation or declining of treatment, providing a prognosis. One main difference between human and veterinary medicine is that physicians typically provide a prognosis directly to the patient (with the exceptions of those who lack capacity or are below the legal age of consent), while veterinarians provide a prognosis to the animal owner on behalf of the patient. In both cases, a prognosis is provided to the individual responsible for decisions about patient care.

What Is a Prognosis?

Ostensibly, the term prognosis has been associated with patient survival times and life expectancy [1, 2] and the delivery of bad news [3]. More accurately, prognosis refers to "communicating what a patient can reasonably expect of the future with respect to a medical condition or its treatment" [4].

Rationale for Providing a Prognosis

The purpose of providing a prognosis is so that animal caregivers can make informed medical decisions about the patient's future and the goals of veterinary care [2, 5]. Note that these objectives overlap those of informed consent. Providing a prognosis can therefore be viewed as a second, more informed stage of educating clients.

What Do Clients Want?

People with serious illnesses want to know, to varying degrees, information about the anticipated course of their condition, life expectancy, the potential benefits of medications, potential symptoms and how to treat them, and anything else that could help guide healthcare decisions [6]. The same desires likely also apply to the owners of veterinary patients.

While some veterinary clinicians may have strong feelings about whether a patient should be treated aggressively, conservatively, or not at all, and may wish to impose their opinion on the client (i.e. paternalism), the preferred paradigm for communicating a prognosis is shared decision-making, involving dialogue with clients. A recent investigation found that pet owners prefer a comprehensive and collaborative approach to information exchange with their veterinarians [7]. Most participants emphasized wanting to know "All of the complexities of how it affects my dog," and a representative comment was "It's my job to make that decision as to what to do next." It was crucial to pet owners that their veterinarians were candid about their pet's prognosis and did not give them "false hope" while discussing options. One of the premier concerns of veterinary clients is "Can you [the clinician] help him/her [the patient]?"

Reluctance to Provide a Prognosis

Multiple reports have concluded that physicians are reluctant to discuss a prognosis with their human patients [2, 5, 8], especially when a terminal illness or serious condition is present, when prognostic information is probably most important [4]. One systematic review found that physicians were inclined to withhold information unless the patient explicitly asked for it [8]. In another investigation, prognosis was discussed in 73% of the interactions between oncologists and patients with advanced cancer [9]. While no data exists focusing on prognostic discussions in veterinary practice, reports documenting that shared decision-making is uncommon suggest that veterinarians may not be meeting their clients' expectations [10–12].

Barriers to Providing a Prognosis

The failure to routinely provide a prognosis despite human patients' and veterinary clients' desire for information suggests there must be powerful barriers to discussing the implications of diagnoses with patients. Many of the obstacles noted by physicians are likely also experienced by veterinarians. Reasons for reluctance to provide prognostic information to veterinary clients are summarized in Table 20.1.

For some clinicians, acknowledging the uncertainty of forecasting by saying "I do not know" may conflict with one's image of the omniscient doctor or may be associated with feelings of shame or humiliation. Such sentiments may arise from a culture of perfectionism in medicine and society, as students are taught to select the "right answers" to exam questions and veterinary clients expect us to find problems and cure them. Perfectionism has been established as a common attribute among veterinary students [15].

As a result of the paucity of data on survival times in veterinary patients, veterinarians are often left either hoping this information is available and accessible or, more likely, are providing clients with their best estimates based on their experience. Novice practitioners would be expected to be challenged by an inadequate capacity to refer to case outcomes and insufficient communication skills compared with experienced clinicians. Insufficient time and accessing and appraising evidence have been identified as the most important barriers to the use of evidence- based veterinary medicine in general practice [16].

Additionally, the interpretation of observational data may be complicated by the practice of euthanasia [17]. Because veterinary patients may be euthanized for reasons unrelated to disease or trauma (i.e. economic limitations, caregiver exhaustion), the potential outcomes and survival times of all patients with particular conditions can only be conjectured. For example, the relative risk of euthanasia associated with non-traumatic hemoabdomen (NTH) treated by interns was 1.5 times that of non-interns, suggesting that experience level may influence the survival times of dogs with this condition [18]. This may become a self-fulfilling prophecy in which frequent euthanasia of patients with NTH reinforces the idea of a poor prognosis [17]. Conversely, for other

Table 20.1 Reasons for reluctance to provide prognostic information to veterinary clients.

Discomfort with the inherent uncertainty of forecasting
Inaccuracy of available evidence or lack of evidence
Fear of being judged for inaccurate predictions
Discomfort with disclosing serious news
Inadequate communication skills training
Lack of time
Fear of diminishing client's hope
Fear of upsetting or causing client distress
Fear of client dissatisfaction
Guilt associated with not being able to offer curative treatments

Source: Adapted from [1, 4, 5, 8, 9, 13, 14].

conditions only patients with the best chances of success may receive treatment while the others are euthanized, which exaggerates the reported survival times associated with treated patients.

I have experienced many of the concerns in Table 20.1. If we offer a prognosis that appears too pessimistic, we may feel guilty that this led to a euthanasia decision and second-guess the accuracy of our explanation, especially if colleagues are routinely having their clients pursue treatment for the same conditions. Also, clients seem to savor the opportunity (sometimes in a derisive fashion) to remind the veterinarian of the patient who exceeded their expectations. Conversely, if our renditions are too optimistic and the patient does not achieve these expectations, we may be concerned that clients may judge us, hold us accountable, or feel guilty that they failed in some way. If our prognosis is ultimately inaccurate, we may fear that our client will be dissatisfied.

Recognition of the importance of prognostic discussions to our clients and the barriers to providing prognoses may allow us to surmount these and find the courage to do our best to accept the inherent uncertainty of forecasting our patients' future.

Formulation of a Prognosis

The ideal components of a prognosis are outlined in Table 20.2.

Let's consider formulating prognoses based on the criteria in Table 20.2 in Case Studies 20.1–20.3.

Table 20.2 Components of a prognosis.

Quality of life

Longevity (quantity of life)

Risks of decline/pain/relapse/side effects

Physical and emotional requirements of patient care

Lifestyle impairments

Frequency of veterinary visits

Need for hospitalization

Costs

Case Study 20.1   A Prognosis for a Large Dog with a Diagnosis of Congestive Heart Failure

What would be the likely prognosis for a large dog with a recent diagnosis of congestive heart failure due to cardiomyopathy? The patient should be able to achieve good physical and mental health while on medications provided PU/PD from diuretics can be managed, but longevity is often in the range of 6–12 months. These patients are at risk of fainting, weakness, or sudden death from arrhythmias, as well as recurrence of labored breathing from heart failure. These circumstances are naturally apt to incur negative emotions in the dog's caretaker. If the dog were to collapse, it may be a physical challenge to carry them into the hospital. Exercise restriction will be warranted. These patients need to be seen for rechecks and medication refills every few weeks at the start of treatment, tapering to every 3–4 months once stable. There is a potential need for hospitalization in the future. The costs of medications, serial lab work, EKGs and chest x-rays can be estimated.

Case Study 20.2   A Prognosis for a Young Dog with Refractory Epilepsy

---

If we consider a prognosis for a young dog with refractory epilepsy, the patient should be able to achieve a reduction in the frequency, severity, and duration of seizures while on medications. Quality of life may be affected by seizures and medication side effects including sedation and excessive urinating; these may limit activity level and there may be a need to get the patient outside more often to urinate. Longevity is uncertain and will be influenced by our capacity to find a balance between minimizing seizures and medication-related side effects. As the medications are not curative, there is a likely risk of ongoing seizures, which may cause emotional upset. Frequent seizures in a 24-hour period may warrant hospitalization; some of these patients need to be carried into the hospital. Routine veterinary visits may be expected every few months or sooner if seizures are not well controlled. The costs of medications, rechecks, and drug monitoring can be estimated.

Case Study 20.3   A Prognosis for a Dog with Multicentric Lymphoma Receiving Chemotherapy

---

What would be a prognosis for a dog with multicentric lymphoma receiving chemotherapy? Remission is achieved in approximately 85% of patients [19]. Physical and mental health should be near normal if remission is achieved, and the median survival time is 12 months. The cancer relapses in all patients, and some patients experience temporary nausea, diarrhea, loss of appetite, or lethargy from chemotherapy, which may be emotionally upsetting. There is a small risk of local ulceration at injection sites on the legs. The client will be expected to give medication regularly and monitor for side effects. There are no lifestyle impairments. Veterinary visits will be required weekly for eight weeks, then every two weeks, and may be discontinued at six months. There is a small risk of hospitalization from infections. Costs of the treatments, consults, and lab tests can be estimated.

Communication of the Prognosis

While it is helpful to have a template for providing a prognosis, it is one thing to know the components of it, and quite another to communicate them to clients in a manner that is accurate, understandable, and compassionate. Because veterinary clinicians often want our clients to pursue treatment (to give the patient a chance for improvement or due to commission bias) and avert euthanasia (which may be viewed as a "failure"), we may unintentionally emphasize the best-case scenario of a patient's outcome and diminish the worst-case scenario.

This optimistic bias is well documented among physicians [4]. In one study, doctors overestimated the chances of survival for terminally ill patients by a factor of five, and the longer the patient–physician relationship, the more optimistic the assessment [20]. In another report of terminal patients whose median survival was only 24 days, 63% of prognoses were excessively optimistic, and survival times were also overestimated by a factor of five [21].

When such discussions do take place, the goal of the client understanding the prognosis may not be met. In a qualitative analysis of human oncologists' language, prognostic descriptions were vague, employing ambiguous terms such as "possibly" or "probably," including euphemisms and jargon, and rarely included a survival estimate [9]. A study of human oncology practice medical records found that 70% of prognosis entries were single words: "excellent, good, fair, poor, or guarded" were the most common [22].

I often used qualitative descriptors for prognoses, including the terms "excellent," "good," "fair," "poor," and "grave." In many cases I discovered that clients did not agree with my optimistic portrayals, as noted in Case Studies 20.4 and 20.5. This creates an awkward setting in which the client may feel coerced to proceed with treatment due to the implication that other clients pursue treatment, or may feel ashamed to decline treatment as this does not align with the clinician's expectations. Conversely, if a grave prognosis is imparted and the client wishes to pursue treatment (Case Study 20.6), they may feel that your negative interpretation may impede treatment outcomes. Additionally, if you perceive the patient is suffering and you are providing futile treatments, this may affect your relationship with the client and cause moral stress [23].

Case Study 20.4   A Large Dog with Hypoadrenocorticism

You see Andi, a two-year-old female Rottweiler with lethargy and vomiting, referred for a diagnosis of acute renal failure. You notice hyponatremia and hyperkalemia on lab work, which supports a diagnosis of hypoadrenocorticism (Addison's disease). This is your first presumptive diagnosis of this disease. You were taught that the prognosis for patients with hypoadrenocorticism receiving treatment is excellent, with a normal lifespan and quality of life. You feel a sense of pride in having made this uncommon diagnosis. You enter the exam room to speak with Andi's owners to inform them of her "excellent" prognosis. When you give them an estimate for lifelong treatment of $200 per month for mineralocorticoid injections after this hospitalization, the owner starts crying and tells you she will have to put Andi to sleep due to the costs.

Case Study 20.5   A Cat with Diabetes Mellitus

You see Jack, a 12-year-old, overweight, aggressive cat who presents for polyphagia and weight loss. Lab testing reveals marked hyperglycemia and glucosuria consistent with a diagnosis of diabetes mellitus. You were taught that this is a very treatable condition with lifelong insulin injections and serial monitoring. You present the diagnosis with a "good" prognosis and describe the need for twice-daily insulin injections and serial monitoring of glucose values. The owner tells you that Jack will not tolerate injections or frequent visits to the hospital, and requests euthanasia.

Case Study 20.6   Provision of Futile Care

You are treating Sandy, a 14-year-old retriever, for metastatic hemangiosarcoma. Sandy had a splenectomy a few months ago and receives chemotherapy monthly. Each time you see Sandy she has lost more weight and seems more lethargic. Prior to her next treatment, you take thoracic radiographs that reveal multifocal pulmonary metastases and a packed cell volume reveals moderate anemia. You discuss a "grave" prognosis for Sandy and advise consideration of euthanasia. Sandy's owner refuses to acknowledge this news and tells you, "I will never consider euthanasia. I want her to continue receiving treatment. If you do not feel you should provide this, please refer me to someone who will."

A challenge for the veterinary practitioner when conveying prognoses is how to balance perceived client desires for both honesty and a sense of hope without misleading those who are emotionally vulnerable. A brief statement conveying concern delivered shortly before a poor prognosis is advised [24]. Incremental disclosure – sharing pieces of information interspersed with checking in with the client – gives the client time to absorb the information.

One author [13] suggests pairing statements of hope and concern simultaneously, such as "While I *hope* that Buster is able to live for a long time with heart disease, I'm *concerned* that time may be measured in months." When working with patients whose short-term survival was uncertain, I asked my clients to "hope for the best and prepare for the worst-case scenario." For example, this lets the client know you are hopeful that her dog with a splenic mass having surgery does not have evidence of metastases, but allows for the acknowledgment that a euthanasia decision may be warranted if metastases are discovered. If we are treating a senior cat with severe kidney failure, we may be hopeful that their azotemia and condition will improve with intravenous fluid diuresis, while preparing for possibly taking the patient home to be euthanized if no improvement is attained. Such an approach acknowledges the uncertainty of prognostication.

Because there is often inadequate data regarding the prognosis for a particular patient's condition(s) or reported survival times are vague (e.g. six months to three years), it is understandable why we use adjectives when discussing a prognosis. Yet, the lack of a standardized or precise vocabulary to describe prognostic information can make what is already unclear even more difficult to understand [25]. For example, does a "grave prognosis" suggest that a veterinary patient has one week, one month, or longer to live? What does a "guarded prognosis" mean? Is it scientific jargon for "I do not know"? Does this term provide any clarity compared to not rendering a prognosis at all? Martin and Widera observe that "Prognostication, like most aspects of clinical medicine, is both an art and a science, with increased accuracy noted when clinical judgment is combined with evidence-based tools" [4].

When communicating a prognosis, veterinary clinicians should strive to use precise language and avoid optimistic bias and the use of ambiguous terms.

Acknowledging Emotions Associated with a Prognosis

Rendering prognoses and prognostic ambiguity likely have a significant impact on veterinarians, patients, and their human families. No one looks forward to having to impart bad news to clients as this inevitably is met with an emotional response, especially if the news is unexpected. Doing so is likely one of the most difficult tasks of caring for patients. Yet, there is evidence suggesting that we can be candid and compassionate, as a poor prognosis is not detrimental to human patients' emotional health or the patient–clinician relationship when it is delivered tactfully and with consideration of the needs of the patient [26, 27]. Martin and Widera [4] offer excellent counsel:

> Upon disclosing prognostic information, clinicians should anticipate that ... [clients] may have an ... emotional response. Although somewhat counterintuitive, a strong emotional reaction often indicates that the information was communicated effectively. Clinicians should allow ... [clients] time to process the new information while remaining attentive to their emotional experience. Attending to emotion can be accomplished through therapeutic silence or responding with empathic statements.

Acknowledging how difficult it must be not to know what will happen to the patient [28] or offering condolences such as "I'm so sorry this has happened to Lola," or "I can see how difficult it must be to see Lola so ill," may be helpful in consoling clients receiving unfavorable prognoses.

Conclusion

The step between acquisition of a diagnosis and initiation of or declining treatment is the provision of a prognosis. Many of the components of a prognosis overlap with those of informed consent. A core competency of a clinical veterinarian is the ability to provide a prognosis that enables animal caretakers to make knowledgeable decisions for both their animal companions and themselves [13]. Evidence from human medicine suggests that there are powerful barriers to discussing the implications of diagnoses with patients. Despite evidence that veterinary clients want to know about their animal's prognosis, shared decision-making is uncommon.

Significant challenges to providing a prognosis include a dearth of information about patient outcomes and lack of veterinary training, unease with uncertainty, and concerns about upsetting clients. Communication of patient prognosis involves a delicate balance of knowledge, empathy, candor, and hope, and should avoid vague adjectives and medical jargon. Addressing client emotions is necessary when relaying an unfavorable prognosis.

References

1 Paladino, J., Lakin, J.R., and Sanders, J.J. (2019). Communication strategies for sharing prognostic information with patients: beyond survival statistics. *Journal of the American Medical Association* 322 (14): 1345–1346.

2 Thomas, J.M., Cooney, L.M., and Fried, T.R. (2019). Prognosis reconsidered in light of ancient insights – from Hippocrates to modern medicine. *JAMA Internal Medicine* 179 (6): 820–823.

3 Thomas, J.M., Cooney, L.M., and Fried, T.R. (2021). Prognosis as health trajectory: educating patients and informing the plan of care. *Journal of General Internal Medicine* 36 (7): 2125–2126.

4 Martin, E.J. and Widera, E. (2020). Prognostication in serious illness. *Medical Clinics* 104 (3): 391–403.

5 Smith, A.K., Williams, B.A., and Lo, B. (2011). Discussing overall prognosis with the very elderly. *New England Journal of Medicine* 365 (23): 2149.

6 Parker, S.M., Clayton, J.M., Hancock, K. et al. (2007). A systematic review of prognostic/end-of-life communication with adults in the advanced stages of a life-limiting illness: patient/caregiver preferences for the content, style, and timing of information. *Journal of Pain and Symptom Management* 34 (1): 81–93.

7 Janke, N., Coe, J.B., Bernardo, T.M. et al. (2021). Pet owners' and veterinarians' perceptions of information exchange and clinical decision-making in companion animal practice. *PLoS One* 16 (2): e0245632.

8 Hancock, K., Clayton, J.M., Parker, S.M. et al. (2007). Truth-telling in discussing prognosis in advanced life-limiting illnesses: a systematic review. *Palliative Medicine* 21 (6): 507–517.

9 Chou, W.Y.S., Hamel, L.M., Thai, C.L. et al. (2017). Discussing prognosis and treatment goals with patients with advanced cancer: a qualitative analysis of oncologists' language. *Health Expectations* 20 (5): 1073–1080.

10 Bard, A.M., Main, D.C., Haase, A.M. et al. (2017). The future of veterinary communication: partnership or persuasion? A qualitative investigation of veterinary communication in the pursuit of client behaviour change. *PLoS One* 12 (3): e0171380.

11 Janke, N., Coe, J.B., Sutherland, K.A. et al. (2021). Evaluating shared decision-making between companion animal veterinarians and their clients using the observer OPTION 5 instrument. *Veterinary Record* 189 (8): e778.

12 DeGroot, A., Coe, J.B., and Duffield, T. (2022). Veterinarians' use of shared decision making during on-farm interactions with dairy and beef producers. *Veterinary Record* 192 (1): e2384.

13 Lakin, J.R. and Jacobsen, J. (2019). Softening our approach to discussing prognosis. *JAMA Internal Medicine* 179 (1): 5–6.

14 Schoenborn, N.L., Bowman, T.L., Cayea, D. et al. (2016). Primary care practitioners' views on incorporating long-term prognosis in the care of older adults. *JAMA Internal Medicine* 176 (5): 671–678.

15 Holden, C.L. (2020). Characteristics of veterinary students: perfectionism, personality factors, and resilience. *Journal of Veterinary Medical Education* 47 (4): 488–496.

16 Haddock, L.A., Baillie, S., Sellers, E.R. et al. (2022). Exploring the motivations, challenges, and barriers for implementing evidence-based veterinary medicine (EBVM) in general practice. *Veterinary Evidence* 8 (1): https://doi.org/10.18849/ve.v8i1.602.

17 Cummings, C.O. and Krucik, D.D. (2023). Not all euthanasias are alike: stratifying treatment effort to facilitate better prognosis prediction. *Veterinary Record* 192 (2): 72–74.

18 Molitoris, A., Pfaff, A., Cudney, S. et al. (2022). Early career clinicians euthanize more dogs with nontraumatic hemoabdomen but not gastric dilatation and volvulus than more experienced clinicians. *Journal of the American Veterinary Medical Association* 260 (12): 1514–1517.

19 Benjamin, S.E., Sorenmo, K.U., Krick, E.L. et al. (2021). Response-based modification of CHOP chemotherapy for canine B-cell lymphoma. *Veterinary and Comparative Oncology* 19 (3): 541–550.

20 Ahalt, C., Walter, L.C., Yourman, L. et al. (2012). "Knowing is better": preferences of diverse older adults for discussing prognosis. *Journal of General Internal Medicine* 27 (5): 568–575.

21 Christakis, N.A., Smith, J.L., Parkes, C.M. et al. (2000). Extent and determinants of error in doctors' prognoses in terminally ill patients: prospective cohort study. Commentary: why do doctors overestimate? Commentary: prognoses should be based on proved indices not intuition. *British Medical Journal* 320 (7233): 469–473.

22 Wilfong, L.S., Ferencik, M., and Neubauer, M.A. (2018). A description of the free text word choices physicians use to describe prognosis in over 50,000 electronic treatment plans. *Journal of Clinical Oncology* 36 (30 Suppl): 219.

23 Jurney, C. and Kipperman, B. (2022). Moral stress. In: *Ethics in Veterinary Practice; Balancing Conflicting Interests*, ch. 22 (ed. B. Kipperman and B.E. Rollin). Hoboken, NJ: Wiley-Blackwell.

24 Clark, J. (2022). Medical errors. In: *Ethics in Veterinary Practice; Balancing Conflicting Interests*, ch. 9 (ed. B. Kipperman and B.E. Rollin). Hoboken, NJ: Wiley-Blackwell.

25 Kelemen, A.M., Kearney, G., Pottash, M. et al. (2017). Poor prognostication: hidden meanings in word choices. *BMJ Supportive & Palliative Care* 7 (3): 267–268.

26 Enzinger, A.C., Zhang, B., Schrag, D. et al. (2015). Outcomes of prognostic disclosure: associations with prognostic understanding, distress, and relationship with physician among patients with advanced cancer. *Journal of Clinical Oncology* 33 (32): 3809–3816.

27 Zwingmann, J., Baile, W.F., Schmier, J.W. et al. (2017). Effects of patient-centered communication on anxiety, negative affect, and trust in the physician in delivering a cancer diagnosis: a randomized, experimental study. *Cancer* 123 (16): 3167.

28 Smith, A.K., White, D.B., and Arnold, R.M. (2013). Uncertainty: the other side of prognosis. *New England Journal of Medicine* 368 (26): 2448.

Section 3

Principles of Treatment

21

Inpatient or Outpatient?

Barry Kipperman

Abstract

For many clinicians, the decision as to whether a patient should be managed as an inpatient or an outpatient can be characterized by uncertainty. This chapter defines the terms inpatient and outpatient in veterinary practice. Clinical guidelines that often warrant inpatient care are provided and the consequences of hospitalization are considered. Patient symptoms and conditions that commonly result in unnecessary hospitalizations are also discussed. Evidence is cited supporting successful outpatient treatment for conditions typically considered to require hospitalization. Options are provided as helpful tools when a clinician remains unsure regarding inpatient or outpatient management despite these clinical guidelines.

Keywords: *inpatient, outpatient, hospitalization, dehydration, pain, caregiver burden*

Once the veterinary clinician has obtained a patient history and informed consent, provided an estimate for any tests, interpreted clinical information into a *useful diagnosis* (see Chapter 16), and provided a prognosis regarding a sick patient (see Chapter 20), a decision must be made about treatment. One of the most fundamental decisions relates to whether the patient is best treated as an inpatient or an outpatient. Let's begin by defining these terms.

Definitions

In human medicine, inpatient status has been defined as "Care in a hospital that requires admission ... and usually requires an overnight stay" [1]. A veterinary inpatient is defined as a patient admitted to the hospital for a minimum of 12 hours, which often entails an overnight stay, either at the admitting practice or at an alternate practice where overnight monitoring is provided. In this chapter, the term "hospitalization" is synonymous with inpatient management. Use of the term hospitalization implies to animal owners that constant supervision of their companion will be provided as in a human hospital. If an animal is sick enough to warrant hospitalization, they are sick enough to justify on-site monitoring to meet their needs, including (for dogs) being walked outside regularly to prevent them from having to void on themselves in their cages.

An outpatient refers to a patient who is treated over a short duration while the owner is present, or who spends less than 12 hours in the hospital while receiving treatment and is sent home.

Examples of outpatients include a vomiting cat receiving subcutaneous fluids during their appointment, a dog staying in the hospital for a few hours while tests are performed and interpreted who receives injections and subcutaneous fluids prior to being sent home, and a dog with lymphoma spending a few hours in the hospital for an examination, a complete blood count, and chemotherapy treatment before being discharged.

Consequences

The decision of whether to treat a sick animal as an inpatient or an outpatient has significant consequences. There are emotional ramifications of a decision to treat as an inpatient, including stress for the patient and the owner as a result of being separated. For many owners, "a house is not a home" until the family is reunited. As inpatient treatment often costs thousands of dollars, there are important financial implications for the owner. Finally, there are potential reputational repercussions for the practitioner. If a decision is made to treat as an outpatient and the animal quickly declines and requires emergency care or dies, this may result in a negative perception of the clinician's competence (Case Studies 21.1 and 21.2). Conversely, if clients sense that any illness results in a request for inpatient status, you may be perceived as insensitive to the emotional aspects of this decision or of being motivated by money.

Let's consider some examples of common patient conditions that typically do and do not benefit from inpatient status to abide by the Principle of Optimizing Patient Outcomes.

Case Study 21.1   A Dog with Snake Bite Envenomation

You see Misty, a two-year-old dog, for facial swelling due to a presumptive snake bite. On examination, Misty has moderate facial swelling and avoids palpation of the face due to pain. Vital signs are stable. You discuss your concern that snake bite envenomation is the likely cause and advise treatment as an inpatient to facilitate pain management and close observation of vital signs and facial swelling. You note a mortality rate of 5–10% to support this recommendation [2]. The owner declines this advice and requests a pain injection and to take Misty home. You provide discharge instructions with discrete warning signs suggesting a declining condition and the need to return to the hospital. The next day, the owner calls to inform you that Misty died at home. The owner berates you for allowing him to take Misty home and for not knowing that Misty would decline, and threatens to post comments on social media that you are unqualified to practice veterinary medicine.

Case Study 21.2   A Dog with Pneumonia

You see Bucky, a 10-year-old golden retriever, for acute onset of coughing. Exam reveals a mild cough, fever, and stable vital signs. Based on these symptoms and thoracic radiographs, you inform the owner of a presumptive diagnosis of pneumonia, which you believe can be successfully treated at home. You dispense an antibiotic and provide discharge instructions requesting Bucky return if weakness, anorexia, or dyspnea is noted. Bucky returns 24 hours later in critical condition from dyspnea, shock, and persistent regurgitation. Thoracic radiographs now suggest severe aspiration pneumonia and megaesophagus. The owner blames your decision to send Bucky home for her emotional trauma and Bucky's poor prognosis.

Patient Criteria Warranting Inpatient Care

Table 21.1 provides patient conditions, owner concerns, and examples that often justify inpatient management.

The most compelling reason to advise inpatient care is that the animal is in a critical condition and at risk of death. It is presumed that this risk is smaller if the patient is treated in the hospital because of care that can (typically) only be provided as an inpatient (i.e. oxygen, intravenous [IV] fluids) and/or because of monitoring (i.e. blood pressure, oxygen saturation) by trained personnel. The most common causes relate to hemodynamic instability, but respiratory distress and neurologic impairment are also potential etiologies.

Another reason for advising hospitalization in critical patients is the belief that if the patient is going to die, it is better for the animal, the owner, and the clinician if this happens in the hospital. The animal can receive symptomatic care that may lessen their pain, nausea, or anxiety; if euthanasia is warranted it can be initiated promptly; the owner is spared the emotional trauma of seeing their companion decline and expire; and the clinician is not blamed for sending a patient home to die. But this perception may be unfounded. Some clients would prefer their animal companion be sent home to die a natural death if they are not going to recover with inpatient treatment. In my experience, this places practitioners in an almost untenable situation, because it is very difficult in many cases to predict who will respond or fail to recover, or when death is inexorable, until a patient is in an agonal condition.

Many patients in stable condition warrant inpatient management. These patients commonly are experiencing significant dehydration or require diuresis and benefit from the capacity to receive IV fluids in a more rapid manner via boluses, or in greater daily volumes than can be administered at home via the subcutaneous route. Patients with anorexia and diabetes mellitus (who often have diabetic ketoacidosis) require insulin to be administered frequently or continuously to reverse metabolic derangements and so need inpatient management and monitoring to hasten their improvement.

Pain is an unpleasant sensory and emotional experience often associated with fear and anxiety (see Chapter 25). Most clinicians are likely familiar with the wailing vocalizations of male cats with urethral obstruction because of pain associated with marked urinary bladder distension. Currently, the most reliable means of abrogating severe pain in companion animals is via use of

Table 21.1 Patient conditions, owner concerns, and examples that often warrant inpatient status.

Conditions and concerns	Examples
Unstable/critical	Shock, dyspnea, status epilepticus, comatose, sepsis
Stable	Vomiting (moderate–severe), diarrhea (intractable), dehydration (moderate–severe), CRF, DKA, anorexia
Pain	Urethral obstruction, ATE, snake bite envenomation, GDV, fracture/polytrauma, degloving wound, pancreatitis, peritonitis, neuropathic (IVDD, root signature), myopathy (acute), postoperative
Emotional/caregiver burden	Epistaxis, facial swelling, seizures, tremors, diarrhea (intractable), non-ambulatory (large patient), pain

ATE, aortic thromboembolism; CRF, chronic renal failure; DKA, diabetic ketoacidosis; GDV, gastric dilatation-volvulus; IVDD, intervertebral disc disease.

opioids/narcotics, and these medications are primarily administered parenterally (often IV), requiring inpatient care and serial evaluation of signs of pain. As most owners understand and can empathize with the experience of pain, they typically feel strongly that they do not want their companion to be in pain.

The final category warranting inpatient management involves conditions that are not medically life-threatening, associated with dehydration, or painful. The rationale for hospitalization in these circumstances is to protect the animal's owner from the emotional or physical trauma that accompanies witnessing seizures or tremors, nose bleeding, the need to clean up watery diarrhea, or having to attempt to carry a large dog that is unable to walk on their own. Owner concern about discomfort and pain in their pet is also associated with caregiver burden [3]. It is often best for the patient to be hospitalized in these circumstances until their condition improves to the point where the caregiver burden at home is minimized.

Clinicians should anticipate owner reluctance to hospitalize patients and be prepared to explain in understandable and compelling language what the benefits of hospitalization are and why these justify the financial and emotional costs relative to sending the patient home: "Mrs. J, I can see how important Buster is to you and I understand why you'd prefer he stay at home. I'm going to explain why I believe that hospitalization is essential for Buster to improve. Most patients with his condition can go home in 36–48 hours when he should feel much better."

Patient Symptoms and Conditions That Result in Unnecessary Hospitalizations

Perhaps because there are so few resources available to guide inpatient versus outpatient decisions, in my experience three common patient symptoms and conditions often result in inappropriate recommendations to hospitalize:

- *Fever of unknown origin*: While many of these patients do not feel well and are not eating well, most are drinking enough water to maintain hydration based on history. Therefore, these patients (provided they are ambulatory, alert, and not severely painful) do not fall into any of the categories in Table 21.1 warranting hospitalization. These patients are most in need of diagnostic testing to find the cause of the fever, for example arthrocentesis to diagnose immune-mediated polyarthritis or ultrasound to confirm neoplasia. Admitting all febrile patients to the hospital routinely for IV fluid support is an inappropriate means of allocating owner resources. This also often limits the owner's financial capacity to pursue required diagnostic strategies beyond the minimum database (see Chapter 17).
- *Anorexia*: As with patients with fever, many patients who are not eating are drinking adequate amounts of water and do not benefit from IV fluid support. Management of stable patients with anorexia of unknown etiology without ongoing gastrointestinal (GI) losses should focus on efforts to find the cause. Owners are often disenchanted with investing over $1000 on supportive care to then receive a subsequent diagnosis of metastatic neoplasia.
- *Icterus*: While some patients with icterus benefit from hospitalization due to the need for monitoring (hemolytic anemia) or because of ongoing water losses (pancreatitis), many patients with icterus do not. For example, anorexic dogs with chronic hepatitis and cats with hepatic lipidosis seldom are markedly dehydrated. As with fever and anorexia, these patients benefit most from a diagnosis and specific treatment tailored to their conditions. The cat with hepatic lipidosis needs liver aspirates and nutritional support via feeding tube placement, and the dog with chronic

hepatitis needs an ultrasound, potentially biopsies, and hepatic supportive therapies, which may include a steroid.

New Evidence Supporting Outpatient Management

A bias is prevalent within veterinary medicine that if all other factors are equal, inpatient management is "better" or is more likely to follow the Principle of Optimizing Patient Outcomes compared with outpatient management. This belief may arise to justify the costs associated with hospitalization, from the enhanced monitoring inpatients can receive, or because we have been trained via the "hidden curriculum" that this is so, despite no evidence-based literature to support this contention. Several recent studies question these time-honored assumptions, finding that over 75% of dogs with parvoviral enteritis survived with outpatient treatment [4, 5], 97% of dogs with pyometra survived to discharge after surgery as outpatients [6], and outpatient care after urethral catheterization succeeded in many cats with urethral obstruction [7].

I am not suggesting that patients with these conditions be preferentially managed as outpatients; in fact, I believe there are many valid reasons to think that inpatient management should yield better patient outcomes. The main value of these studies is to ensure that clinicians acknowledge an outpatient path for patients with these and other conditions whose care may be limited by economic constraints, and not limit options to either inpatient care or euthanasia.

Borderline Cases: To Hospitalize or Not to Hospitalize?

Despite the guidelines in this chapter, it is inevitable that a clinician may be uncertain as to whether a patient should be managed as an inpatient or an outpatient (see Case Study 21.3), especially if this is their first time seeing the patient.

In Case Study 21.3, the number of reported vomiting episodes is concerning and would suggest dehydration that may warrant hospitalization and IV fluid support. Yet, you find little evidence of systemic illness, lethargy, or dehydration based on examination. When you feel unsure as to whether to advise inpatient or outpatient management, I advise being candid with the animal's owner about your doubt over what is best for the patient and explain the case for and against hospitalization for supportive care. In these borderline cases, I advise consideration of the following ancillary tools:

- *Ask the owner if the patient's demeanor is normal*: There have been many times when I felt a patient seemed bright and alert, yet the owner has told me when I specifically asked, "He's very subdued compared to his normal demeanor when he's at the vet."

Case Study 21.3   A Dog with Acute Vomiting

You see JD, a two-year-old Labrador retriever, for acute onset of vomiting. He has vomited six times today. The owner believes he may have eaten some debris in the yard. On physical examination, he seems bright and responsive with normal skin turgor and capillary refill time and is wagging his tail. Abdominal radiographs are normal. Should JD be managed as an inpatient or an outpatient?

- *Ask the referring veterinarian or a colleague more familiar with the patient if the patient's demeanor is normal*: I recall seeing a dog named Dusty for a similar presentation as in Case Study 21.3. Because I was uncertain of the right treatment decision, I called Dusty's primary veterinarian. He asked me, "Is Dusty jumping all over you?" When I replied that he was not, my colleague said, "He's sick. Better hospitalize."
- *If the first two options are not helpful or applicable, advise laboratory testing*: As numerous factors such as patient age, breed, body condition, and temperature can influence the reliability of examination parameters, many owners will approve minimal lab testing for blood urea nitrogen (BUN), creatinine, electrolytes, and urine specific gravity to more reliably determine evidence of dehydration and/or electrolyte imbalances that may warrant hospitalization. I have found that even when these are normal, owners (and I) are relieved and feel better about the decision to send the patient home.

References

1 HealthCare.gov (n.d.). Hospitalization. https://www.healthcare.gov/glossary/hospitalization (accessed May 31, 2023).

2 Bolon, I., Finat, M., Herrera, M. et al. (2019). Snakebite in domestic animals: first global scoping review. *Preventive Veterinary Medicine* 170: 104729.

3 Spitznagel, M.B., Jacobson, D.M., Cox, M.D. et al. (2018). Predicting caregiver burden in general veterinary clients: contribution of companion animal clinical signs and problem behaviors. *Veterinary Journal* 236: 23–30.

4 Perley, K., Burns, C.C., Maguire, C. et al. (2020). Retrospective evaluation of outpatient canine parvovirus treatment in a shelter-based low-cost urban clinic. *Journal of Veterinary Emergency and Critical Care* 30 (2): 202–208.

5 Sarpong, K.J., Lukowski, J.M., and Knapp, C.G. (2017). Evaluation of mortality rate and predictors of outcome in dogs receiving outpatient treatment for parvoviral enteritis. *Journal of the American Veterinary Medical Association* 251 (9): 1035–1041.

6 McCobb, E., Dowling-Guyer, S., Pailler, S. et al. (2022). Surgery in a veterinary outpatient community medicine setting has a good outcome for dogs with pyometra. *Journal of the American Veterinary Medical Association* 260 (S2): S36–S41.

7 Seitz, M.A., Burkitt-Creedon, J.M., and Drobatz, K.J. (2018). Evaluation for association between indwelling urethral catheter placement and risk of recurrent urethral obstruction in cats. *Journal of the American Veterinary Medical Association* 252 (12): 1509–1520.

22

The Therapeutic Trial

Barry Kipperman

Abstract

This chapter considers the therapeutic trial, a commonly performed procedure in veterinary practice. A therapeutic trial is defined and contributing factors for this practice are proposed. The merits, risks, and optimal and unfavorable conditions associated with therapeutic trials are outlined. Case studies are utilized to illustrate these principles. A checklist of guidelines is provided for clinicians to consider before proceeding with therapeutic trials. A therapeutic trial should commence only after discussion explaining the rationale and potential benefits, costs, and risks of testing as well as the trial, so that the animal's owner can make an informed decision.

Keywords: *therapeutic trial, merits, risks, patient outcomes, costs, diagnoses, response, treatment, checklist, treat for the treatable*

A therapeutic trial is a medical procedure where a clinician prescribes medication(s) to achieve a desired clinical outcome without a definitive diagnosis and/or uses the patient's response to treatment to indirectly deduce a diagnosis, guide future testing, or establish a prognosis. Although veterinarians are taught to make a diagnosis prior to initiating therapy, the realities of clinical practice often require us to stray from this ideal path. One study identified that the median frequency with which small animal practitioners perform therapeutic trials instead of diagnostic testing is a few times a week [1]. Therapeutic trials can be conducted on an inpatient or outpatient basis (see Chapter 21).

Reasons for proceeding with therapeutic trials in veterinary practice vary from mundane (cannot obtain urine), to practical (limited resources), to paternalistic (the practitioner assumes that the owner prefers to try medication first). Other contributing factors to choosing therapeutic trials instead of testing or a more definitive intervention include risk aversion, ageism (see Chapter 4), an optimistic bias of the benefits of treatments, and commission bias (see Chapter 19).

Veterinarians are under considerable pressure to proceed with therapeutic trials due to the pervasive influence of economics on decisions affecting patient care (see Chapter 8). When faced with the choice between performing testing to attempt to make a diagnosis or initiating treatment, clients may prefer to pursue the therapeutic trial, especially if they believe that these two alternatives have equivalent outcomes, perceiving the trial as a less costly and more direct path to improvement in their animal's condition.

Clients may be more critical of the veterinarian for errors of commission (recommending tests that yield negative or inconclusive results) than errors of omission (not recommending testing when it was necessary). Practitioners may feel awkward offering testing that clients may refuse to pursue, and it would be a natural response when clients regularly decline our advice to stop offering diagnostic testing to all owners of sick animal companions [2]. As a result, over time veterinarians may develop a conservative diagnostic approach and consider therapeutic trials as a starting point to meet client expectations. Yet, such a common and seemingly benign endeavor can have profound consequences.

A therapeutic trial, like all other medical procedures, should be initiated only after discussion of the rationale, benefits, risks, and costs of both the trial and testing, so the animal's owner can make an informed decision. The merits and risks of therapeutic trials are outlined in Tables 22.1 and 22.2.

In practice, it is common for the clinician to feel pressure to resolve the patient's problem; this "burden transfer" is often commensurate with the anxiety level of the client [3]. The greater the sense of urgency you feel, the less deliberate and thoughtful the trial may become. Tables 22.3 and 22.4 describe ideal and unfavorable conditions for proceeding with therapeutic trials.

Case Studies 22.1–22.7 illustrate the information in Tables 22.1–22.4.

Table 22.1 Merits of therapeutic trials.

Easy and rapid to initiate
Lower cost to client than testing
May avoid risky or invasive interventions
Sometimes successful
Satisfy many clients who perceive that "something" is being done

Table 22.2 Risks and drawbacks of therapeutic trials.

Client may perceive benefit from a placebo effect
May interfere with subsequent diagnostic testing
May delay onset of effective therapy
May increase risk of effective therapies
May worsen patient prognosis
May provide false hope to client if terminal/non-responsive condition
May prolong patient suffering if terminal/non-responsive condition

Table 22.3 Ideal conditions to proceed with therapeutic trials.

Treatment is safe and inexpensive
Rapid response is expected (1–3 days)
Treatment will not interfere with potential tests or other therapies
Potential tests or alternative interventions are costly, invasive, or risky

Table 22.4 Unfavorable conditions to proceed with therapeutic trials.

Treatment is costly or risky
Prolonged course to assess response
Treatment may interfere with potential tests or other therapies
Tests are inexpensive, low risk, and non-invasive
Young patient and lifelong therapy

Case Study 22.1 A Dog with Pollakiuria and Stranguria

Pickles, a 12-year-old female spayed mixed-breed dog, is seen for acute onset of frequent urinations and straining to urinate. Appetite and energy are normal. You are unable to obtain urine as her urinary bladder is empty due to frequent voiding. You dispense an antibiotic for five days for a presumptive urinary tract infection (UTI). You ask the client to schedule another visit if Pickle's signs are not improved in 48 hours.

The most likely cause of Pickle's symptoms is a UTI. Uroliths and urinary tract neoplasms would not be expected to have an acute onset. You consider asking to keep Pickles for observation in the hope of being able to obtain urine, but hospitalization is still no assurance that you can obtain a urine sample via cystocentesis.

Benefits of this trial:

- High success rate.
- Low cost/low risk.
- Timely contingency plan for poor response.

Risks/drawbacks of this trial:

- Signs may persist if due to uroliths or a urinary bladder mass.
- Selection of antibiotic is empirical without a urine culture.

An important component of an effective therapeutic trial is ensuring a contingency plan or "Plan B" (in this case the advised recheck) in case the trial fails to achieve the desired response. These should be advised within a time frame that limits significant patient decline. The benefit–risk ratio in this patient supports this common therapeutic trial in the face of inability to procure a urinalysis.

Case Study 22.2 A Dog with Fever and Polyarthritis

You see Gretel, a three-year-old female spayed golden retriever, for acute onset of lethargy, stiffness, and pain. Fever is noted on examination. You suspect polyarthritis, perform arthrocentesis, and diagnose suppurative inflammation in multiple joints. Considering historical tick exposure and her stable condition (ambulatory, drinking), you dispense doxycycline for tick-borne disease and advise the owner to monitor serial temperatures at home and call you in 48 hours for a progress report. You suspect Gretel has either tick-borne/rickettsial or immune-mediated polyarthritis.

Benefits of this trial:

- High success rate (50%) based on likely diagnoses.
- Low cost/low risk.
- Timely progress report advised.
- Ability to rapidly pursue alternate therapy (steroid) as diagnosis is already made.

Risks/drawbacks of this trial:

- Signs may persist if immune-mediated disease.
- Condition may worsen during the trial.

This appears to be a reasonable therapeutic trial. The client should be informed that if Gretel does not respond signs could worsen, and this could possibly require a hospital stay if fever is very high, or if she cannot walk. Alternatively, one could dispense steroid to begin at some predetermined time if the trial fails or Gretel declines. Provided the client understands these risks, this seems to carry a good benefit–risk ratio.

Case Study 22.3   A Dog with Fever and Stiffness

You see Gretel, a three-year-old female spayed golden retriever, for acute onset of lethargy, stiffness, and pain. Fever is noted on examination. You perform blood testing, which shows an inflammatory leukogram, and dispense a non-steroidal anti-inflammatory drug (NSAID) for the pain and fever.

Benefits of this trial:

- Some chance that lethargy and fever will improve after NSAID administration.
- If patient improves, a rapid response is expected.

Risks/drawbacks of this trial:

- Cause of fever is unknown.
- Condition will likely decline due to disease progression.
- NSAID therapy may impede future diagnostics.
- NSAID therapy increases risk if steroids are needed.
- No progress report advised.

Although NSAIDs are anti-pyretics, this therapeutic trial is myopic in that the elevated white blood cell count and fever suggest a serious, inflammatory disorder. As NSAIDs are never the primary means of treating fever due to infectious, neoplastic, or immune-mediated conditions, this trial puts Gretel at significant risk in that appropriate diagnostic samples such as joint taps and spinal taps may be affected by the therapy, and if Gretel requires immunosuppressive steroid for immune-mediated disease, the juxtaposition with the NSAID puts her at high risk for gastrointestinal (GI) ulcers.

Given the signs of pain, fever, and Gretel's young age being inconsistent with degenerative arthritis, it is compelling to make a diagnosis in this patient. Either further testing or referral is warranted. The therapy may have provided short-term benefits but carried significant and detrimental long-term risks.

Case Study 22.4   A Boxer with Acute Onset of Coughing

A 10-year-old boxer dog presents for acute onset of coughing. Appetite, attitude, and temperature are normal. Examination reveals an occasional cough, mild tachycardia without a heart murmur, and no evidence of dyspnea. You dispense an antibiotic for kennel cough for a week and an anti-tussive to use as needed. Thoracic radiographs are not advised. You advise a progress report in one week.

Benefits of this trial:

- Therapy may palliate the cough.
- Medications have a low cost and side effect profile.

Risks/drawbacks of this trial:

- Masking of the cough with an anti-tussive may allow underlying disease to progress without owner recognition.
- Patient may develop dyspnea and pulmonary infiltrates if in congestive heart failure and require costly emergency interventions.
- Timing of progress report delayed.

The assumption of kennel cough was not reasonable in this patient without a history of kenneling. Thoracic radiographs should be advised for *all* patients with the clinical complaint of cough or dyspnea. This is a dangerous therapeutic trial that often results in a dyspneic patient in an oxygen chamber.

Case Study 22.5   A Large Dog with Acute Onset of Anorexia

You see Chumly, an 11-year-old male mastiff, on Friday afternoon for acute onset of lethargy and anorexia. Examination reveals a mild fever. You advise blood work, which is sent out to the lab, and dispense an antibiotic and appetite stimulant over the weekend. Chumly is seen again on Monday for progressive decline; no food intake was noted all weekend. Abdominal radiographs reveal ascites. Centesis retrieves turbid fluid and Chumly is referred for further evaluation. A diagnosis of septic peritonitis is made at the referral hospital and Chumly dies during surgery to discern the cause.

The most common causes of this presentation are infectious, metabolic, and anatomic (GI obstruction, neoplasia). It was irrational to assume that prescribing an oral antibiotic to a senior, anorexic patient would provide a good chance of success. In addition, the client delayed presenting Chumly to an emergency hospital over the weekend despite his decline, because she was told that the medications would take effect sometime over the weekend. Clients may become so hopeful that therapy will succeed that they are often reluctant to acknowledge failure of the trial; the patient may decline during this period, often to the point where it becomes too late to achieve a positive outcome. In some respects, no therapy is better than unsuccessful therapy, as any therapy may lead to delay in owner recognition of the patient's lack of response.

In my experience, large dogs are far less likely to have radiographs performed compared to smaller dogs, perhaps due to the logistical difficulties of lifting these dogs onto the x-ray table and the number of staff needed to properly restrain them. This is not an acceptable reason to perform therapeutic trials.

It is common for clinicians to perform therapeutic trials with antibiotics, antiemetics, and/or appetite stimulants during the weekend on the premise that "This will get him [the patient] through the weekend." The recognition of your practice's limited weekend hours should encourage referrals to hospitals providing full services during this period rather than a tendency to conduct therapeutic trials to bridge this gap. Either imaging or referral should have been strongly advised. Had Chumly presented on a weekday, then a three-day period of decline could have potentially been avoided via a timely progress report or recheck. This trial is a reminder that the day of the week matters (see Chapter 13).

Case Study 22.6   A Geriatric Cat with Chronic Weight Loss

You see Tinker, a 15-year-old male cat, for acute onset of collapse and weakness. The owner reports that Tinker has been losing weight for a year and has had poor appetite and diarrhea for months. He is profoundly underweight at 5 lb (2.25 kg). Examination reveals an obtunded condition and weak pulses. Tinker's alertness improves after intravenous fluid boluses. A CBC and chemistry panel are unremarkable. Abdominal ultrasound and low serum vitamin B_{12} results suggest chronic enteropathy. You discuss the merits of anesthesia and endoscopic biopsies to confirm your suspicion of intestinal disease, but instead advise placement of a feeding tube for nutritional support under mild sedation and a steroid trial. A callback is scheduled in 48 hours and a recheck appointment is advised in one week.

Benefits of this trial:

- High rate of short-term success.
- Avoids high risk of anesthesia given Tinker's debilitated condition.
- Timely progress report and recheck appointment.

Risks/drawbacks of this trial:

- Cannot provide a precise long-term prognosis without staging of the intestinal disease to distinguish inflammatory from neoplastic cause.
- Uncertainty whether Tinker's survival time would be optimized by oral chemotherapy.

This scenario is common in practice. "A diagnosis at any cost" cannot be justified if the mortality rate of the diagnostic test is deemed too high (see Chapter 16). Although the long-term merits of accruing a histopathologic diagnosis for staging were discussed, the risk of death or setback in Tinker's condition from anesthesia supported this therapeutic trial. The feeding tube was removed after three weeks, and Tinker gained weight over the next few months (up to 8.5 lb!) and was still doing well 12 months later, on oral steroid.

Case Study 22.7   A Cat with Severe Dyspnea

You see Rascal, an eight-year-old cat, for acute onset of dyspnea. Marked labored breathing, gasping, and cyanosis are noted, and Rascal is placed into an oxygen cage. Thoracic radiographs reveal pulmonary infiltrates, but the etiology is not apparent. You advise and initiate treatment for asthma, pneumonia, and heart failure, with steroid, antibiotic, and a diuretic, respectively. Rascal recovers over the ensuing 24 hours. Referral to a specialist is then advised to make a diagnosis.

Benefits of this trial:

- Aggressive action was taken to treat for treatable causes of dyspnea.
- Medications were inexpensive and low risk.
- High-risk diagnostics were averted.

Risks/drawbacks of this trial:

- It is uncertain what medication (if any) Rascal responded to.
- The diagnosis must be attained after stabilization, which may make it more difficult.

It is common for patients to present in such distress or advanced states of illness that their condition risks their surviving the necessary or preferred diagnostic tests. Prior to digital radiography, the risk of "radiograph mortalities" in cats with dyspnea was considerable. In these situations, prioritizing the most likely causes and "treating for the treatable" becomes a reasonable strategy. It is better to have a live patient without a diagnosis than to have a critical patient expire from the stress of a cardiac ultrasound or venipuncture while delaying initiation of a potentially helpful therapy. Generally, the more perilous the patient's condition, the more reasonable a "polypharmacy" approach becomes.

Considerations Before Performing a Therapeutic Trial

To adhere to the Principle of Optimizing Patient Outcomes, the veterinary clinician should consider the questions in Table 22.5 as a checklist before beginning a therapeutic trial.

- *Can the animal's owner reliably administer medication to the patient?* Owners are often reluctant or unable to administer medications by mouth unless the patient is eating. Cats are notoriously difficult to medicate by mouth. As reduced appetite and anorexia are among the most common reasons for initiating a therapeutic trial, ask your client how they feel about being able to give medication to the patient. Watch for both verbal and non-verbal cues in interpreting a response. Consider injectable medication if appropriate.
- *Can the patient tolerate the medication?* It is common for anorexic patients to develop vomiting after receiving commonly used medications such as antibiotics. In small patients, side effects are more common due to the potential for exceeding the therapeutic dose.
- *Is the medication safe in the face of dehydration or anorexia?* If the trial fails, therapy should "do no harm." Administering NSAIDs to a patient that is not eating or drinking all weekend could result in the development of acute renal failure and/or gastroduodenal ulcers. Ensure that your clients have written instructions regarding when medication should be discontinued.
- *Is the medication costly?* The more costly the medication, the less reasonable the trial becomes relative to confirming a diagnosis via testing.

Table 22.5 Questions to consider before proceeding with a therapeutic trial.

Can the animal's owner reliably administer medication to the patient?	☐
Can the patient tolerate the medication?	☐
Is the medication safe in the face of dehydration or anorexia?	☐
Is the medication costly?	☐
Monotherapy or combination therapy?	☐
Could the medication(s) interfere with subsequent testing or increase the risk associated with other treatments?	☐
What should the duration of the trial be?	☐
What are the chances the patient may decline significantly during the trial?	☐
How will success or failure of the trial be determined?	☐
How long should therapy be continued if the trial succeeds?	☐
Could the patient's response be unrelated to treatment?	☐

- *Monotherapy or combination therapy?* For a therapeutic trial to serve the purpose of determining a likely diagnosis, only one medication should be prescribed. There is nothing more frustrating than having a client spill six different medications on the exam table and proclaim to the practitioner, "One of these definitely helped!" Emergent patients in critical condition may necessitate a "polypharmacy" approach, but combination therapy is difficult to justify in stable patients and reduces the value of the therapeutic trial. In addition, if the patient develops a new problem such as vomiting while on combination therapy, it may require trial and error to determine which medication is responsible. If multiple medications are being considered, sequential monotherapy is best. For example, prescribing a short course of furosemide to ascertain whether a cough is cardiogenic in origin before adding pimobendan.
- *Could the medication(s) interfere with subsequent testing or increase the risk associated with other treatments?* Steroid therapy has the potential to impede a diagnosis of lymphoma and other immune-mediated diseases. The administration of NSAIDs will increase patient risk factors for GI ulceration if high-dose steroids are ultimately necessary (see Case Study 22.3). Use your differential diagnosis list and the possible treatments to assess this concern.
- *What should the duration of the trial be?* In most cases, a 2–3-day duration is preferred to determine success or failure of therapy. In conjunction with a contingency plan for a recheck or progress report, this provides a safety net that limits the potential for significant decline in patient condition. The exception would be a stable patient undergoing a novel protein diet trial for food allergy.
- *What are the chances the patient may decline significantly during the trial?* Although this may at first glance seem impossible to predict, in many cases evaluation of the differential diagnoses allows a fair guess. The greater the potential for patient decline during the trial, the less reasonable the trial becomes. This is especially pertinent near the weekend when most practices are closed for 2–3 days (see Case Study 22.5).
- *How will success or failure of the trial be determined?* In many cases, practitioners rely on the client's verbal reports regarding patient appetite and activity to assess the success or failure of a therapeutic trial (see Chapter 23). The client's opinion is not an objective arbiter, as they want the trial to succeed and may not want to acknowledge that their animal companion may require testing or is not responding to the trial. Ideally, a recheck visit should be scheduled prior to pronouncing success of the trial. We should strive for evaluating objective data whenever possible such as temperature, PCV, body weight, etc.
- *How long should therapy be continued if the trial succeeds?* This should be determined by the most likely diagnosis based on patient response. For example, an uncomplicated UTI only requires a 3–5-day course of treatment, while treatment of pneumonia may require 2–3 weeks to resolve. Generally, the longer the period of treatment, the more compelling a diagnosis becomes, and the less reasonable a prolonged therapeutic trial is.
- *Could the patient's response be unrelated to treatment?* Because of an optimistic bias about the benefits of medication, practitioners may attribute patient response to our interventions and may not consider that many of our patients get better irrespective of our treatment. Although we are trained to appreciate that a temporal association does not prove a cause-and-effect relationship (correlation is not causation), our clients often will attribute the desired outcome to the medication(s) because of the placebo effect. The most common example is the cat with idiopathic lower urinary tract disease who "responds to antibiotic." Respect the possibility that your patient may simply respond to time.

References

1 Kipperman, B., Morris, P., and Rollin, B. (2018). Ethical dilemmas encountered by small animal veterinarians: characterisation, responses, consequences and beliefs regarding euthanasia. *Veterinary Record* 182 (19): 548. https://doi.org/10.1136/vr.104619.

2 Kipperman, B.S., Kass, P.H., and Rishniw, M. (2017). Factors that influence small animal veterinarians' opinions and actions regarding cost of care and effects of economic limitations on patient care and outcome and professional career satisfaction and burnout. *Journal of the American Veterinary Medical Association* 250 (7): 785–794.

3 Spitznagel, M.B., Ben-Porath, Y.S., Rishniw, M. et al. (2019). Development and validation of a burden transfer inventory for predicting veterinarian stress related to client behavior. *Journal of the American Veterinary Medical Association* 254 (1): 133–144.

23

Interpreting Therapeutic Outcomes

Barry Kipperman

Abstract

One of the primary means of assessing treatment outcomes is the "callback," where a team member calls the animal's owner and inquires about the patient's progress. This chapter considers evidence regarding telephone communication in human medicine, including caregiver assessments and patient-reported outcomes. The merits and drawbacks of the callback in veterinary practice are discussed. Categorizations are proposed to guide which patients should receive callbacks, when, and from which team members. Practices should create written protocols addressing callbacks. Early telephone contact after hospital discharge should be considered as a routine practice.

Keywords: *callback, telephone communication, compliance, caregiver assessments, proxy, patient-reported outcomes, bias, priority, follow-up*

One of the primary means of assessing treatment outcomes in veterinary practice is the "callback," in which a team member calls the animal's owner or caretaker and inquires about the patient's progress. This may include open-ended questions such as "How is Buster feeling today?" or closed-ended questions including "When did Clancy last vomit?" or "What was Clancy's last temperature?" There is typically no uniformity both within and between practices regarding the methods used to conduct these assessments, or whether these are best performed by veterinarians, veterinary technicians, or customer service team members. While technology now allows for video calls, typical callbacks as discussed in this chapter do not utilize this feature.

The rationale for the callback is to evaluate whether the patient's response to an intervention was positive, neutral, or negative, which can also guide recommendations to continue, terminate, or modify the treatment protocol. Clinicians hypothesize that the information received reflects an accurate representation of our patient's condition. Most clinicians also believe that the callback creates a positive perception of the practice as caring about the patient. From the perspective of our clients, the callback is often viewed as an informal consultation obviating the need for the patient to visit the hospital.

Before we consider the merits and liabilities of using the callback as a method of assessing veterinary patient outcomes, let's examine comparable evaluations used in human medicine as a guide.

Decision-Making in Veterinary Practice, First Edition. Barry Kipperman.
© 2024 John Wiley & Sons, Inc. Published 2024 by John Wiley & Sons, Inc.

Telephone Follow-up in Human Medicine

The period just after discharge from the hospital has been noted as having a high incidence of miscommunications and errors resulting in compromise of patient safety. It is estimated that 20–30% of medical patients experience an adverse event at this time leading to unfavorable outcomes [1]. Telephone calls post discharge are a potential means of improving continuity in the transition from hospital to home-based care, which may improve compliance with discharge instructions and with scheduled recheck appointments [2, 3].

Almost all studies evaluating the success of these follow-ups are based on nurses (who may or may not have worked directly with the patient) making calls. A systematic review of controlled studies found no benefits to older patients discharged from an emergency department from a call from a trained nurse regarding return visits, hospitalization, acquisition of prescribed medication, and compliance with follow-up appointments [4]. Other studies also do not support improvement in patient readmission, mortality, or return visits to the emergency department within 30 days of discharge after telephone follow-ups [5, 6]. While one report found that a scripted call from nurses had no benefits in compliance with instructions [4], another investigation discovered that a revised program consisting of a scripted phone call from a trained nurse volunteer at 72–96 hours post discharge improved patient compliance with follow-up and reduced rates of repeat visits to the emergency department within a week of discharge [3].

One interesting study hypothesized that clinicians might be more proficient in identifying problems and assisting patients after hospital discharge [1]. The trial evaluated clinicians who cared for the patient during their hospitalization making phone calls based on a structured assessment 2–3 days after discharge from an internal medicine service. New or progressive symptoms were discovered in 56% of these callbacks. Most of these problems were addressed on the phone and did not require additional visits or resources. The authors concluded that physicians were more successful in identifying problems compared to nurses and customer service representatives (CSRs) calling patients in a similar time frame [7, 8]. Possible reasons for this are that patients may be more comfortable discussing symptoms with their treating physicians or because of the knowledge of the physician and/or their familiarity with the patient.

There is convincing evidence that postoperative [9] and post-discharge [5] telephone follow-ups have been associated with patient satisfaction in numerous disciplines. Patients report advantages of telephone communication including availability, convenience, and potential for serial conversations [10].

Caregiver Assessments

One of the significant differences between telephone callbacks in human and veterinary medicine is that veterinary team members are speaking to the caregivers of patients rather than to the patients themselves. This proxy relationship may influence the reports veterinary staff receive about patients. In human medicine, proxy reports provided by family members are often utilized to evaluate the health and wellbeing of older patients [11]. Multiple studies confirm that caregivers consistently report greater suffering and poorer quality of life than are reported by patients associated with numerous conditions [11–14]. In addition, investigations also identify that caregiver burden strongly correlates with the degree of caregiver–patient discrepancy [11, 14]. The authors of one of these studies caution clinicians to consider that when the caregiver's own wellbeing is compromised, their assessments may be negatively biased, which may result in inaccurate interpretations and inappropriate interventions for the patient [11].

Human Patient-Reported Outcomes

Formal assessments of illness symptoms or treatment-related toxicity by acquiring the patient's perspective have received little attention until recently. Traditional methods were based on clinician-assessed outcome measures [15]. A patient-reported outcome (PRO) is an assessment of a patient's health status that originates directly from the patient without interpretation of the patient's response by a healthcare professional [16]. PRO measures are structured and validated questionnaires that yield quantitative results. While patient satisfaction with PROs is high [15–17], a systematic review indicates inconclusive evidence regarding whether routine assessment of PROs in clinical practice improves patients' health outcomes [18]. Two studies concluded that use of PROs enhanced shared decision-making and facilitated clinical assessment, diagnosis, and monitoring of issues [16, 17].

Given the relative infancy of the use of PROs in human medicine, the need to use valid instruments, and the uncertain benefits, the rest of this chapter will be devoted to the callback in veterinary practice.

The Callback in Veterinary Practice

Merits

The potential merits of the callback in veterinary practice are outlined in Table 23.1.

Some of the most common issues when patients are transitioning from hospital-based to home-based care are the development of new problems such as vomiting or anorexia from receiving oral medications including antibiotics, poor patient compliance with receiving medication or subcutaneous fluids (i.e. fearful or hiding under the bed), or patient intolerance of medication (i.e. salivating due to bitter taste). Early identification of these concerns via the callback should allow for remedies that may include temporary or permanent discontinuation of medication, a different approach to administering medication, or a different formulation of medication.

Table 23.1 Merits of the callback in veterinary practice.

Identify new or progressive problems

Improve compliance with treatments and care

Reduce caregiver burden

Preclude need for recheck or subsequent visits

Improve compliance with recheck appointments

Determine if treatments or rechecks require modification

Improve client satisfaction

Convenience/ease

Address new questions and enhance understanding

Team feels positive about performing a valued service

Regarding issues with patient compliance, if you have never had to administer oral medications or subcutaneous fluids to a cat by yourself, I can assure you ... it's hard! The callback in these settings allows the caller both to be a problem-solver and to express empathy for the client, since owners of sick animal companions experience caregiver burden [19]. This is an opportune time for client coaching and support, as many clients understandably become discouraged rather quickly when your prescribed plan is not proceeding well. Try to impart a sense of optimism whenever possible and let the client know they are not alone in navigating at-home care and that your team is always available to provide support. Additional training (whether via videos or in person) may also be warranted.

If the patient is doing better than expected, canceling a recheck appointment may be appropriate, while if the patient is declining, advising a visit before the scheduled recheck may be necessary. If the patient is progressing as expected, the callback is an opportunity to remind the client of the scheduled recheck. In my experience, clients often had questions that they had not asked before or did not understand despite a previous explanation. Callbacks are a great opportunity to enhance client understanding of their companion's condition or needs.

Timely callbacks performed by qualified team members should ideally enhance client satisfaction as noted in human medicine, but also should improve the morale of the hospital staff conducting the calls, as clients so often express their appreciation for this gesture. I never received a callback from my doctor's office after two separate epidural injections under anesthesia in the past year, which may explain why so many veterinary clients are pleasantly surprised to receive callbacks!

Disadvantages

The potential disadvantages of the callback in veterinary practice are outlined in Table 23.2.

While many veterinary clients have mobile phones, which mitigates the inability to speak with the patient's caregiver, these also increase the likelihood that the callback may be accepted when the caregiver is distracted or when there is excessive background noise causing a distraction. Veterinary team members should be mindful of this when calling a mobile phone number and ask if it is a good time to discuss the patient's condition. Technical issues such as dropped calls may also occur. A frustrating scenario arises when a staff person spends time discussing the patient's condition and answering questions, only to receive a call later from another family member requesting that the information be repeated because the previous call was accepted by someone who is not the patient's primary caretaker. This happened often enough in my career that when I called, I politely asked if I was speaking with the primary decision-maker if I was uncertain or if multiple family members were involved.

The callback may limit meaningful communication due to language barriers or because owners have difficulty comprehending new information when it is only conveyed verbally rather than both verbally and in writing. Without being able to respond to visual cues that indicate emotional upset [20], clinicians may fail to recognize these and therefore may not give clients adequate time before imparting additional information or may not know to move the conversation in a different

Table 23.2 Disadvantages of the callback in veterinary practice.

Inability to speak with any caregiver
Inopportune time to receive thorough evaluation
May not speak to primary caretaker
Inability to communicate
Inability to recognize emotions
Inability to provide written guidance
Caregiver bias and/or unqualified team member may lead to misinterpretation

direction. Language barriers, misunderstanding, or lack of recognition of the client's emotional state on the phone may contribute to lack of compliance with veterinary recommendations.

Finally, as documented in human medicine, a pessimistic or negative caregiver bias toward the patient's condition may be associated with caregiver burden and may lead to misinterpretation and inappropriate intervention, negative patient outcomes, and higher costs. It has been my experience that the converse problem often prevails in veterinary practice: the caretaker portrays an optimistic bias that may lead to failure to recognize a patient in need of additional evaluation or care. Several contributing factors for false-positive patient reports may include that the client does not want to emotionally accept that their companion is not responding or may have a serious problem; the client may not want to disappoint you and disclose that your treatment plan is failing; the client does not want to have to make another trip with their companion to the hospital; or the client is concerned about the financial ramifications of a modified plan resulting in additional tests or treatments.

Which Patients Should Receive a Callback and When?

Early telephone contact after hospital discharge should be considered a routine practice. Table 23.3 prioritizes the need and timing for a callback based on patient conditions, treatments, and settings. This list is by no means exhaustive and is intended to offer guidance to the clinician for some of the

Table 23.3 Prioritization of the need and timing for a callback based on patient conditions, treatments, and settings.

High priority – call within 24 hours post discharge
Owner is considering euthanasia or patient may expire at home
Postoperative
Painful condition
Urethral obstruction
Prolonged hospitalization
Costly hospitalization or procedure
Corneal ulcers
Paresis/paralyzed/non-ambulatory
Splints/bandages
Feeding tube management
Subcutaneous fluids/insulin injections
Moderate priority – call within 48 hours post discharge
Gastroenteritis/pancreatitis
Vestibular disease
Endocrinopathies – diabetes mellitus, Cushing's disease, hyperthyroidism
High-dose steroid therapy in dogs
Chemotherapy
Cone or collar placement
Low priority
Abscess/minor wounds
Toxin ingestion – asymptomatic
Dermatologic/otic conditions
Vaccines

most common problems seen in veterinary practice. A callback should ideally be performed within 48 hours from patient discharge, and within 24 hours for high-priority patients. Hospitals should establish a written protocol for which patients are to receive callbacks and at what interval post discharge. Blocking out a time slot during the workday should be considered to ensure staff availability to accomplish this important task. While it is increasingly difficult to have a human physician accept or return a telephone call, and the trend is for physicians to charge fees for responding to patient emails and queries via patient portals, whether to charge fees for the callback must be left to the discretion of the veterinary practice owner(s).

High priority cases are those in which the risks of death, euthanasia, complications, recurrence, or disease progression are greatest. If an owner's emotional state is fragile, euthanasia is more likely to be considered, or you believe that the patient is likely to die at home, these patients should be considered as a high priority regardless of disease condition. All patients undergoing major surgery should be considered as postoperative and high priority. These calls should address anesthetic recovery and pain. As the gap in efficacy between parenteral and oral analgesics is considerable, all painful patients should receive prompt callbacks to ensure that the patient seems comfortable or to consider alternate analgesics as needed. Patients who have experienced a prolonged hospital stay or a very expensive procedure should be considered high priority if for no other reason than to provide excellent service to justify the costs incurred.

Patients with corneal ulcers are painful, require frequent treatments, and are at risk of vision loss justifying their high-priority status. Non-ambulatory or weakly ambulatory patients may require being carried or supported, which can be a burden commensurate with the size of the patient. Patients with splints and bandages are at risk of distal limb swelling and local necrosis if the bandage is not properly cared for. Many anorexic patients will develop vomiting at the outset of being fed via a tube, and tube feedings cause significant client burden, so all these patients should receive prompt follow-up, as should patients receiving subcutaneous fluids or insulin injections for the first time.

Moderate-priority cases are those in which the risks of death, euthanasia, complications, recurrence, disease progression, or caregiver burden are less concerning compared with high-priority cases. Most routine cases of gastroenteritis, pancreatitis, and vestibular disease would fit into this category. Patients beginning treatment for hyperadrenocorticism, diabetes mellitus, hyperthyroidism, and immune-mediated diseases are subject to numerous side effects from treatment, so these patients should receive prompt callbacks. Patients receiving serial chemotherapy as outpatients should be considered moderate priority except those receiving a medication for the first time, which should make them high priority.

Many patients may not eat well, walk normally, or play when wearing a cone or collar, while others may be able to access the wound or incision despite wearing them. A recent report found that 77% of pet owners reported a poorer quality of life in their animal companion while wearing an Elizabethan collar [21]. Judicious removal with observation at mealtimes and/or transition to alternative methods to prevent self-trauma may be warranted.

Low-priority cases are those in which the attendant risks and concerns are unlikely. Patients receiving vaccinations would be included in this category. Clients should be apprised to expect transient, mild lethargy for up to 48 hours post vaccine.

Who Should Perform the Callback?

In addition to deciding which patients should receive callbacks and when, the final important decision is to assign staff members to make the calls. Case Study 23.1 may be instructive.

Case Study 23.1   A Labrador with Poor Appetite

Shane is a four-year-old Labrador seen yesterday at your practice for vomiting and poor appetite. He was treated as an outpatient with an appetite stimulant and antiemetic medication. The next day, a CSR performs a callback:

CSR: "Hello, Mrs. X, how is Shane feeling today?"

MRS. X: "I think he's doing better. Yesterday he didn't eat at all, but this morning I coaxed him to eat a small bit of hamburger and chicken, and he's only vomited once."

CSR: "That's great news, Mrs. X! Do feel free to call us if you have any further questions and I'm so happy that Shane is feeling better."

The CSR documents a summary of the call into Shane's medical record. Shane is referred to an internist six days later and a small intestinal obstruction from corn cob ingestion is diagnosed.

The outcome of Shane's callback reflects both a client with an optimistic bias and a veterinary team member not discerning or knowledgeable enough to recognize that a Labrador who needs to be coaxed to eat is a very sick dog. Ideally, the CSR would have advised an immediate recheck appointment or moved the call to a veterinary technician or clinician.

All staff members conducting callbacks should be cognizant of the potential for an optimistic bias in caretaker reports and should be trained to ask closed-ended questions to better characterize patient condition. Such questions include:

- How much food is the patient eating relative to their normal intake?
- Is the patient eating their normal food?
- How many episodes of vomiting or diarrhea have occurred since discharge?
- Is the patient able to sleep and rest normally?

Categorization of patient priority should determine who performs the callback. As physicians were more successful in identifying problems compared to nurses [1] (and this coincides with my experience in veterinary practice), high-priority cases should be called by clinicians, moderate-priority cases should be called by technicians, and low-priority cases can be called by CSRs. As these categories are simply guidelines and many patients may not fit into one specific category, training programs and protocols should encourage that calls be moved to more suitable team members as needed. For example, in Case Study 23.1, the call should have been diverted to a technician or clinician. If a clinician is on a call and finds that the client needs assistance with how to medicate their companion, the call can be transferred to a technician who may be better qualified to address this concern.

Conclusion

Callbacks to assess patient response to treatment are an integral component of veterinary practice. Ideally, the callback should ensure a smooth transition between hospital and home care, improve patient outcomes, and enhance client and veterinary team satisfaction. With an appreciation of the advantages and liabilities, each practice should create a protocol establishing who should call which patients at what interval post discharge.

References

1 Stella, S.A., Keniston, A., Frank, M.G. et al. (2016). Post-discharge telephone calls by hospitalists as a transitional care strategy. *American Journal of Managed Care* 22 (10): e338–e342.

2 Bahr, S.J., Solverson, S., Schlidt, A. et al. (2014). Integrated literature review of postdischarge telephone calls. *Western Journal of Nursing Research* 36 (1): 84–104.

3 Luciani-McGillivray, I., Cushing, J., Klug, R. et al. (2020). Nurse-led call back program to improve patient follow-up with providers after discharge from the emergency department. *Journal of Patient Experience* 7 (6): 1349–1356.

4 van Loon-van Gaalen, M., van Winsen, B., van der Linden, M.C. et al. (2021). The effect of a telephone follow-up call for older patients discharged home from the emergency department on health-related outcomes: a systematic review of controlled studies. *International Journal of Emergency Medicine* 14 (1): 1–9.

5 Woods, C.E., Jones, R., O'Shea, E. et al. (2019). Nurse-led postdischarge telephone follow-up calls: a mixed study systematic review. *Journal of Clinical Nursing* 28 (19–20): 3386–3399.

6 van Loon-van Gaalen, M., van der Linden, M.C., Gussekloo, J. et al. (2021). Telephone follow-up to reduce unplanned hospital returns for older emergency department patients: a randomized trial. *Journal of the American Geriatrics Society* 69 (11): 3157–3166.

7 Tang, N., Fujimoto, J., and Karliner, L. (2014). Evaluation of a primary care-based post-discharge phone call program: keeping the primary care practice at the center of post-hospitalization care transition. *Journal of General Internal Medicine* 29 (11): 1513–1518. https://doi.org/10.1007/s11606-014-2942-6.

8 Epstein, K., Juarez, E., Loya, K. et al. (2007). Frequency of new or worsening symptoms in the posthospitalization period. *Journal of Hospital Medicine* 2 (2): 58–68.

9 Vance, S., Fontecilla, N., Samie, F.H. et al. (2019). Effect of postoperative telephone calls on patient satisfaction and scar satisfaction after Mohs micrographic surgery. *Dermatologic Surgery* 45 (12): 1459–1464.

10 Car, J. and Sheikh, A. (2003). Telephone consultations. *British Medical Journal* 326 (7396): 966–969. https://doi.org/10.1136/bmj.326.7396.966.

11 Schulz, R., Cook, T.B., Beach, S.R. et al. (2013). Magnitude and causes of bias among family caregivers rating Alzheimer disease patients. *American Journal of Geriatric Psychiatry* 21 (1): 14–25.

12 Janssen, D.J., Spruit, M.A., Wouters, E.F. et al. (2012). Symptom distress in advanced chronic organ failure: disagreement among patients and family caregivers. *Journal of Palliative Medicine* 15 (4): 447–456.

13 Oechsle, K., Goerth, K., Bokemeyer, C. et al. (2013). Symptom burden in palliative care patients: perspectives of patients, their family caregivers, and their attending physicians. *Support Care Cancer* 21 (7): 1955–1962. https://doi.org/10.1007/s00520-013-1747-1.

14 Hsu, T., Loscalzo, M., Ramani, R. et al. (2017). Are disagreements in caregiver and patient assessment of patient health associated with increased caregiver burden in caregivers of older adults with cancer? *Oncologist* 22 (11): 1383–1391.

15 Chang, E.M., Gillespie, E.F., and Shaverdian, N. (2019). Truthfulness in patient-reported outcomes: factors affecting patients' responses and impact on data quality. *Patient Related Outcome Measures* 10: 171–186.

16 Carfora, L., Foley, C.M., Hagi-Diakou, P. et al. (2022). Patients' experiences and perspectives of patient-reported outcome measures in clinical care: a systematic review and qualitative meta-synthesis. *PLoS One* 17 (4): e0267030.

17 Bull, C., Byrnes, J., Hettiarachchi, R. et al. (2019). A systematic review of the validity and reliability of patient-reported experience measures. *Health Services Research* 54 (5): 1023–1035.

18 Campbell, R., Ju, A., King, M.T. et al. (2021). Perceived benefits and limitations of using patient-reported outcome measures in clinical practice with individual patients: a systematic review of qualitative studies. *Quality of Life Research* 31 (6): 1597–1620.

19 Spitznagel, M.B., Jacobson, D.M., Cox, M.D. et al. (2017). Caregiver burden in owners of a sick companion animal: a cross-sectional observational study. *Veterinary Record* 181 (12): 321.

20 Cary, J.A., Farnsworth, K.D., and Kurtz, S. (2010). Telephone communication in emergency cases: a training program for veterinary students. *Journal of Veterinary Medical Education* 37 (2): 130–135. https://doi.org/10.3138/jvme.37.2.130.

21 Shenoda, Y., Ward, M.P., McKeegan, D. et al. (2020). "The cone of shame": welfare implications of Elizabethan collar use on dogs and cats as reported by their owners. *Animals* 10 (2): 333.

24

Setting Goals and Therapeutic Endpoints

Barry Kipperman

Abstract

This chapter considers the importance of setting goals when treating patients. The concept of therapeutic endpoints is introduced, defined as criteria that warrant discontinuation or modification of the therapeutic plan, referral, or euthanasia in failing patients or that represent success in others. Such endpoints are goals that should be clearly understood and agreed to by the clinician and client. Examples of common therapeutic endpoints are outlined. Veterinary clinicians must balance the therapeutic and health-related outcomes of patients that we are trained to value as indicative of wellbeing with client concerns to provide goal-oriented care. Case studies illustrate challenges in navigating these considerations.

Keywords: *goals, goals of care, therapeutic endpoints, endpoints, responder, non-responder, goal-oriented care, humane endpoints*

Setting Goals

Society views setting goals as an important step toward achieving desired outcomes. The classic example is New Year's resolutions, often centered on being a better person, being kinder, losing weight, etc. If one sets goals that are considered too ambitious (such as when my guidance counselor in high school advised me to consider another career because becoming a veterinarian was too difficult), disappointment and frustration may ensue. Conversely, if you set a goal that is too easy to achieve (i.e. "I will not be found guilty of being cruel to any of my patients this year"), personal growth and evolution and societal benefits are unlikely.

Provided that the basis of clinician decisions is founded in the Principle of Optimizing Patient Outcomes rather than in pursuit of economic gain or self-interest, the idea of setting goals when working with patients seems logical and desirable. Yet, in my experience, it was very uncommon to see the word "goals" in veterinary medical records. Perhaps this is because the goals are inherently obvious or implicitly understood. For example, it's assumed that the goal of gastroscopic foreign body retrieval is to find and remove the foreign body. But what if the foreign object is not identified or cannot be removed?

Chapter 9 addressed the importance of having a "Plan B," documenting this, and ensuring the client is aware of the nature of the backup plan. In the case of the patient with a gastric foreign body, the medical record entry might state: "Transition to laparotomy/gastrotomy if foreign body is identified but cannot be retrieved in <30 minutes." In other cases, the goal of intervention may be less clearly defined. What is the goal of surgery to repair a ruptured cruciate ligament in a lame dog? Is it 100% resolution of lameness? Or 90%? Over what time frame should this outcome be expected? Is this information important and, if so, is it commonly noted in medical records? Let's consider some data from human medicine evaluating goals of care (GOC).

Goals of Care in Human Medicine

While human clinicians frequently use the term GOC, there is a lack of uniformity regarding what it means. GOC has been defined as "the *overarching aims* of medical care for a patient that are informed by *patients' underlying values and priorities* ... and [are] used to *guide decisions* about the use of or limitation on specific *medical interventions*" [1]. The objectives of GOC are to enhance patient autonomy and patient-centered care and prevent the provision of unnecessary care [1]. Of course, considering GOC in veterinary practice involves substituting the word "clients" for "patients" (with patient-centered care being a common goal in both fields).

One study found that the term GOC was omnipresent in the health records of critical patients admitted to an ICU [2]. This may be explained by the need to discuss advanced healthcare directives with these patients and whether life-prolonging measures were desired. While it is possible that veterinary emergency clinicians commonly document GOC, this was not my experience working in hospitals providing emergency care. What is becoming more common in veterinary practice is documenting whether clients wish their animal to be resuscitated (CPR [cardiopulmonary resuscitation] or DNR [do not resuscitate] orders) if the patient arrests, which can be viewed as a specific type of GOC. In a recent report of veterinarians working in specialty practice, 75% confirmed that their hospital assigned such codes to patients [3]. Yet, even among those who reported a policy requiring patients to have a code, only 50% indicated that a code is always assigned.

A study of stable patients may better reflect what should be done to consider using GOC in veterinary practice. In one human study at a clinic providing primary or specialty care for seriously ill patients, three methods were used to assess the incidence of a GOC discussion – patient reports, clinician reports, and documentation in the electronic health records [4]. While 66% of clinicians reported such discussions taking place, only 52% of patients reported this, and only 42% of medical records documented GOC discussions. This suggests that some clinicians believe that GOC were discussed but this was not documented in the medical record. Lawyers would caution us that "If it's not in the medical record, it never happened."

Humane Endpoints in Animals

The concept that there should be limits placed on the amount of suffering, pain, or distress that animals used in research and testing endure is founded on moral, scientific, and legal grounds. Clinical signs and behaviors highly indicative of imminent death among animals in these settings, known as humane endpoints, are routinely used to terminate or modify the experiment or to perform euthanasia [5]. There is an ethical tension between the compelling need to end suffering and the desire of the scientist to attain the study objectives.

Therapeutic Endpoints in Veterinary Practice

I propose the utilization of *therapeutic endpoints* in veterinary practice, defined as predetermined criteria that warrant discontinuation or modification of the therapeutic plan, referral, or euthanasia in failing patients or that represent therapeutic success in others. Such endpoints are goals that should be clearly understood and agreed to by the clinician and the client and recorded in the medical record to ensure that other clinicians also caring for the patient will adhere to the plan, which facilitates continuity of care. Two categories of therapeutic endpoints apply to veterinary patients: (i) to define non-responders (equivalent to humane endpoints); and (ii) to define responders.

Non-responders

Quain et al. [6] have astutely noted the lack of formal protections to limit suffering in veterinary patients relative to animals used in research:

> Unlike laboratory animals, the veterinary treatment of companion animals is not limited by predetermined humane endpoints. This may lead to a situation where a … companion animal … may suffer more at the end of their lives than a laboratory animal undergoing an experiment. In the light of concerns about companion animals being subjected to essentially unregulated experiments in some situations … humane endpoints should be established and agreed upon in advance of commencing treatment, and owner consent appropriately documented.

Table 24.1 provides examples of therapeutic endpoints for non-responders in veterinary practice.

The rationale for establishing therapeutic endpoints for non-responders is that these will prompt either discontinuing or modifying the therapy or diagnostic plan, referral, initiation of hospice care, or euthanasia. These also address diagnostic momentum bias (see Chapter 19), whereby clinicians are reluctant to modify a patient's existing treatment plan. Such endpoints should protect patients from futile care because a client is reluctant to accept a poor response or because a clinician wishes to continue treatment to acquire data, generate income, or satisfy their curiosity.

If you are treating a dog with azotemia with high-dose intravenous fluids for suspected hypoadrenocorticism pending adrenocorticotropic hormone (ACTH) stimulation test results, the record could state, "If Stim results are not consistent with Addison's or no improvement in azotemia after 24 hours, inform owner of poor response and prognosis and consider ultrasound and screening for causes of acute kidney failure, referral, hospice care, or euthanasia." If you are treating a patient

Table 24.1 Examples of therapeutic endpoints for non-responders in veterinary practice.

No improvement in symptoms after predetermined time frame
Progression of symptoms
Medication intolerance
Compliance issues
Lesion is non-resectable
Poor quality of life
Metastases

with a diuretic for congestive heart failure, the record may note, "If no improvement in or progression of dyspnea in next 24 hours, inform owner of poor response and prognosis and consider non-cardiogenic causes vs. increase diuretic dose × 12 hours vs. referral vs. euthanasia."

Medication intolerance and compliance concerns are common causes for unsatisfactory patient responses, which may be simple (different formulation) or impossible to remedy (such as a cat with hyperthyroidism who cannot be medicated by mouth whose owner cannot afford radioactive iodine). If a large tumor causing poor quality of life cannot be excised or a patient develops distant metastases, these are poor prognostic indicators.

Responders

Table 24.2 provides examples of therapeutic endpoints for responders in veterinary practice.

The rationale for establishing therapeutic endpoints for inpatient responders is that these will prompt sending the patient home. One of the most fundamental behaviors signifying a desired patient response is eating normal amounts of food. As many anxious or nervous patients (especially cats) may be reluctant to eat in the hospital, clinicians should consider alternate endpoints in these patients. For example, if fever in a feline patient has resolved but the cat will not eat, consider seeing if the patient will eat with the owner present, or simply consider trialing the patient at home. The medical record for this patient could state, "Goal is to establish good appetite or resolve fever × 12 hours."

Table 24.2 Examples of therapeutic endpoints for responders in veterinary practice.

Inpatient
- Eating
- Fever resolved × 12 h
- Resolution of pain
- No vomiting or diarrhea × 12 h
- Resolution of dyspnea
- Urinating voluntarily
- Azotemia improved and plateaued

Outpatient
- Eating
- Owner reports acceptable quality of life
- Resolution of fever
- Resolution of pain symptoms
- Improvement in pruritis
- Wound/incision healed
- Resolution of lymph node enlargement
- Weight stabilization or weight gain
- Resolution of cough
- Heart rate <160/min
- Systolic blood pressure <160 mmHg
- PCV >30%

For many inpatients, resolution of symptoms such as pain, vomiting, diarrhea, or dyspnea should be cited as the therapeutic endpoint. As resolution of pain symptoms in a patient receiving opioids may or may not indicate that pain has resolved, discharge should be considered when pain symptoms have resolved off analgesics or on the same analgesic that will be used at home. For a cat with urethral obstruction whose indwelling urinary catheter has been removed, spontaneous urination would be noted as the desired endpoint, with the caveat that some anxious or sedate cats may not urinate in the hospital for 12–24 hours or longer and may need to be sent home to void. When treating a patient with kidney failure, the record could note, "Continue diuresis until no further improvement in azotemia."

The rationale for establishing therapeutic endpoints for outpatient responders is that these will prompt modifying, tapering, or discontinuing therapy in some patients or justify the need for continued treatment in others. These endpoints may be confirmed via recheck appointment (i.e. lymphoma) or from home (i.e. appetite). It's important to be cognizant of the potential liabilities of using the callback to interpret therapeutic endpoints and outcomes (see Chapter 23), especially if metrics are not applicable to monitoring the patient's condition.

A patient should be eating normal or near-normal amounts to be considered a responder. For many outpatients, resolution of symptoms should be cited as the therapeutic endpoint. Pruritis is a common cause of poor welfare, as is ocular and otic pain. Treatment of patients with these conditions must focus on resolving these symptoms. For treating many chronic diseases, the goal is to achieve remission rather than cure. Remission may be indicated by resolution of lymph node enlargement in a patient with lymphoma, by weight stabilization in a cat with chronic enteropathy, or by resolution of cough in a patient with bronchitis. For a patient being treated for a tachyarrhythmia, the endpoint may be a heart rate of less than 160 beats per minute, or for a patient with hypertension a systolic blood pressure below 160 mmHg.

As examples, the medical record for a patient with immune-mediated hemolytic anemia may note, "Remission = packed cell volume (PCV) > 30%. After day 10 recheck, begin prednisone taper by 25% when PCV > 30%." When treating idiopathic epilepsy, the record could state, "Recheck two weeks. Goals are improved seizure frequency, acceptable quality of life and pheno level = 25 μg/ml. If pheno level < 25 μg/ml, increase dose prn and recheck blood levels in two weeks. If pheno level = 25–30 μg/ml, continue present dose and recheck in two months."

Goal-Oriented Care

One of the liabilities of using therapeutic endpoints is that the veterinary clinician may emphasize health-related outcomes that we are trained to value as indicative of wellbeing and diminish the importance of the patient's quality of life as perceived by the animal's owner. Early in my career, I often made the mistake of placing more importance on data (which I perceived as more objective and scientific) than on owner perceptions (which I viewed as more subjective and prone to bias). Boeykens et al. [7] eloquently describe this concern in human medicine:

> The healthcare system is oriented towards a disease-oriented paradigm. As a result, treatment goals can be in contrast with what patients value. The focus on single disease guidelines might distract providers from what really matters to the patient. A possible way to overcome many of the challenges is to shift care back from "what's the matter with the patient" to "what matters to the patient".

Collaboration between the animal owner and the clinician is the foundation of goal-oriented care and shared decision-making, which requires listening to our clients' needs and preferences [7, 8]. Case Studies 24.1–24.4 illustrate circumstances where clinicians faced challenges balancing therapeutic endpoints with goal-oriented care.

Case Study 24.1   A Dog with Hemolytic Anemia

You are treating Max, a six-year-old dog with immune-mediated hemolytic anemia. Max is sent home on prednisone at a dose of 2 mg/kg/day. The medical record states, "Continue immunosuppressive dose of pred until PCV = 30%, then taper dose by 25%." At the first week recheck, Max's appetite is good, the PCV is 22%, but the owner reports marked lethargy and excessive water drinking and urinating. At the second week recheck, Max's PCV is 25%, and the owner reports increasing concerns with steroid side effects. You inform Max's owner that you are concerned that tapering the steroid dose too soon will risk remission of the disease and to continue the steroid for another two weeks. Max does not return, and you discover that his owner requested Max's records be transferred to another practice.

Case Study 24.2   A Dog with Hypoadrenocorticism

You are a new graduate treating Butter, a four-year-old dog recently diagnosed with hypoadrenocorticism. Butter is sent home on prednisone at a dose of 0.2 mg/kg/day. The medical record states, "Continue physiologic dose of steroid indefinitely." At a callback two weeks post discharge from the hospital, her appetite is reported to be very good, but the owner complains that Butter is lethargic and is drinking and urinating excessively. The owner attributes these symptoms to the steroid and requests a modified dose.

Based on the literature, you cannot document a dose this low as causing these symptoms. You inform the owner that it is very unlikely that a physiologic dose of steroid would cause these symptoms, which are typically induced by much higher doses. You advise repeat laboratory testing and urine culture. These results reveal elevated alkaline phosphatase (ALP) and isosthenuria. At recheck four weeks post discharge to receive her monthly mineralocorticoid injection, the concerns regarding Butter's symptoms persist. You reduce the steroid dose by 50%, which resolves the concern with no decline in Butter's activity or appetite. The owner calls your employer to request a refund for the most recent laboratory testing.

Case Study 24.3   A Dog with Epilepsy

You are treating Herman, a three-year-old border collie, for idiopathic epilepsy and cluster seizures. Your medical record denotes, "Rx phenobarbital 2.2 mg/kg/day and recheck blood levels in two weeks. Modify dose to achieve pheno levels = 25 μg/ml." At the initial recheck, the owner is pleased to report no seizures, but complains that Herman is lethargic and is drinking and urinating excessively. The phenobarbital level is 22.5 μg/ml. Your associate reviews the test results and your record notes and advises increasing the medication dose by 20%.

You see Herman two weeks later and while you are pleased that no seizures have been seen, his quality of life is reported to be unacceptable as he sleeps all day and does not want to play. You inform the owner that this is the tradeoff for adequate seizure control and that Herman should adapt over time to the medication. Herman's owner requests referral to a neurologist, who adds a second medication without these side effects and tapers Herman off the phenobarbital. Herman's owner requests continued care for the seizures with the neurologist.

Case Study 24.4   A Cat with Diabetes Mellitus

You see Grace, a 10-year-old cat with newly diagnosed diabetes mellitus. You prescribe insulin injections twice daily. Your medical record states, "Modify insulin dose prn to achieve glucose values of 90–180 mg/dl." Glucose evaluations at the first recheck are all greater than 300 mg/dl, and you double the insulin dose. One week later, glucose values are between 220 and 270 mg/dl. You increase the insulin dose by 50%. One week later, glucose values are between 200 and 240 mg/dl. You increase the insulin dose by 66% and advise recheck in two weeks. During this period Grace is gaining weight, has a good appetite, and water intake is reported as normal. You inform the owner that you want to abide by the therapeutic goals you have set to optimize her diabetic regulation.

One week later, Grace presents to an emergency hospital for seizures. Her glucose concentration was 40 mg/dl. After incurring a 48-hour hospital stay, Grace is sent home on an insulin dose that is 25% of what you last prescribed. Grace's owner calls you and is quite upset. She feels you "treated the numbers and not my cat" and requests a refund for the emergency visit and referral to an internal medicine specialist.

Conclusion

Setting goals via using and documenting therapeutic endpoints provides clarity for clinicians and animal owners and should inform treatment decisions. Ideally, these would support discharge from the hospital, treatment adjustments, or confirmation of remission when patients respond, and encourage modifications to treatment plans and prevent non-beneficial care when treatment goals are not met. Using the prognostic model of "hope for the best and prepare for the worst," the clinician may document in the medical record of a patient with severe kidney failure: "If the azotemia improves after 48 hours, continue diuresis until no further improvement. If no improvement in azotemia at that time, discuss poor response/prognosis and consider hospice care, referral for dialysis, or euthanasia." Veterinary clinicians should balance endpoint criteria and patient-generated data with client concerns and expectations to provide goal-oriented care and to follow the Principle of Optimizing Patient Outcomes.

References

1 Secunda, K., Wirpsa, M.J., Neely, K.J. et al. (2020). Use and meaning of "goals of care" in the healthcare literature: a systematic review and qualitative discourse analysis. *Journal of General Internal Medicine* 35: 1559–1566.

2 Kruser, J.M., Benjamin, B.T., Gordon, E.J. et al. (2019). Patient and family engagement during treatment decisions in an ICU: a discourse analysis of the electronic health record. *Critical Care Medicine* 47 (6): 784.

3 Cabral, K.E., Rozanski, E.A., Cabral, H.J. et al. (2019). Does do not resuscitate (DNR) always mean DNR? Exploring DNR orders in small animal veterinary medicine. *Canadian Veterinary Journal* 60 (12): 1331.

4 Modes, M.E., Engelberg, R.A., Downey, L. et al. (2019). Did a goals-of-care discussion happen? Differences in the occurrence of goals-of-care discussions as reported by patients, clinicians, and in the electronic health record. *Journal of Pain and Symptom Management* 57 (2): 251–259.

5 Humane Endpoints (n.d.). Humane endpoints in laboratory animal experimentation. https://www.humane-endpoints.info/en (accessed February 8, 2023).

6 Quain, A., Ward, M.P., and Mullan, S. (2021). Ethical challenges posed by advanced veterinary care in companion animal veterinary practice. *Animals* 11 (11): 3010.

7 Boeykens, D., Boeckxstaens, P., De Sutter, A. et al. (2022). Goal-oriented care for patients with chronic conditions or multimorbidity in primary care: a scoping review and concept analysis. *PLoS One* 17 (2): e0262843.

8 Barbato, A., D'Avanzo, B., Cinquini, M. et al. (2022). Effects of goal-oriented care for adults with multimorbidity: a systematic review and meta-analysis. *Journal of Evaluation in Clinical Practice* 28 (3): 371–381.

25

Pain Management

Barry Kipperman

Abstract

Although the veterinary profession has made strides in treating pain, many animals in pain still do not receive analgesics, receive therapy that is inappropriate relative to their pain, or are not treated for an adequate duration. Practical recommendations and guidelines for managing pain are provided in this chapter. Literature evaluating acute pain management in small animal practice is examined. Contributing factors to undertreatment of pain include the common practice of sending patients home a few hours after surgery when most hospitals close, and the fact that technicians play an ancillary role in pain management. Steps forward in the evolution of pain management are proposed.

Keywords: *pain, recommendations, guidelines, opioids, local anesthetics, pain scales, oligoanalgesia, veterinary technician, overnight supervision*

As noted in Chapter 24, recognizing and treating pain and ensuring it is resolved are among the most important therapeutic endpoints in veterinary practice. This chapter focuses on the management of acute and perioperative pain. Practical recommendations and guidelines for managing pain are provided and steps forward in the evolution of pain management are proposed.

What Is Pain?

The International Association for the Study of Pain defines pain as "an unpleasant sensory and emotional experience associated with . . . actual or potential tissue damage" [1]. The sensory component of pain refers to *"what it feels like"* (i.e. perceptual qualities such as mild, severe, burning, tingling, etc.). The emotional component of pain refers to *"how it makes one feel"* (i.e. fearful, frustrated, anxious) [2].

Consequences of Pain

Pain induces systemic changes that can influence response to therapy and patient outcomes. Detrimental consequences of pain include activation of the sympathetic nervous system, increased secretion of stress hormones, immunosuppression, decreased food intake, altered function (e.g. lameness), impaired healing, and increased morbidity [3, 4].

Pain burden refers to the harmful effects of pain for the animal and the owner/caregiver. For the animal, pain has a negative impact on physical health and function, nutrition, behavior, socialization, and mental state [4]. Pain causes negative emotions and negative emotions enhance pain perception [5, 6]. The animal–owner relationship may be strained or ruined, i.e. animals with chronic pain require significant economic, time, and physical commitments from owners, and caring for them can be emotionally taxing [7, 8]. An overlooked issue is the impact that witnessing and/or hearing painful animals can have on veterinary team members, including emotional distress, compassion fatigue [2], or desensitization to or normalization of pain.

The Case for Managing Pain

Veterinarians have an ethical and medical duty to prevent, diagnose, and treat pain. Although the word "pain" is not explicitly used in the American Veterinary Medical Association Veterinarian's Oath, it is implied within the concept of "suffering": "prevention and relief of animal suffering" [9]. The medical obligation relates to the fact that pain has undesirable consequences for animal welfare [3, 4]. Finally, society is increasingly aware of pain and owners may ask the practitioner whether and how their animal's pain will be addressed.

Recommendations for Managing Pain

Recommendations for managing pain in animals include the following:

- *Be empathic*: The anthropomorphic adage "What would be painful for us is likely painful for them" is a good rule to abide by. Patients should never have to prove they are in pain to receive therapy. While some patients with acute pain may vocalize, most suffer in silence. We should always be open to learning more about recognizing signs of pain in animals and means of treating it. As an example, for much of my career I did not recognize or treat presumed muscle pain in my patients recovering from frequent seizures due to status epilepticus or tremors from metaldehyde toxicosis. I focused on the neurologic manifestations. I then noticed that some of these patients had a stiff gait as they were leaving to be discharged, which I presume reflected myalgia from the severity of muscular activity. I also (regrettably) neglected to recognize and treat pain in many patients with dermatitis, otitis, and corneal ulcers (I wasn't taught to do so decades ago) until I saw recent graduates prescribe analgesics for these conditions.
- *Treat early*: Also known as *preemptive analgesia*. Pain is far easier to prevent than to manage once signs manifest. Therapy should be given prior to the painful procedure if possible. The classic example of this approach occurs when the pain is planned and iatrogenic in nature, being a result of surgery or other invasive procedure.
- *Use a multimodal approach*: This refers to the use of different classes of analgesics acting at different locations in the pain pathway. This results in improved pain control, reduced doses of each drug, and fewer side effects [2]. One example may include use of local anesthetics, opioids, and sedatives/anxiolytics. This should include utilization of non-drug approaches such as addressing urine retention, consolidating cage visits, and providing a quiet environment to facilitate sleep, minimizing needle sticks and probes, and provision of soft and clean bedding.

- *Use an analgesic that is suited to the degree of pain*: Administering a weak opioid such as butorphanol to a cat with severe pain from aortic thromboembolism would be inappropriate and ineffective. Clinicians should become familiar with multiple analgesics to mitigate limitations associated with lack of access to one's preferred choice.
- *Ensure the timing of administration will provide analgesia during a planned procedure*: Simply administering an analgesic is not tantamount to effective pain relief. I cannot count how many times in my career I heard a surgical technician proclaim "The [opioid name] is on board!" immediately after it was injected. Such declarations were often an indication that the team could consider induction of anesthesia. The peak effect of buprenorphine given via intravenous (IV) administration is at least 30–60 minutes [10].
- *Treat often*: Do not deny an uncomfortable patient analgesic therapy because the next scheduled dose is not yet due to be administered.
- *Adjust analgesic type or dose until signs of pain have resolved*: Suitable indicators of pain should be monitored to ensure the desired therapeutic outcome is achieved.
- *Treat for an adequate duration*: The long-standing tradition in veterinary practice of sending patients home on oral analgesics a few hours after surgery precludes use of the most potent analgesics (opioids) as rescue agents to alleviate pain.

Guidelines for Managing Pain

Guidelines from the International Society of Feline Medicine (ISFM) advise: "The first step of acute pain treatment involves the administration of opioids, local anaesthetics and NSAIDs [non-steroidal anti-inflammatory drugs]" [11]. The World Small Animal Veterinary Association (WSAVA) guidelines state that opioids have been "the cornerstone of acute pain management in veterinary medicine" [12]. In support of the importance of opioids to manage acute pain, studies have confirmed that when using an opioid-free multimodal pain management protocol including ketamine, dexmedetomidine, meloxicam, and intraperitoneal bupivacaine, most adult cats undergoing ovariohysterectomy still needed a single preoperative dose of an opioid to ensure optimal pain control [13, 14].

Regarding use of local anesthesia, the ISFM guidelines note that "Locoregional anesthesia is an important part of multimodal analgesia and should be incorporated into a pain management plan whenever possible" [11]. The WSAVA guidelines recommend "intraperitoneal and incisional anaesthesia for the management of pain, particularly as adjuvant techniques in dogs and cats undergoing abdominal surgery" [12]. The American Animal Hospital Association (AAHA) guidelines state that "Local anesthetics are the most effective analgesic available in small animal practice, and they should be used in every surgery" [15]. In a recent report of cats undergoing ovariohysterectomy, local anesthesia combined with an opioid provided superior analgesia than opioid alone [16]. The AAHA guidelines observe that the availability of resources to learn how to use them, the development of more advanced methods to ensure reliable administration, and the availability of a long-acting bupivacaine preparation (Nocita™), should enhance the routine use of local anesthesia.

Both the WSAVA and AAHA guidelines encourage use of pain scales to assess pain in dogs and cats [12, 15]. Multidimensional composite pain scales for assessing postoperative pain in cats are available and a Feline Grimace Scale© that relies on facial expressions as an indication of pain has been recently introduced [17, 18]. Now that we have a sense of what should be done, let's look at evidence on what is done regarding monitoring and treating pain in small animal practice.

Pain Management in Small Animal Practice

In an investigation evaluating acute pain management in cats in Australia, 85% and 80% of veterinarians administered NSAIDs and opioids, respectively, but only 55% reported regularly using local anesthetics [19]. The authors concluded that more than half of the practitioners may be providing an inadequate duration of postoperative pain management. For example, the WSAVA recommendation for postoperative pain relief for ovariohysterectomy is of up to 72 hours [12].

In a survey of New Zealand veterinarians, opioids were used in 88% of cats and 95% of dogs before undergoing an ovariohysterectomy [20]. In dogs, NSAIDs were most commonly administered as an oral medication for three days after surgery. In cats, NSAIDs and opioids were usually administered as a single injection following surgery. Approximately 90% of patients were sent home the day of surgery. In a report of US veterinarians in general practice treating dogs undergoing ovariohysterectomies, 79% used NSAIDs, 70% used opioids, and only 45% used local anesthetics [21] (Case Study 25.1). Most dogs (88%) were discharged the day of surgery.

Case Study 25.1 Esophagostomy Tube Placement in a Cat

You give all the interns at your practice a lecture on pain management during the first month of their program with an emphasis on the value of, and indications for, local anesthesia. A few months later, you visit the hospital over the weekend and find one of the interns placing an esophagostomy tube in a cat. You are pleased they have learned the procedure and are incorporating this into their practice. When you inquire about pain management you are told, "We gave an opioid about 20 minutes ago." When you inquire about use of a local anesthetic at the site of the incision, you are met with a sheepish grin.

Regarding use of pain scales, one investigation found that only 15% of veterinarians reported using validated pain scales [19], another study reported that only 10% of 30 Canadian veterinary clinics routinely used standardized objective pain scales to identify postoperative pain in cats and dogs [22], and another report found that almost 50% of small animal practices in the United States reported the routine use of pain scales [23].

Contributing Factors to Undertreatment of Pain in Small Animal Practice

There is a significant and concerning disparity between best practices and what is being done to identify and treat pain in small animal practice. Although our profession has made significant strides in acknowledging and managing pain in animals over the past few decades, some animals in pain still do not receive analgesics, receive therapy that is inappropriate relative to their degree of pain, or are not treated for an adequate duration.

Oligoanalgesia is defined as failure to provide analgesia in patients with acute pain [24]. One of the major contributing factors to oligoanalgesia relates to the common practice of sending patients home a few hours after surgery when most hospitals close (Case Study 25.2). Such decisions are justified by the fact that these patients appear alert and are ambulatory. Administering an injection

---

Case Study 25.2   A Dog Recovering from an Enucleation

My friend's dog Elle was scheduled for an enucleation due to intractable ocular disease at a general practice. I saw her a few days after the procedure and asked how Elle had recovered from surgery. She replied, "She had a rough first night at home, but she's doing fine now." When I inquired, I was told that Elle was sent home four hours after her procedure.

---

of most opioids to a surgical patient at or before closing time and informing the client at discharge that the patient should be comfortable for the night is disingenuous and has no basis in pharmacokinetics, as the duration of action of almost all parenteral opioids is less than six hours [25], and treatment does not assure analgesia.

In one study, cats receiving an ovariectomy via a midline laparotomy who received an opioid (morphine 0.1 mg/kg) and medetomidine as premedication were evaluated up to 12 hours after endotracheal extubation using pain scales [26]. At 12 hours, approximately 50% of the cats still exhibited moderate pain requiring opioid rescue. In another report evaluating cats undergoing ovariohysterectomy, all cats received either methadone (0.28 mg/kg) or buprenorphine (0.01 mg/kg) combined with ketamine, midazolam, and medetomidine 20 minutes before surgery [27]. Pain scores were evaluated for up to eight hours postoperatively. Rescue analgesia with methadone was needed in 39% of the cats, including cats in both groups. All doses were provided within the first six hours after premedication.

In another investigation, dogs undergoing ovariohysterectomy received either nalbuphine (0.5 or 1 mg/kg), butorphanol (0.4 mg/kg), or morphine (0.2 mg/kg) 25 minutes before induction of anesthesia [28]. Pain scores were evaluated for up to six hours postoperatively. Rescue analgesia with morphine was required in 71% of dogs. The authors concluded that no preoperative treatments provided satisfactory analgesia. In a similar study of dogs undergoing ovariohysterectomy receiving a higher dose of morphine (0.5 mg/kg) before anesthesia who were monitored for three hours post extubation, 77% required rescue analgesia with morphine [29].

Another study evaluated the effect of local anesthesia in dogs undergoing elective ovariohysterectomy [30]. All dogs received dexmedetomidine and hydromorphone (0.1 mg/kg) as premedication. Pain scores were evaluated for up to 96 hours postoperatively. Among the dogs not receiving local anesthesia, 78% required rescue treatment with hydromorphone 3–4 hours after aseptic abdominal preparation. Of the dogs who received the local anesthetic, 39% needed analgesic rescue at ≤6 hours after preparation. One report concluded that cats undergoing multiple dental extractions required rescue analgesia with hydromorphone for up to 72 hours [31].

These studies document that dogs and cats likely experience significant pain for at least 6–12 hours after laparotomy and even longer for more painful procedures. As most surgical procedures are performed after 12 p.m. and most practices close at 6 p.m., ensuring a minimum 6 hour interval of monitoring pain after surgery cannot be accomplished via current practices.

Rationales for sending patients home the evening of surgery may include the presumptions that the surgical procedure elicits a minimal or short duration of pain [32], that clients expect this based on precedent with other animals or practitioners, and that this decision reduces client expense. Yet, there is ample evidence disputing the premise that laparotomy causes only minimal or transient pain. Veterinarians are the experts: our counsel should be guided by evidence-based medicine rather than by client expectations or a presumption to conserve client resources. It appears that current pain management practices are designed to coincide with hospital hours rather than with a Principle of Optimizing Patient Outcomes posture that acknowledges that post-operative pain does not end at 6 p.m.

At many hospitals, the staff veterinarians are responsible for overseeing pain management. In this model, veterinary technicians or nurses are expected to administer analgesics to patients and follow the orders of the veterinarian. The problem with this approach is that in most hospitals the veterinary technician rather than the practitioner observes an animal's behaviors prior to anesthesia and cares for the patient after surgery. Since our animal patients cannot ring for the nurse to increase their rate of opioid IV infusion, the veterinary technician is in the most suitable position to detect when their patient is uncomfortable and to request the initiation or modification of analgesic therapy.

Technicians can and should exert significant influence on the analgesic protocol regarding the types, timing, route, and dose of analgesics administered to their patients [33]. Reports have documented a perceived lack of autonomy among veterinary technicians [34, 35], which likely discourages assuming a leadership role in pain management. In my experience, technicians are often reluctant to raise concerns that a patient may be in discomfort to the veterinary surgeon (especially if they are in the operating room), as this may be perceived as questioning the surgeon's authority.

Other impediments to managing pain successfully include a lack of education or training, failure to establish and disseminate validated, standardized pain scales, and no mechanism of accountability for undertreatment of pain [36].

A Way Forward

Recognizing, treating, and monitoring pain in our patients are among the most fundamental callings of our profession. Yet, there was a time during my career when veterinarians did not treat pain at all and when practitioners gave owners the option of whether they consented to pay for analgesics for patients having surgery (including onychectomy!). The reader may find this history lesson inconceivable and/or anachronistic. It is now time for veterinary clinicians to take additional steps forward in the evolution of pain management lest we be viewed through the same lens by those who follow us.

It has been my experience that veterinary practitioners seldom disclose that a surgical or dental procedure is painful when communicating with clients. This is supported in human medicine, as a meta-analysis concluded that caregivers significantly underestimated patients' pain [37]. This falsely reassures clients that their companion will not be in pain and precludes them from being partners in shared decisions regarding pain management. How can we expect clients to approve proper pain management if they do not know that the procedure is painful? This is also inconsistent with scientific evidence and discourages following the principles of pain management discussed in this chapter. Acknowledging that veterinary surgeries and particular dental procedures are painful and reassuring clients that all efforts will be made to minimize pain are honest and compassionate and should not be perceived as shameful or malevolent or raise concerns that clients will decline the procedure or question your competence.

Adhering to the Principle of Patient Advocacy would entail advising that *all* patients experiencing major surgery be monitored for a minimum of six hours (and ideally overnight) for continued pain management so that rescue analgesics can be provided based on patient behaviors and pain scores. When performing procedures in the afternoon, either the practice would provide this monitoring or refer the patient to another hospital (where such is available) for overnight care.

Alternatively, practices could choose to modify their surgical schedules so that major procedures are all completed in the morning.

One may reasonably contend that the stress to the animal of continued hospitalization or transport after surgery is more detrimental to its welfare than being painful. Balancing these two welfare concerns should be discussed with clients prior to surgery so that an informed decision regarding postoperative care for each patient can be made. Clients can be reassured that anxiolytic treatment will be provided to address this concern. In some cases, the client may elect to have the procedure performed in a 24-hour hospital (if available) to avoid the need for transferring the patient after surgery. Studies have found that almost all pet owners surveyed affirmed that "being assured that all necessary analgesic drugs/techniques will be used" [38] and "adequate pain management" [39] were important or very important, and owner concern about discomfort and pain in their pet was associated with caregiver burden [7], suggesting that many clients may prefer a slightly longer separation from their pet rather than worrying that their companion is in pain at home.

A paradigm shift that empowers the veterinary technician to a far greater degree of involvement with pain management is needed. It is in the patient's best interest for the veterinary technician to be the first responder in determining their pain level, as the technician typically spends more time cage-side than any other member of the healthcare team. In this partnership approach, the veterinarian proposes a suitable analgesic plan and the veterinary technician reviews this and offers suggestions, administers the medications, and provides frequent and valued feedback to the veterinarian regarding whether the protocol is providing adequate pain relief.

The technician who can anticipate and recognize pain, effectively communicate the success or failure of the treatment plan to the veterinarian, and is aware of options for modification, including pharmacologic and anxiety-relieving nursing care, is a tremendous asset to their patients. Veterinarians must discourage conveying the impression that such advocacy efforts are an annoyance, threat to their autonomy, or personal indictment, and should instead express their appreciation to encourage this partnership.

Finally, local anesthetics should be administered to *all* patients having surgery, as they are effective and low cost, have virtually no contraindications, and may reduce the need for rescue analgesia [30]. These should be added to the anesthetic or surgical checklists used by the practice.

There are more analgesics available than ever before, including long-acting opioids (Simbadol™, Zorbium®) and local anesthetics (Nocita®), and medications administered via variable-rate infusions (i.e. fentanyl, dexmedetomidine, ketamine) that can achieve rapid onset of effect and can be immediately titrated or discontinued. To take advantage of these advances and to follow the Principle of Optimizing Patient Outcomes, veterinary practices should institute pain management protocols in accord with evidence-based medicine supporting multimodal analgesia and documenting that significant pain is present for at least 6–12 hours after ovariohysterectomy and presumably after many other surgical procedures.

References

1 Raja, S.N., Carr, D.B., Cohen, M. et al. (2020). The revised International Association for the Study of Pain definition of pain: concepts, challenges, and compromises. *Pain* 161 (9): 1976–1982.

2 Monteiro, B. and Robertson, S. (2022). Animal pain. In: *Ethics in Veterinary Practice: Balancing Conflicting Interests*, ch. 19 (ed. B. Kipperman and B.E. Rollin). Hoboken, NJ: Wiley-Blackwell.

3 Steagall, P.V. and Monteiro, B.P. (2019). Acute pain in cats: recent advances in clinical assessment. *Journal of Feline Medicine and Surgery* 21 (1): 25–34.

4 Steagall, P.V., Bustamante, H., Johnson, C.B. et al. (2021). Pain management in farm animals: focus on cattle, sheep and pigs. *Animals* 11 (6): 1483.

5 Finan, P.H. and Garland, E.L. (2015). The role of positive affect in pain and its treatment. *Clinical Journal of Pain* 31 (2): 177–196.

6 Hanssen, M.M., Petters, M.L., Boselie, J.J. et al. (2017). Can positive affect attenuate (persistent) pain? State of the art and clinical implications. *Current Rheumatology Reports* 19 (12): 80.

7 Spitznagel, M.B., Jacobson, D.M., Cox, M.D. et al. (2018). Predicting caregiver burden in general veterinary clients: contribution of companion animal clinical signs and problem behaviors. *Veterinary Journal* 236: 23–30.

8 Spitznagel, M.B., Patrick, K., Gober, M.W. et al. (2022). Relationships among owner consideration of euthanasia, caregiver burden, and treatment satisfaction in canine osteoarthritis. *Veterinary Journal* 286: 105868.

9 American Veterinary Medical Association (AVMA) (n.d). Veterinarian's Oath. https://www.avma.org/resources-tools/avma-policies/veterinarians-oath (assessed February 15, 2023).

10 Robertson, S.A., Lascelles, B.D.X., Taylor, P.M. et al. (2005). PK-PD modeling of buprenorphine in cats: intravenous and oral transmucosal administration. *Journal of Veterinary Pharmcology and Therapeutics* 28 (5): 453–460. https://doi.org/10.1111/j.1365-2885.2005.00677.x.

11 Steagall, P.V., Robertson, S., Simon, B. et al. (2022). 2022 ISFM consensus guidelines on the management of acute pain in cats. *Journal of Feline Medicine and Surgery* 24 (1): 4–30.

12 Monteiro, B.P., Lascelles, B.D.X., Murrell, J. et al. (2022). WSAVA guidelines for the recognition, assessment and treatment of pain. *Journal of Small Animal Practice* 64 (4): 177–254. https://doi.org/10.1111/jsap.13566.

13 Rufiange, M., Ruel, H.L., Monteiro, B.P. et al. (2022). A randomized, prospective, masked clinical trial comparing an opioid-free vs. opioid-sparing anesthetic technique in adult cats undergoing ovariohysterectomy. *Frontiers in Veterinary Science* 9: 1002407.

14 Diep, T.N., Monteiro, B.P., Evangelista, M.C. et al. (2020). Anesthetic and analgesic effects of an opioid-free, injectable protocol in cats undergoing ovariohysterectomy: a prospective, blinded, randomized clinical trial. *Canadian Veterinary Journal* 61 (6): 621–628.

15 Gruen, M.E., Lascelles, B.D.X., Colleran, E. et al. (2022). 2022 AAHA pain management guidelines for dogs and cats. https://www.aaha.org/globalassets/02-guidelines/2022-pain-management/resources/2022-aaha-pain-management-guidelines-for-dog-and-cats_updated_060622.pdf (accessed February 15, 2023).

16 Garbin, M., Ruel, H.L.M., Watanabe, R. et al. (2023). Analgesic efficacy of an ultrasound-guided transversus abdominis plane block with bupivacaine in cats: a randomised, prospective, masked, placebo-controlled clinical trial. *Journal of Feline Medicine and Surgery* 25 (2): 1098612X231154463.

17 Université de Montréal (2019). Feline Grimace Scale. www.felinegrimacescale.com (accessed February 18, 2023).

18 Evangelista, M.C., Watanabe, R., Leung, V.S.Y. et al. (2019). Facial expressions of pain in cats: the development and validation of a feline grimace scale. *Scientific Reports* 9: 19128.

19 Rae, L., MacNab, N., Bidner, S. et al. (2022). Attitudes and practices of veterinarians in Australia to acute pain management in cats. *Journal of Feline Medicine and Surgery* 24 (8): 715–725.

20 Gates, M.C., Littlewood, K.E., Kongara, K. et al. (2020). Cross-sectional survey of anaesthesia and analgesia protocols used to perform routine canine and feline ovariohysterectomies. *Veterinary Anaesthesia and Analgesia* 47 (1): 38–46.

21 Kramer, B.M., Hellyer, P.W., Rishniw, M. et al. (2022). Anesthetic and analgesic techniques used for dogs undergoing ovariohysterectomies in general practice in the United States. *Veterinary Anaesthesia and Analgesia* 49 (6): 556–562.

22 Dawson, L.C., Dewey, C.E., Stone, E.A. et al. (2017). Evaluation of a welfare assessment tool to examine practices for preventing, recognizing, and managing pain at companion-animal veterinary clinics. *Canadian Journal of Veterinary Research* 81 (4): 270–279.

23 Costa, R.S., Hassur, R.L., Jones, T. et al. (2023). The use of pain scales in small animal veterinary practices in the USA. *Journal of Small Animal Practice* 64 (4): 265–269. http://dx.doi.org/10.1111/jsap.13581.

24 Simon, B.T., Scallan, E.M., Carroll, G. et al. (2017). The lack of analgesic use (oligoanalgesia) in small animal practice. *Journal of Small Animal Practice* 58 (10): 543–554.

25 Dyson, D.H. (2008). Perioperative pain management in veterinary patients. *Veterinary Clinics of North America Small Animal Practice* 38 (6): 1309–1329.

26 Gauthier, O., Holopherne-Doran, D., Gendarme, T. et al. (2015). Assessment of postoperative pain in cats after ovariectomy by laparoscopy, median celiotomy, or flank laparotomy. *Veterinary Surgery* 44 (S1): 23–30.

27 Shah, M., Yates, D., Hunt, J. et al. (2019). Comparison between methadone and buprenorphine within the QUAD protocol for perioperative analgesia in cats undergoing ovariohysterectomy. *Journal of Feline Medicine and Surgery* 21 (8): 723–731.

28 Gomes, V.H., Barbosa, D.D.J., Motta, A.S. et al. (2020). Evaluation of nalbuphine, butorphanol and morphine in dogs during ovariohysterectomy and on early postoperative pain. *Veterinary Anaesthesia and Analgesia* 47 (6): 803–809.

29 Marquez, M., Boscan, P., Weir, H. et al. (2015). Comparison of NK-1 receptor antagonist (maropitant) to morphine as a pre-anaesthetic agent for canine ovariohysterectomy. *PLoS One* 10 (10): e0140734. https://doi.org/10.1371/journal. pone.0140734.

30 Campoy, L., Martin-Flores, M., Boesch, J.M. et al. (2022). Transverse abdominis plane injection of bupivacaine with dexmedetomidine or a bupivacaine liposomal suspension yielded lower pain scores and requirement for rescue analgesia in a controlled, randomized trial in dogs undergoing elective ovariohysterectomy. *American Journal of Veterinary Research* 83 (9): ajvr.22.03.0037.

31 Watanabe, R., Doodnaught, G., Proulx, C. et al. (2019). A multidisciplinary study of pain in cats undergoing dental extractions: a prospective, blinded, clinical trial. *PLoS One* 14 (3): e0213195.

32 Farnworth, M.J., Adams, N.J., Keown, A.J. et al. (2014). Veterinary provision of analgesia for domestic cats (Felis catus) undergoing gonadectomy: a comparison of samples from New Zealand, Australia and the United Kingdom. *New Zealand Veterinary Journal* 62 (3): 117–122.

33 Kipperman, B. (2012). Pain and its management. In: *Small Animal Internal Medicine for Veterinary Technicians and Nurses* (ed. L. Merrill), 433–448. Ames, IA: Wiley-Blackwell.

34 Kogan, L.R., Wallace, J.E., Schoenfeld-Tacher, R. et al. (2020). Veterinary technicians and occupational burnout. *Frontiers in Veterinary Science* 7: 328.

35 Liss, D.J., Kerl, M.E., and Tsai, C.L. (2020). Factors associated with job satisfaction and engagement among credentialed small animal veterinary technicians in the United States. *Journal of the American Veterinary Medical Association* 257 (5): 537–545.

36 Carvalho, A.S., Martins Pereira, S., Jácomo, A. et al. (2018). Ethical decision making in pain management: a conceptual framework. *Journal of Pain Research* 11: 967–976.

37 Ruben, M.A., Blanch-Hartigan, D., and Shipherd, J.C. (2018). To know another's pain: a meta-analysis of caregivers' and healthcare providers' pain assessment accuracy. *Annals of Behavioral Medicine* 52 (8): 662–685.

38 Steagall, P.V., Monteiro, B.P., Ruel, H.L.M. et al. (2017). Perceptions and opinions of Canadian pet owners about anaesthesia, pain and surgery in small animals. *Journal of Small Animal Practice* 58 (7): 380–388.

39 Simon, B.T., Scallan, E.M., Von Pfeil, D.J. et al. (2018). Perceptions and opinions of pet owners in the United States about surgery, pain management, and anesthesia in dogs and cats. *Veterinary Surgery* 47 (2): 277–284.

Index

Note: Page numbers followed by *f* indicates figures and *t* indicates tables.